Trauma and Psychosis

Trauma and Psychosis provides a valuable contribution to the current understanding of the possible relationships between the experience of trauma and the range of phenomena currently referred to as psychosis.

Warren Larkin and Anthony P. Morrison bring together contributions from leading clinicians and researchers in a range of fields including clinical psychology, mental health nursing and psychiatry. The book is divided into three parts, providing comprehensive coverage of the relevant research and clinical applications. **Part I Research and theoretical perspectives** provides the reader with a broad understanding of current and developing theoretical perspectives. **Part II Specific populations** examines the relationship between trauma and psychotic experiences in specific populations. **Part III From theory to therapy** draws together current knowledge and investigates how it might be used to benefit individuals experiencing psychosis.

This book will be invaluable for clinicians and researchers interested in gaining a greater insight into the interaction between trauma and psychosis.

Warren Larkin is Lead Consultant Clinical Psychologist in a specialist early intervention service for young people who experience psychosis. He is also an Honorary Lecturer at Lancaster University and is engaged in an ongoing research programme examining the theme of trauma and psychosis.

Anthony P. Morrison is a Professor of Clinical Psychology at the University of Manchester and coordinates early intervention services for Bolton, Salford and Trafford Mental Health Trust. In addition, he has edited and authored several books on the subject of cognitive therapy for psychosis.

Contributors: Paul Bebbington, Sarah Bendall, Richard P. Bentall, Max Birchwood, Pauline Callcott, Sandra D. M. Escher, Susie Farrelly, David Fowler, Ruth Fox, Daniel Freeman, Philippa Garety, Andrew I. Gumley, Corrina Hackman, Paul Hammersley, Amy Hardy, Chris Jackson, M. Kay Jankowski, Helen Krstev, Elizabeth Kuipers, Warren Larkin, Angus MacBeth,

Patrick McGorry, Anthony P. Morrison, Kim T. Mueser, John Read, Rebecca Rollinson, Marius A. J. Romme, Stanley D. Rosenberg, Thom Rudegeair, Ben Smith, Craig Steel, Douglas Turkington.

Trauma and Psychosis

New directions for theory and therapy

Edited by Warren Larkin and Anthony P. Morrison

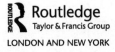
Routledge
Taylor & Francis Group

LONDON AND NEW YORK

First published in 2006 by Routledge
27 Church Road, Hove, East Sussex BN3 2FA

Simultaneously published in the USA and Canada
by Taylor & Francis
711 Third Avenue, New York NY 10017

First issued in paperback 2015

Routledge is an imprint of the Taylor & Francis Group, an informa business

Typeset in Times by
RefineCatch Limited, Bungay, Suffolk

Cover design by Sandra Heath

British Library Cataloguing in Publication Data
A catalogue record for this book is available from the British Library

Library of Congress Cataloging-in-Publication Data
    Trauma & psychosis : new directions for theory and therapy /
edited by Warren Larkin & Anthony P. Morrison.
        p. cm.
    Includes bibliographical references and index.
    ISBN–13: 978–1–58391–820–3 (hbk)
    ISBN–10: 1–58391–820–5 (hbk)
    1. Psychoses—Etiology.   2. Psychic trauma.   3. Post-traumatic
stress disorder.   I. Larkin, Warren.   II. Morrison, Anthony P.,
1969–.   III. Title: Trauma and psychosis.
    [DNLM: 1. Psychotic Disorders—etiology.   2. Stress
Disorders, Post-Traumatic—complications.   3. Psychotic
Disorders—therapy.   4. Stress Disorders, Post-Traumatic—
therapy.   5. Cognitive Therapy—methods.
    WM 200 T777 2006]
    RC512.T735 2006
    616.85′21—dc22

                                                                2006025822

ISBN 13: 978-1-138-87189-2 (pbk)
ISBN 13: 978-1-5839-1820-3 (hbk)

Contents

Figures and tables

Figures

Tables

Foreword

Many times, books are edited to provide a useful update of existing paradigms in research and clinical practice. More rarely, a book appears that for the first time comprehensively brings together data from different sources that combine into a true paradigm shift with major implications for clinicians, patients and researchers.

This book does exactly that. It describes a new way of understanding the experience of psychosis by focusing on a powerful environmental influence that since the early 1990s, as the dominant techno-optimistic view that psychosis equalled the passive reflection of a diseased brain rose and fell, struggled to get into view. The authors demonstrate that the evidence linking trauma, in particular in childhood, and psychosis not only is scientifically sound, but also provides a means of tracing the psychological mechanisms of the phenomena of psychosis, its onset in young adulthood, the relapses that patients present with, and the relationship between PTSD and psychosis. The book rightly dedicates ample space to the therapeutic implications of uncovered cognitive mechanisms, and the approaches that can be used to help patients discuss their experiences.

The editors have done a remarkable job in bringing together the foremost experts in the field, providing a clear structure for and coherence between the chapters, thus helping the reader to effortlessly understand the context, the aetiological evidence, cognitive mechanisms and therapeutic approaches in that order. The most important issue, however, and the one the authors ought to be congratulated on most, is the fact that they were capable of spotting and developing the new paradigm in the first place. This book deserves widespread reading.

Jim van Os

Acknowledgement

The concept for the book cover was created by service users at the Moorside Unit, Trafford General Hospital. Part of a series of art projects delivered by blueSCI.

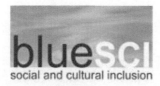

blueSCI is a not-for-profit organisation based at Broome House, Trafford which promotes wellbeing through social engagement and creative opportunities. blueSCI works with individuals to achieve their goals and aspirations, promoting recovery, self-management and social inclusion in partnership with other agencies and mainstream organisations.

For more information contact stuart@bluesci.org.uk or visit www.bluesci.org.uk

Introduction

Warren Larkin and Anthony P. Morrison

This volume is intended to provide clinicians, academics and students with an understanding of the possible relationships between the experience of trauma (early sexual, physical and emotional abuse for the most part, although it is recognised that revictimisation and traumatic stressors in adulthood are also important) and the range of phenomena currently referred to as psychosis. The contributors to this volume are clinicians and researchers recognised as leaders in the field of trauma and psychosis. The contributors represent a variety of professional backgrounds, including clinical psychology, mental health nursing and psychiatry. The majority of the contributors write from a cognitive psychological perspective, while others are more eclectic in their theoretical orientation.

The editors requested that authors carefully considered the use of language in their contributions in light of the obvious psychosocial orientation of the book and the broad range of current perspectives for understanding psychotic experiences. Our own view is that the language we use to describe mental health problems and 'unusual' or 'culturally unacceptable' experiences is important. Describing the experience of hearing voices as a 'mental illness', or viewing such experiences as a likely sign of a brain disease such as 'schizophrenia', is to collude with a 'scientific delusion', to quote Mary Boyle. That is not to say that some service users and professionals do not find an 'illness/disease model' helpful, but rather, that in our experience of talking to and working with consumers of mental health services (both as clients and colleagues), many prefer a more normalising, descriptive or experience-focused approach to their difficulties.

The book is divided into three parts, the first providing the reader with a broad understanding of current and developing theoretical perspectives. The potential relationships between trauma and psychosis are examined with particular attention being given to three predominant viewpoints: that trauma may lead to the development and play a role in the maintenance of psychosis in some individuals, that the experience of psychosis is, in some circumstances, so traumatic that posttraumatic stress disorder (PTSD) emerges, and that psychosis and PTSD are both part of a spectrum of possible responses to traumatic life events. Evidence in support of all of these pathways is presented.

Richard P. Bentall's chapter sets the scene in Part I, examining the role of physical and psychological stressors in psychosis and arguing that environmental influences have for many years been severely underestimated by psychiatric researchers. The following chapters in Part I guide the reader through the predominant viewpoints regarding the possible relationships between trauma and psychosis. John Read, Thom Rudegeair and Susie Farrelly's chapter reviews the evidence supporting the role of childhood sexual abuse in the subsequent development of psychosis. Sarah Bendall, Patrick McGorry and Helen Krstev review the literature on PTSD as a result of psychotic experience and hospitalisation and go on to integrate this with current understandings of PTSD. Finally, M. Kay Jankowski, Kim T. Meuser and Stanley D. Rosenberg draw upon recent research to support the notion that PTSD is a common comorbid feature of psychosis and other severe mental health difficulties, and present a model which hypothesises that PTSD mediates the course of these difficulties, contributing to a worse outcome as a consequence of both direct and indirect mechanisms. The chapter by David Fowler, Daniel Freeman, Craig Steel, Amy Hardy, Ben Smith, Corrina Hackman, Elizabeth Kuipers, Philippa Garety and Paul Bebbington proposes a hypothesis which attempts to explain how psychological processes associated with reactions to trauma and threat memories, might sometimes play a role in the maintenance of psychotic symptoms.

In Part II, there are chapters that examine the relationship between trauma and psychotic experiences in specific populations. In the first of these, Chris Jackson and Max Birchwood explore the link between trauma and first episode psychosis. They propose a model which examines the role of mediating variables such as cognitive appraisals and coping style. They argue that the relationship between early trauma and the first episode of psychosis is influenced by a complex array of interacting psychobiosocial factors, which arise as a result of disruption to a person's developmental trajectory. They go on to make practical suggestions for intervention. Following this, Paul Hammersley and Ruth Fox examine the importance of childhood trauma on the experience of psychosis in the context of bipolar mood difficulties and major depression. The third chapter in this part focuses specifically on the experience of hearing voices. Marius A. J. Romme and Sandra D. M. Escher suggest that traumatic life events can be a precipitating factor and influence on the content of voices for both adults and children. They draw upon the literature that links trauma to the voice hearing experience, as well as describing their own research in detail. They go on to make practical suggestions for working therapeutically with voice hearers who have a history of trauma.

Part III is an attempt to draw together the currently available knowledge in this area in a practical way and to make some suggestions as to how we might use it to benefit individuals with psychotic experiences who are help-seeking and experience trauma-related difficulties. In the first chapter of this part, John Read discusses the fundamental issue of why, when and how to ask about trauma. He offers practical suggestions and guidelines based on his considerable experience of both talking to service users about abuse and trauma and his experience of training other professionals in this approach. Pauline Callcott and Douglas Turkington's chapter outlines a formulation-driven approach that draws together well-established cognitive therapy interventions for PTSD and psychosis. Similarly, Ben Smith, Craig Steel, Rebecca Rollinson, Daniel Freeman, Amy Hardy, Elizabeth Kuipers, Paul Bebbington, Philippa Garety and David Fowler illustrate how understanding and validating the experience of traumatic events, and incorporating them into individualised formulations of psychosis, can shape cognitive behavioural therapy (CBT) interventions. In our own chapter, we outline a theoretical approach to understanding the relationship between the experience of traumatic life events and the development and maintenance of psychotic experiences. We also illustrate with the aid of case material how such a cognitive model can be utilised to guide the assessment process and to develop idiosyncratic case conceptualisations, which, in turn, determine the selection of intervention strategies.

Appropriately, in the last chapter in Part III, Andrew I. Gumley and Angus MacBeth describe a trauma-based model of relapse in psychosis. They argue that risk of relapse and recurrence is heightened by excessively negative danger-based appraisals of relapse. They also propose that disruption in early developmental and attachment experiences are linked to poorer outcome in psychosis and are a vulnerability factor for future relapse. The clinical implications of this model are discussed and illustrated with case examples.

This book is intended as a starting point for clinicians and researchers who seek a greater insight into the interaction between trauma and psychosis. It is clear that there is already a significant volume of research and therapy that has been conducted in this area, including the development of testable models, and the application of such ideas in the real world. It is our hope that this book will serve to add to the momentum of new ideas, perspectives and therapeutic approaches and to ultimately benefit individuals who have experienced trauma and are living with unusual, distressing experiences that attract stigma because they fall outside of what is regarded as 'normal' in our society.

The enthusiasm with which we have approached the development of this book, and the formation of the ideas within it, have been influenced by many people. These include colleagues who we work closely with on a daily basis, service users from our local services, and clinicians and researchers from the fields of both trauma and psychosis. Most of the latter have actually contributed chapters to this book. Among the many trauma-related influences, most noteworthy is the approach developed by Anke Ehlers, David Clark and colleagues, as well as the work of Chris Brewin, Emily Holmes and Ann Hackmann. We would also like to acknowledge the important contribution of our colleagues in the IMPACT/EDIT early intervention psychology services. They have collaborated in research, participated in peer supervision and collectively contributed to the evolution of a normalising approach to working with individuals with psychosis that we feel lucky to be a part of. These are Samantha Bowe, Paul French, David Glentworth, Ian Lowens, Nicola Marshall, Graeme Reid, Gary Sidley and Mary Welford. Other colleagues have worked closely with us in the development of our work in the area of trauma and psychosis: Lucy Frame, Aoiffe Kilcommons, Michelle Campbell, Clare Calvert, Louise Cumbley, David Lee and Tanya Petersen. We have also valued the opportunity to work with service users as colleagues and discuss our ideas with them, particularly Martina Kilbride, Liz Pitt and Rory Byrne.

A special tribute must be paid to all those individuals who consented to their stories being used in the preparation of this book. It is paramount that we continue to collaborate with the people who use our services. We would be wise to draw upon and utilise the wealth of knowledge and expertise offered to us by service users every time we sit down to begin a therapy session, plan a service or develop a research study.

Part I

Research and theoretical perspectives

Chapter 1

The environment and psychosis
Rethinking the evidence

Richard P. Bentall

Many researchers studying the psychoses believe that the field is currently undergoing a paradigm shift. Long-held assumptions about the nature and origins of conditions such as 'schizophrenia' and 'bipolar disorder' are being questioned and new research strategies are being employed to examine old questions in new ways. One assumption that is long overdue for re-examination is the idea that severe psychiatric disorders are hardly at all influenced by the physical and psychological environment, for example, by where one is born, how one is raised or whether or not one has the misfortune to experience various kinds of adverse events.

This idea has a long history. During the late nineteenth and first half of the twentieth centuries, a period which the historian Edward Shorter (1997) has described as the first era of biological psychiatry, the psychoses were widely regarded as neurodegenerative diseases, the result of cerebral pathology that was almost certainly inherited. It is true that, during the 1950s and 1960s, this idea became briefly unfashionable when American psychiatry, under the influence of émigré psychoanalysts, attributed 'schizophrenia' to 'double-bind' patterns of interactions between parents and children (Bateson et al. 1956) or malevolent, 'schizophrenogenic' mothers (Fromm-Reichmann 1950). However, in the second era of biological psychiatry, ushered in by the publication of the third edition of the American Psychiatric Association's *Diagnostic and Statistical Manual* (DSM-III: American Psychiatric Association 1980), environmental theories were once more rejected, and psychosis was again seen as exclusively a product of some kind of endogenous pathological process. From that time until the present day, it has usually been assumed that the search for environmental determinants, briefly stimulated by psychoanalytic theorising, has led only to negative results, and that further investigations of environmental influences are therefore unwarranted.

In this chapter I will argue that this prejudice has been ill founded, and that the role of environmental influences in psychosis has almost certainly been severely underestimated by psychiatric researchers in recent years. My argument will proceed in two stages. First, I will attempt to identify some impediments to thinking clearly about this issue, which may have contributed to the historical bias against environmental hypotheses, and second, I will briefly review some recent evidence that addresses the issue empirically, and which challenges traditional assumptions.

Some reasons why environmental influences on psychosis have been underestimated

It is possible to identify a number of serious conceptual, methodological and ideological impediments to understanding how the environment can affect the risk of severe mental health problems.

'Schizophrenia' as an explanandum

Undoubtedly, one serious problem has been researchers' reliance on psychiatric diagnoses that have questionable scientific validity, particularly the diagnosis of 'schizophrenia'. I have discussed the limitations of this concept at length elsewhere (Bentall 1990b, 1998, 2003) and therefore will provide only a brief overview of the relevant issues here.

In order to be useful, diagnoses have to meet two main criteria (Blashfield 1984; Kendell 1975). First of all, they have to be *reliable*, which is to say that different clinicians must use the diagnoses consistently (different clinicians should diagnose the same patients as 'schizophrenic'). Second, they have to be *valid*, which is to say that they have to perform the functions for which they are designed, such as grouping together patients with similar symptoms and whose problems have similar aetiologies, or predicting outcome (what will happen to patients in the future) and response to treatment (for example, which kinds of drugs will work).

The diagnostic systems employed by modern psychiatry were based on clinical concepts developed by early German psychiatrists, particularly Emil Kraepelin (1899/1990), who believed he had identified a small number of discrete disorders, notably dementia praecox (later known as 'schizophrenia') and manic depression (now often known as 'bipolar disorder') (see Bentall 2003, for a historical review). Kraepelin believed that each of these disorders produced a particular cluster of symptoms (hallucinations, delusions and cognitive deterioration in the case of schizophrenia, extreme mood states in the case of manic depression) and had a particular outcome (poor versus good). Later researchers came to believe that schizophrenia responded well to dopamine receptor agonist drugs (the 'neuroleptics' or 'antipsychotics') whereas manic depression responded to mood stabilizers, particularly lithium carbonate.

In fact, none of these assumptions have stood the test of time. The reliability of psychiatric diagnoses, even using modern 'operational' definitions, remains unacceptably low (Kirk and Kutchins 1992) and moreover, as several different definitions have been proposed for each of the major diagnoses, different patients tend to be given each diagnosis depending on which criteria are employed (Brockington 1992). Patients with a mixture of schizophrenic and manic depressive symptoms are common (Kendell and Gourlay 1970), and the symptoms of patients with either diagnosis (however defined) fall into a number of separate clusters (positive symptoms, symptoms of cognitive disorganisation, negative symptoms), which do not observe traditional diagnostic borders (Liddle 1987; Toomey et al. 1998). Both diagnoses are associated with a wide range of outcomes (Ciompi 1984; Tsuang et al. 1979) and, more alarmingly for clinicians, appear to be poor predictors of response to different types of psychotropic medication (Johnstone et al. 1988). Overall, it is difficult to avoid the impression that the categorical diagnoses employed in modern psychiatry have much in common with astrological star signs, a diagnostic system that is also widely held to say something about the characteristics of individuals and what will happen to them in the future.

The poor validity of psychiatric diagnoses has profound scientific and clinical implications that are well beyond the scope of this chapter (see Bentall 2003). In the present context it is sufficient to note that the widespread use of meaningless diagnoses in research has impeded the identification of aetiological factors that might be responsible for severe psychiatric problems. How can it be possible to determine whether any particular factor (biological or environmental) influences the development of psychiatric conditions when the diagnoses employed in the research group together people with widely differing problems, undoubtedly with widely differing aetiologies?

Misunderstanding the genetic evidence

A second impediment has been over-reliance on genetic evidence that seemed to suggest that the psychotic disorders are under strong genetic control. According to this line of reasoning, disorders such as 'schizophrenia' are highly heritable, high heritability excludes the possibility of important environmental influences, and therefore the environment cannot play a crucial role in the development of psychosis. The conclusion of this argument is undermined by the fact that both of its premises are false.

In recent years it has become clear that early genetic studies exaggerated the heritability of psychiatric disorders, partly because researchers treated the genetic determination of psychosis as an axiom rather than a hypothesis to be rigorously tested (Marshall 1990). Numerous methodological problems beset widely disseminated studies carried out by investigators who believed that genetic influences could be demonstrated without giving consideration to confounding factors. For example, in the famous series of Danish-American adoption studies carried out by Kety et al. (1975) and Rosenthal et al. (1974), significant results in favour of the genetic hypothesis could be found only by adopting an impossibly broad definition of schizophrenia, by carrying out the wrong statistical analyses (Joseph 2003), and by including 'interview' data from participants who sceptical observers later discovered had been dead at the time of the alleged interview (Rose et al. 1985). Although the data from these studies is almost scientifically worthless, they continue to be widely cited. Moreover, some of these bad practices have persisted in the new era of molecular genetics. For example, the first investigators to report a linkage between a particular gene and 'schizophrenia' were only able to obtain significant results by including as cases of the disorder persons suffering from phobias and alcoholism (Sherington et al. 1988). Small wonder that, until recently, replicable associations between particular genes and schizophrenia have proven elusive (Crow 1997; Moldin 1997). Even when at last, such associations have been found, the genes identified appear to be ones of very small effect (for example, the gene neuregulin-1 is found in approximately 15 per cent of patients with a diagnosis of schizophrenia and about 7 per cent of unaffected members of the population (Sigurdsson 2004) which, because the patients are a very small proportion of the population, means that it is present in many more non-patients than patients) and not specifically associated with a particular diagnosis (Bramon and Sham 2004; Craddock et al. 2005).

A more subtle problem with the genetic objection to environmental influences concerns common misunderstandings about the implications of heritability estimates. These give values (between 0 and 1) indicating the proportion of the variance between individuals that can be attributed to genes. However, these values depend on the extent to which there is variability in the environment. If individuals all experience the same environment, variation in the occurrence of a disorder can only be accounted for by genetic differences, so important environmental determinants will not be recognised. For example, if everyone smoked, whether or not a particular person succumbs to lung cancer would presumably depend on genetic vulnerability alone, and researchers who paid too much attention to heritability estimates would suffer the illusion that an important environmental influence – exposure to tobacco smoke – plays no causal role whatsoever (Joseph 2003).

A further complication is that heritability estimates, even when environmental influences are understood and measured, pay no heed to gene–environment correlations (the tendency of individuals with particular genetic constitutions to experience particular environments). In fact, correlations of this kind are the norm in nature because individuals (even plants!) tend to create their own environments (Lewontin 1993). As a consequence, the occurrence of a trait such as intelligence, which is under very strong genetic control, may still depend on environmental influences such as exposure to an emotionally supportive and stimulating environment in the first few years of life. In a mathematical treatment of this issue, Dickins and Flynn (2001) use sporting prowess as a readily understandable hypothetical example illustrating the effect. As certain physical characteristics (for example, height) predispose individuals to excellence in sport, whether one becomes a world champion undoubtedly depends on the possession of particular genes. However, actual success also crucially depends on receiving the right coaching, an environmental influence. This apparent paradox is resolved when it is recognised that professional coaches seek out individuals with particular physical characteristics, and hence the relevant genes.

Overall, these arguments show that genetic research has very few implications for the possible contribution of the environment to psychosis. The only way of establishing whether particular environmental factors play a role is by studying them.

Misunderstanding the neurobiological evidence

Similar misunderstandings have beset the interpretation of neurobiological data. As in the case of the genetic evidence, much of the evidence is less clear cut than biological psychiatrists have been prepared to admit. For example, while it is true that a proportion of 'schizophrenia' patients have enlarged cerebral ventricles, the magnitude of this effect is much less than initially thought, and the phenomenon has also been found in patients with bipolar disorder and psychotic depression (Raz and Raz 1990). Hypofrontality (reduced activity in the frontal lobes), once touted as a clear biological concomitant of schizophrenia, is not found in the resting state and observed only when patients are asked to perform tasks that engage the frontal lobes (Liddle 1996), tasks which are highly sensitive to motivation (Green et al. 1992). Most remarkably of all, the dopamine hypothesis (which proposed that 'schizophrenia' is caused by some kind of overactivity of pathways employing the neurotransmitter dopamine), once the front-running biological theory of schizophrenia, has been abandoned by many researchers because of numerous failures to find evidence of dopamine abnormalities in the brains of patients (Carlsson 1995; McKenna 1994). (Two studies which have implicated the dopamine system suggest that it may be implicated only during acute psychotic crises (Laruelle and Abi-Dargham 1999) or in psychotic responses to trauma (Hamner and Gold 1998).)

However, it is not the weakness of the biological findings that concerns us here (given that minds are ultimately brains it would be nothing short of amazing if no neurobiological differences could be detected between patients and other people: Rose 1984) but, once again, the inferences that have been drawn from them. Numerous studies have demonstrated that experience quite literally shapes the structure of the brain. For example, animals separated from their parents early in life show neurotransmitter abnormalities in adulthood (Suomi 1997) and human females who have been sexually abused in childhood show reduced hypocampal volume when adults (Stein et al. 1997) whereas the size of the hypocampus increases the longer London taxi drivers remain in their profession (Maguire et al. 2000). Structural and neurotransmitter differences between patients and others might therefore be taken as evidence of environmental causation rather than evidence against it. This is precisely the argument developed by Read et al. (2001), who have noted similarities between the brain abnormalities reported in 'schizophrenia' patients and those observed in victims of childhood sexual abuse.

Politics

A final, more difficult to document set of explanations for the relative neglect of environmental determinants of psychosis can be loosely labelled 'political', and to some extent subsumes the sources of misunderstanding that we have already considered. Under this rubric we can include various ideological and economic forces that have conspired, over recent decades, to encourage simplistic reductionistic, biological explanations of psychosis, to discourage investigation of social influences such as the family environment and sexual abuse, and to foster those misconceptions about the biological evidence that we have already noted.

The historical development of these forces is complex, but they came together in the early 1970s, when the battle between biological psychiatry and the antipsychiatry movement was widely regarded as having being won by the former group (Shorter 1997). At this time, organised psychiatry in North America and Britain was seeking to reinforce its identity as a branch of medicine, partly as a reaction to the ideas expressed by psychiatric dissidents such as Laing (1967) and Szasz (1960), which threatened to undermine any rationale for the profession's existence. DSM-III (American Psychiatric Association 1980) was one product of this renewed enthusiasm for biological approaches, and was authored by psychiatrists who saw themselves as returning to their Kraepelinian roots (Klerman 1978). Two further influences that reinforced the dominance of biological approaches were the drug companies, which had a financial stake in the widespread belief that psychiatric disorders are medical conditions (Healy 1997) and which have since continued to make staggering profits from their sale of psychiatric drugs (Angell 2004), and also some family support groups (Sedgwick 1982), who objected to the crude way in which they had been maligned by early environmental theorists. As a consequence, the idea that families might influence the development of psychosis became almost taboo during the 1980s and 1990s (Johnstone 1999).

Overview of known environmental influences

Despite these impediments to understanding the aetiological significance of the environment for psychosis, in recent years a small amount of evidence has emerged that does address the issue. Some of the data has been collected by die-hard advocates of a social psychiatry approach, who have struggled on during the second era of biological psychiatry, and some has been collected adventitiously during studies designed to address other issues, for example the inheritance of psychosis. One substantial line of research into the effects of migration on psychosis has been stimulated by an observation (high rates of psychosis in African Caribbeans living in the United Kingdom) that puzzled biological investigators, and which turned out to be best accounted for by environmental factors. The quality of the research has varied. Perhaps the strongest evidence comes from prospective investigations, in which some aspect of the social environment (family environment, exposure to sexual abuse or some other kind of victimisation) has been measured in advance of the development of symptoms but, for practical reasons, these kinds of investigations have been rare. Other researchers have therefore been forced to investigate environmental influences retrospectively, for example, by asking patients whether they have experienced victimisation or abuse. It is easy, given the zeitgeist that has prevailed since the mid-1970s, to apply double standards and require greater levels of methodological rigour for poorly funded environmental research than for richly endowed biological investigations (to assume, for example, that associations between ventricular enlargement and symptoms mean that brain damage *causes* symptoms while, at the same time, rejecting any association between retrospectively assessed family environment and psychosis as evidence of causality). However, to do so would be muddle-headed. Not only would such an attitude discourage potentially important future lines of investigation, but also it would amount to mistaking the trees for the wood. A balanced appraisal of the evidence demands that we look at the consistencies in data collected using many different methods. When we do this, we find that the results of investigations of the social origins of psychosis have been surprisingly consistent.

Family relationships

Much of the evidence on the role of family relationships in psychosis is retrospective. For example, adult psychotic patients, when interviewed, have reported insecure attachment relationships with their parents (Dozier and Lee 1995; Dozier et al. 1991). Two studies have also reported an association between insecure attachment and psychotic symptoms in population samples (Cooper et al. 1998; Mickelson et al. 1997). Fortunately, these findings are supported by the results obtained from a number of prospective investigations. In the Copenhagen high-risk study, it was found that those children born to patients diagnosed as 'schizophrenic' who later became psychotic were especially likely to have experienced separation from their parents during early childhood (Cannon et al. 1990). Moreover, reports of adverse relationships with their parents by the participants in the study when interviewed during adolescence were associated with the onset of psychosis in later years (Schiffman et al. 2002). As a similar effect was not found in the children of psychologically healthy parents, this finding suggests that genetically vulnerable children may be especially sensitive to adverse family environments.

Similar evidence of a gene–environmental interaction was reported in the only adoption study of psychosis to include measurement of environmental variables, carried out in Finland. Briefly, it was found that the adopted-away offspring of psychotic parents were more likely than control adoptees to develop thought disorder in adulthood, but only if the adoptive parents showed evidence of communication deviance (a style of speaking that is vague and inconsistent) (Wahlberg et al. 1997).

Further evidence on family influences emerged from the only prospective study so far designed specifically to examine this possibility. Carried out in California, the UCLA high-risk study interviewed the parents of children attending a child guidance clinic for non-psychotic disorders, and then followed-up the children fifteen years later (Goldstein 1987, 1998). Two characteristics of parenting style, communication deviance and high expressed emotion (a tendency to be critical and over-controlling, previously shown to predict relapse in patients living with their parents) were found to predict schizophrenia-spectrum symptoms at follow-up. This study has been criticised for the small numbers involved (only four out of fifty-two participants followed-up met the criteria for probable or definite schizophrenia) and because the children were experiencing non-psychotic psychological difficulties at the outset. Once again, however, the results are consistent with those from the other prospective investigations that we have considered.

One final prospective study which is also worthy of consideration in this context is a birth cohort study carried out in Finland, in which the mothers of 11,000 children born in 1966 were interviewed and the children followed-up at regular intervals into adulthood. Studies of this sort are usually designed to answer questions about the medical needs of the population and therefore tend to be short on psychiatric or psychological measures. Nonetheless, it was found that the children of unwanted pregnancies (as judged by the mothers' self-reports when interviewed during pregnancy) had a four-fold increased risk of psychosis twenty-six years later (Myhrman et al. 1996). Interestingly, the authors of this study chose to discuss possible biological explanations for this association (for example, that mothers carrying schizophrenia genes might be more likely to have an unplanned pregnancy) and completely neglected more obvious psychological explanations.

Trauma

Studies of the relationship between psychosis and trauma are the main topic of this book, and therefore will be dealt with only briefly here. Suffice it to say that the evidence consistently points to a high prevalence of trauma, especially sexual abuse, in the histories of patients suffering from severe psychiatric disorder (Bentall 2003; Goodman et al. 1997). For example, one epidemiological study found that the risk of meeting the diagnostic criteria for schizophrenia is increased by a factor of fifteen in individuals who had experienced childhood sexual abuse (Bebbington et al. 2004). This is an effect of much greater magnitude than any so far detected in genetic studies.

Most of the studies are, of course, retrospective – it is very hard indeed to carry out prospective studies of sexual abuse. However, one study found high rates of reported abuse in patients admitted to hospital for the first time (Neria et al. 2002) and there is consistent indication that sexual abuse is implicated particularly in hallucinations (Hammersley et al. 2003; Read et al. 2003; Ross et al. 1994).

Discrimination and victimisation

The high rate of psychosis observed in UK African Caribbeans has been found in community samples (Harrison et al. 1988) and therefore is unlikely to be the consequence of selective admissions to hospital. Those African Caribbeans growing up in predominantly white neighbourhoods appear to be especially vulnerable (Boydell et al. 2001). Moreover, African Caribbeans living in the Caribbean do not have especially high rates of psychosis (Bhugra et al. 1996; Bhugra et al. 1999) whereas other immigrant groups in other countries do (Selten et al. 2001; Zolkowska et al. 2001). It is difficult to escape the conclusion that racial discrimination and/or social marginalisation are the critical factors involved. Consistent with this hypothesis, a longitudinal epidemiological study of psychiatric symptoms conducted in the Netherlands reported that participants who reported experiences of discrimination at the beginning of the study were especially likely to develop paranoid symptoms by the time of a follow-up assessment several years later (Janssen et al. 2003).

Types of victimisation other than discrimination are also likely to contribute to psychosis. Several studies have reported that psychotic episodes can be provoked by intrusive life events, such as arrests or evictions (Day et al. 1987; Harris 1987). The high probability of such events in urban environments may help to explain why children raised in cities are more likely to become psychotic than children raised in rural areas (Mortensen et al. 1999). In a population-level survey of the inhabitants of Juarez in Mexico and El Passo in the United States, Mirowsky and Ross (1983) reported that paranoid beliefs, as assessed by questionnaire, were associated with social circumstances (poverty, lack of education) indicative of powerlessness. They suggested that an external locus of control (a tendency to attribute all events to external forces) might be a psychological mediator between such circumstances and paranoid beliefs. This hypothesis is consistent with evidence that paranoid patients have an external locus of control (Kaney and Bentall 1989; Rosenbaum and Hadari 1985), and tend to make excessively external attributions for negative events (Bentall et al. 2001). (In this context, it is also of some interest that one high-risk study reported that an external locus of control, assessed in adolescence, predicted psychosis in adulthood: Frenkel et al. 1995.)

The future: a developmental psychology perspective?

I want to finish this chapter by briefly considering how I think research into the role of environmental influences on psychosis might proceed in the future. There is currently much enthusiasm for the idea that psychosis is the end-point of some kind of abnormal developmental pathway. This idea has been stimulated by the observation that children who later become psychotic often show subtle psychological and physiological abnormalities many years before they become unwell; for example, in infancy they are often abnormally clumsy (Walker 1994), have delayed developmental milestones (Jones and Done 1997) and show high levels of negative emotion (Walker et al. 1993). Later in childhood they may be abnormally suspicious (Cannon et al. 2001). However, these observations are typically explained exclusively in neurobiological terms, for example by assuming that early damage to the brain or problems in cerebral maturation are responsible for the emergence of psychotic symptoms (see Keshavan and Murray 1997). Some evidence is clearly consistent with this assumption, for example the observation that children born in the winter or early spring are at increased vulnerability to psychosis (Torrey et al. 1997), the (not entirely consistent) finding that obstetric birth complications are associated with vulnerability to psychosis (Geddes and Lawrie 1995) and the observation that children born during periods of famine are also especially likely to develop severe mental health problems in later life (Susser and Lin 1992). However, given the evidence we have already considered, neurodevelopment cannot be the whole story. Psychotic symptoms seem to be the product of cognitive abnormalities that are the end-point of developmental pathways, which in turn are shaped by both environmental and maturational forces. It appears that some of the environmental influences involved may be quite subtle – for example, it is not necessary to believe that the parents of psychotic patients are either monstrous or malicious in order to believe that they play some causal role in psychosis.

In fact, psychologists studying both normal and abnormal child development have found that the early environment influences the growth of the very cognitive processes that seem to be involved in the positive symptoms of psychosis. For example, many psychotic patients have an impaired ability to understand the mental states of other people (sometimes called 'theory of mind' skills) (Corcoran 2000). Some studies have shown that securely attached children develop these skills more readily than insecurely attached children (Fonagy and Target 1997; Meins 1997). As we have already seen, an external locus of control and a tendency to make external attributions for negative events appears to be a characteristic of patients with paranoid delusions (Bentall et al. 2001); studies of both healthy children (Durkin 1995) and young adults vulnerable to depression (Alloy et al. 2001) suggest that interactions with parents and caregivers tend to shape children's attributional styles throughout childhood. Hallucinations, by contrast, seem to be the consequence of deficits in the ability to distinguish between self-generated thoughts and external stimuli (Bentall 1990a), a process known as 'source-monitoring'. The process by which this skill is acquired in childhood is not entirely understood but it appears that particular circumstances provide opportunities for this skill to develop (Fernyhough and Russell 1997).

These observations suggest that a full understanding of the origins of psychosis will require a sophisticated integration of theoretical concepts from psychopathology and developmental psychology. It is only by understanding the processes involved in normal cognitive, emotional and social development that we can hope to understand why some people arrive at adulthood handicapped by delusions, hallucinations and other psychotic experiences. In order to test the specific hypotheses that will inevitably flow from this kind of integration, it will be necessary to design a new generation of longitudinal investigations which will explore the origins of psychosis in early life, taking full account of the kind of environmental influences considered here and in other chapters of this book.

References

Alloy, L. B., Abramson, L. Y., Tashman, N. A., Berrebbi, D. S., Hogan, M. E., Whitehouse, W. G., et al. (2001) Developmental origins of cognitive vulnerability to depression: Parenting, cognitive and inferential feedback styles of the parents of individuals at high and low cognitive risk for depression. *Cognitive Therapy and Research, 25*, 397–423.

American Psychiatric Association (APA) (1980) *Diagnostic and statistical manual of mental disorders – 3rd edition*. Washington, DC: APA.

Angell, M. (2004) *The truth about the drug companies*. New York: Random House.

Bateson, G., Jackson, D. D., Haley, J., and Weakland, J. (1956) Towards a theory of schizophrenia. *Behavioral Science, 1*, 251–264.

Bebbington, P., Bhugra, D., Bruhga, T., Singleton, N., Farrell, M., Jenkins, R., et al. (2004) Psychosis, victimisation and childhood disadvantage: Evidence from the second British National Survey of Psychiatric Morbidity. *British Journal of Psychiatry, 185*, 220–226.

Bentall, R. P. (1990a) The illusion of reality: A review and integration of psychological research on hallucinations. *Psychological Bulletin, 107*, 82–95.

Bentall, R. P. (1990b) The syndromes and symptoms of psychosis: Or why you can't play 20 questions with the concept of schizophrenia and hope to win. In R. P. Bentall (ed.) *Reconstructing schizophrenia* (pp. 23–60). London: Routledge.

Bentall, R. P. (1998) Why there will never be a convincing theory of schizophrenia. In S. Rose (ed.) *From brains to consciousness: Essays on the new sciences of the mind* (pp. 109–136). London: Penguin.

Bentall, R. P. (2003) *Madness explained: Psychosis and human nature*. London: Penguin.

Bentall, R. P., Corcoran, R., Howard, R., Blackwood, R., and Kinderman, P. (2001)

18 Richard P. Bentall

Persecutory delusions: A review and theoretical integration. *Clinical Psychology Review, 21*, 1143–1192.

Bhugra, D., Hilwig, M., Hossein, B., Marceau, H., Neehall, J., Leff, J. P., et al. (1996) First contact incidence rates of schizophrenia in Trinidad and one-year follow-up. *British Journal of Psychiatry, 169*, 587–592.

Bhugra, D., Leff, J., Mallett, R., and Mahy, G. E. (1999) First-contact incidence rate of schizophrenia on Barbados. *British Journal of Psychiatry, 175*, 28–33.

Blashfield, R. K. (1984) *The classification of psychopathology: NeoKraepelinian and quantitative approaches*. New York: Plenum.

Boydell, J., van Os, J., McKenzie, J., Allardyce, J., Goel, R., McCreadie, R., et al. (2001) Incidence of schizophrenia in ethnic minorities in London: Ecological study into interactions with environment. *British Medical Journal, 323*, 1–4.

Bramon, E., and Sham, P. (2004) The shared genetic architecture which underlies schizophrenia and bipolar disorder. In C. McDonald, K. Schulze, R. M. Murray and P. Wright (eds) *Schizophrenia: Challenging the orthodox* (pp. 173–181). London: Taylor and Francis.

Brockington, I. (1992) Schizophrenia: Yesterday's concept. *European Psychiatry, 7*, 203–207.

Cannon, M., Walsh, E., Hollis, C., Kargin, M., Taylor, E., Murray, R. M., and Jones, P. B. (2001) Predictors of later schizophrenia and affective psychosis among attendees at a child psychiatry department. *British Journal of Psychiatry, 178*, 420–426.

Cannon, T. D., Mednick, S. A., and Parnas, J. (1990) Two pathways to schizophrenia in children at risk. In L. Robins and M. Rutter (eds) *Straight and devious pathways from childhood to adulthood* (pp. 328–350). Cambridge: Cambridge University Press.

Carlsson, A. (1995) The dopamine theory revisited. In S. R. Hirsch and D. R. Weinberger (eds) *Schizophrenia* (pp. 379–400). Oxford: Blackwell.

Ciompi, L. (1984) Is there really a schizophrenia? The longterm course of psychotic phenomena. *British Journal of Psychiatry, 145*, 636–640.

Cooper, M. L., Shaver, P. R., and Collins, N. L. (1998) Attachment style, emotion regulation, and adjustment in adolescence. *Journal of Personality and Social Psychology, 74*, 1380–1397.

Corcoran, R. (2000) Theory of mind in other clinical samples: Is a selective 'theory of mind' deficit exclusive to schizophrenia. In S. Baron-Cohen, H. Tager-Flusberg and D. Cohen (eds) *Understanding other minds: Perspectives from developmental neuroscience* (2nd edn). Oxford: Oxford University Press.

Craddock, N., O'Donovan, M. C., and Owen, M. J. (2005) The genetics of schizophrenia and bipolar disorder: Dissecting psychosis. *Journal of Medical Genetics, 42*, 193–204.

Crow, T. J. (1997) Current status of linkage for schizophrenia: Polygenes of vanishingly small effect or multiple false positives? *American Journal of Medical Genetics (Neuropsychiatric Genetics), 74*, 99–103.

Day, R., Neilsen, J. A., Korten, A., Ernberg, G., Dube, K. C., Gebhart, J., et al. (1987) Stressful life events preceding the onset of acute schizophrenia: A cross-national study from the World Health Organization. *Culture, Medicine and Psychiatry, 11*, 123–206.

Dickins, W. T., and Flynn, J. R. (2001) Heritability estimates versus large environmental effects: The IQ paradox resolved. *Psychological Review, 108*, 346–369.

Dozier, M., and Lee, S. W. (1995) Discrepancies between self and other-report of psychiatric symptomatology: Effects of dismissing attachment strategies. *Development and Psychopathology, 7*, 217–226.

Dozier, M., Stevenson, A. L., Lee, S. W., and Velligan, D. I. (1991) Attachment organization and familiar overinvolvement for adults with serious psychopathological disorders. *Development and Psychopathology, 3*, 475–489.

Durkin, K. (1995) *Developmental social psychology*. Oxford: Blackwell.

Fernyhough, C., and Russell, J. (1997) Distinguishing one's own voice from those of others: A function for private speech? *International Journal of Behavioral Development, 20*, 651–665.

Fonagy, P., and Target, M. (1997) Attachment and reflective function: Their role in self-organization. *Development and Psychopathology, 9*, 679–700.

Frenkel, E., Kugelmass, S., Nathan, M., and Ingraham, L. J. (1995) Locus of control and mental health in adolescence and adulthood. *Schizophrenia Bulletin, 21*, 219–226.

Fromm-Reichmann, F. (1950) *Principles of intensive psychotherapy*. Chicago, IL: University of Chicago Press.

Geddes, J. R., and Lawrie, S. M. (1995) Obstetric complications and schizophrenia: A meta-analysis. *British Journal of Psychiatry, 167*, 786–793.

Goldstein, M. J. (1987) The UCLA high-risk project. *Schizophrenia Bulletin, 13*, 505–514.

Goldstein, M. J. (1998) Adolescent behavioral and intrafamilial precursors of schizophrenia spectrum disorders. *International Clinical Psychopharmacology, 13 (suppl. 1)*, 101.

Goodman, L. A., Rosenberg, S. D., Mueser, K., and Drake, R. E. (1997) Physical and sexual assault history in women with serious mental illness: Prevalence, correlates, treatment, and future research directions. *Schizophrenia Bulletin, 23*, 685–696.

Green, M. F., Satz, P., Ganzell, S., and Vaclav, J. F. (1992) Wisconsin Card Sorting Test performance in schizophrenia: Remediation of a stuborn deficit. *American Journal of Psychiatry, 149*, 62–67.

Hammersley, P., Dias, A., Todd, G., Bowen-Jones, K., Reilly, B., and Bentall, R. P. (2003) Childhood trauma and hallucinations in bipolar affective disorder: A preliminary investigation. *British Journal of Psychiatry, 182*, 543–587.

Hamner, M. B., and Gold, P. B. (1998) Plasma dopamine beta-hydroxylase activity in psychotic and non-psychotic post-traumatic stress disorder. *Psychiatry Research, 77*, 175–181.

Harris, T. (1987) Recent developments in the study of life events in relation to psychiatric and physical disorders. In B. Cooper (ed.) *Psychiatric epidemiology: Progress and prospects* (pp. 81–102). London: Croom Helm.

Harrison, G., Owens, D., Holton, A., Neilson, D., and Boot, D. (1988) A prospective study of severe mental disorder in Afro-Caribbean patients. *Psychological Medicine, 18*, 643–657.

Healy, D. (1997) *The anti-depressant era*. Cambridge, MA: Harvard University Press.

Janssen, I., Hanssen, M., Bak, M., Bijl, R. V., De Graaf, R., Vollenberg, W., et al. (2003) Discrimination and delusional ideation. *British Journal of Psychiatry, 182*, 71–76.

Johnstone, E. C., Crow, T. J., Frith, C. D., and Owens, D. G. C. (1988) The Northwick

Park 'functional' psychosis study: Diagnosis and treatment response. *Lancet, ii*, 119–125.

Johnstone, L. (1999) Do families cause 'schizophrenia'? Revisiting a taboo subject. *Changes*, 77–90.

Jones, P. B., and Done, D. J. (1997) From birth to onset: A developmental perspective of schizophrenia in two national birth cohorts. In M. S. Keshavan and R. M. Murray (eds) *Neurodevelopment and adult psychopathology* (pp. 119–136). Cambridge: Cambridge University Press.

Joseph, J. (2003) *The gene illusion: Genetic research in psychology and psychiatry under the microscope*. Ross-on-Wye: PCCS Books.

Kaney, S., and Bentall, R. P. (1989) Persecutory delusions and attributional style. *British Journal of Medical Psychology, 62*, 191–198.

Kendell, R. E. (1975) *The role of diagnosis in psychiatry*. Oxford: Blackwell.

Kendell, R. E., and Gourlay, J. A. (1970) The clinical distinction between the affective psychoses and schizophrenia. *British Journal of Psychiatry, 117*, 261–266.

Keshavan, M. S., and Murray, R. M. (eds) (1997) *Neurodevelopment and adult psychopathology*. Cambridge: Cambridge University Press.

Kety, S., Rosenthal, D., Wender, P. H., Schulsinger, F., and Jacobsen, B. (1975) Mental illness in the biological and adoptive families of adopted individuals who have become schizophrenic: A preliminary report based on psychiatric interviews. In R. Fieve, D. Rosenthal and H. Brill (eds) *Genetic research in psychiatry*. Baltimore, MD: Johns Hopkins University Press.

Kirk, S. A., and Kutchins, H. (1992) *The selling of DSM: The rhetoric of science in psychiatry*. Hawthorne, NY: Aldine de Gruyter.

Klerman, G. L. (1978) The evolution of a scientific nosology. In J. C. Shershow (ed.) *Schizophrenia: Science and practice* (pp. 99–121). Cambridge, MA: Harvard University Press.

Kraepelin, E. (1899/1990) *Psychiatry: A textbook for students and physicians. Volume 1: General psychiatry*. Canton, MA: Watson Publishing International.

Laing, R. D. (1967) *The politics of experience and the bird of paradise*. London: Penguin.

Laruelle, M., and Abi-Dargham, A. (1999) Dopamine as the wind in the psychotic fire: New evidence from brain imaging studies. *Journal of Psychopharmacology, 13*, 358–371.

Lewontin, R. C. (1993) *The doctrine of DNA: Biology as ideology*. London: Penguin.

Liddle, P. F. (1987) The symptoms of chronic schizophrenia: A reexamination of the positive-negative dichotomy. *British Journal of Psychiatry, 151*, 145–151.

Liddle, P. F. (1996) Functional imaging in schizophrenia. In S. Lewis and N. Higgins (eds) *Brain imaging in psychiatry* (pp. 215–226). Oxford: Blackwell.

McKenna, P. J. (1994) *Schizophrenia and related syndromes*. Oxford: Oxford University Press.

Maguire, E. A., Gadian, D. G., Johnsrude, I. S., Good, C. D., Ashburner, J., Frackowiak, R. S. J., and Frith, C. D. (2000) Navigation-related structural changes in the hippocampi of taxi drivers. *Proceedings of the National Academy of Science*.

Marshall, R. (1990) The genetics of schizophrenia: Axiom or hypothesis? In R. P. Bentall (ed.) *Reconstructing schizophrenia* (pp. 89–117). London: Routledge.

Meins, E. (1997) *Security of attachment and the social development of cognition*. Hove: Psychology Press.

Mickelson, K. D., Kessler, R. C., and Shaver, P. R. (1997) Adult attachment in a nationally representative sample. *Journal of Personality and Social Psychology, 73*, 1092–1106.

Mirowsky, J., and Ross, C. E. (1983) Paranoia and the structure of powerlessness. *American Sociological Review, 48*, 228–239.

Moldin, S. O. (1997) The maddening hunt for madness genes. *Nature Genetics, 17*, 127–129.

Mortensen, P. B., Pedersen, C. B., Westergaard, T., Wolfahrt, J., Ewald, H., Mors, O., et al. (1999) Effects of family history and place and season of birth on the risk of schizophrenia. *New England Journal of Medicine, 340*, 603–608.

Myhrman, A., Rantakallio, P., Isohanni, M., Jones, P., and Partanen, U. (1996) Unwantedness of preganancy and schizophrenia in the child. *British Journal of Psychiatry, 169*, 637–640.

Neria, Y., Bromet, E. J., Sievers, S., Lavelle, J., and Fochtmann, L. J. (2002) Trauma exposure and posttraumatic stress disorder in psychosis: Findings from a first-admission cohort. *Journal of Consulting and Clinical Psychology, 70*, 246–251.

Raz, S., and Raz, N. (1990) Structural brain abnormalities in the major psychoses: A quantitative review of the evidence. *Psychological Bulletin, 108*, 93–108.

Read, J., Perry, B. D., Moskowitz, A., and Connolly, J. (2001) The contribution of early traumatic events to schizophrenia in some patients: A traumagenic neurodevelopmental model. *Psychiatry: Interpersonal and Biological Processes, 64*, 319–345.

Read, J., Agar, K., Argyle, N., and Aderhold, V. (2003) Sexual and physical abuse during childhood and adulthood as predictors of hallucinations, delusions and thought disorder. *Psychology and Psychotherapy: Theory, Research and Practice, 76*, 1–22.

Rose, S. (1984) Disordered molecules and diseased minds. *Journal of Psychiatric Research, 18*, 351–360.

Rose, S., Kamin, L. J., and Lewontin, R. C. (1985) *Not in our genes*. Harmondsworth: Penguin.

Rosenbaum, M., and Hadari, D. (1985) Personal efficacy, external locus of control, and perceived contingency of parental reinforcement among depressed, paranoid and normal subjects. *Journal of Abnormal Psychology, 49*, 539–547.

Rosenthal, D., Wender, P. H., Kety, S. S., Welner, J., and Schulsinger, F. (1974) The adopted away offspring of schizophrenics. In S. A. Mednick, F. Schulsinger, J. Higgins and B. Bell (eds) *Genetics, environment and psychopathology*. Amsterdam: North Holland.

Ross, C. A., Anderson, G., and Clark, P. (1994) Childhood abuse and the positive symptoms of schizophrenia. *Hospital and Community Psychiatry, 42*, 489–491.

Schiffman, J., LaBrie, J., Carter, J., Tyrone, C., Schulsinger, F., Parnas, J., and Mednick, S. (2002) Perception of parent-child relationships in high-risk families, and adult schizophrenia outcome of offspring. *Journal of Psychiatric Research, 36*, 41–47.

Sedgwick, P. (1982) *Psychopolitics*. London: Pluto Press.

Selten, J.-P., Veen, N., Feller, W., Blom, J. D., Schols, D., Camoenie, W., et al. (2001) Incidence of psychotic disorders in immigrant groups to The Netherlands. *British Journal of Psychiatry, 178*, 367–372.

Sherington, R., Brynjolfsson, J., Perturrson, H., Potter, M., Dudleston, K., Barraclough, B., et al. (1988) Localization of a susceptibility locus for schizophrenia on chromosome 5. *Nature, 336*, 164–167.

Shorter, E. (1997) *A history of psychiatry*. New York: Wiley.

Sigurdsson, E. (2004) Genomics and genealogy provide an Icelandic springboard into the human gene pool. *Journal of Mental Health, 13*, 1–21.

Stein, M. B., Koverola, C., Hanna, C., Torchia, M. G., and McClarty, B. (1997) Hippocampal volume in women victimized by child sexual abuse. *Psychological Medicine, 27*, 951–959.

Suomi, S. J. (1997) Long-term effects of different early rearing experiences on social, emotional, and physiological development in nonhuman primates. In M. S. Keshavan and R. M. Murray (eds) *Neurodevelopment and adult psychopathology* (pp. 104–116). Cambridge: Cambridge University Press.

Susser, E. S., and Lin, S. P. (1992) Schizophrenia after prenatal exposure to the Dutch hunger winter of 1944–1945. *Archives of General Psychiatry, 49*, 938–988.

Szasz, T. S. (1960) The myth of mental illness. *American Psychologist, 15*, 564–580.

Toomey, R., Faraone, S. V., Simpson, J. C., and Tsuang, M. T. (1998) Negative, positive and disorganized symptom dimensions in schizophrenia, major depression and bipolar disorder. *Journal of Nervous and Mental Disease, 186*, 470–476.

Torrey, E. F., Miller, J., Rawlings, R., and Yolken, R. H. (1997) Seasonality of births in schizophrenia and bipolar disorder: A review of the literature. *Schizophrenia Research, 28*, 1–38.

Tsuang, M., Woolson, R. F., and Fleming, J. A. (1979) Long-term outcome of major psychoses: I. Schizophrenia and affective disorders compared with psychiatrically symptom-free surgical conditions. *Archives of General Psychiatry, 36*, 1295–1301.

Wahlberg, K.-E., Wynne, L. C., Oja, H., Keskitalo, P., Pykalainen, L., Lahti, I., et al. (1997) Gene-environment interaction in vulnerability to schizophrenia: Findings from the Finnish Adoptive Family Study of Schizophrenia. *American Journal of Psychiatry, 154*, 355–362.

Walker, E. F. (1994) Neurodevelopmental precursors of schizophrenia. In A. S. David and J. C. Cutting (eds) *The neuropsychology of schizophrenia*. Hove: Erlbaum.

Walker, E. F., Grimes, K. E., Davis, D. M., and Smith, A. J. (1993) Childhood precursors of schizophrenia: Facial expressions of emotion. *American Journal of Psychiatry, 150*, 1654–1660.

Zolkowska, K., Cantor, G. E., and McNeil, T. F. (2001) Increased rates of psychosis among immigrants to Sweden: Is migration a risk factor for psychosis? *Psychological Medicine, 31*, 669–678.

Chapter 2

The relationship between child abuse and psychosis

Public opinion, evidence, pathways and implications

John Read, Thom Rudegeair and Susie Farrelly

Bad things do happen and they really can drive you crazy

While Freud and others were developing their theories that adult psycho-pathology is rooted in adverse childhood experiences, Kraepelin was promulgating very different ideas (Bentall 2003; Read 2004b). The second half of the twentieth century saw a new player enter the fray in this age-old debate about whether the failings of our genes or the slings and arrows of outrageous fortune are primarily responsible for driving some of us crazy. The pharmaceutical industry tipped the balance decisively in favour of the bio-genetic view (Mosher et al. 2004), reflecting the power, throughout recorded history, of social, economic and political forces in shaping our understanding of disturbed people (Read 2004a, 2005). In August 2005 Dr Steven Sharfstein, the president of the American Psychiatric Association, in an article entitled 'Big Pharma and American psychiatry: The good, the bad, and the ugly', was both honest and brave in stating:

> There is widespread concern at the over-medicalization of mental disorders and the overuse of medications. Financial incentives and managed care have contributed to the notion of a 'quick fix' by taking a pill and reducing the emphasis on psychotherapy and psychosocial treatments. There is much evidence that there is less psychotherapy provided by psychiatrists than 10 years ago. This is true despite the strong evidence base that many psychotherapies are effective used alone or in combination with medications. ... If we are seen as mere pill pushers and employees of the pharmaceutical industry, our credibility as a profession is compromised.
>
> (Sharfstein 2005: 3)

Armed with intriguing new technologies for understanding the biological concomitants of the workings of the mind, bio-genetic viewpoints eclipsed pre-existing psychosocial understandings of psychosis, while undercutting funding of, and respect for, new research about the social causes of madness (Aderhold and Gottwalz 2004; Read et al. 2004c). The relative roles of science and ideology in the nature–nurture debate about madness are more fully discussed elsewhere (Read and Hammersley 2006).

This dominance of a reductionist paradigm has been camouflaged since the 1970s as an apparent conceptual integration, the so-called 'bio-psychosocial' model. Central to this illusion has been the 'vulnerability-stress' idea that acknowledges a role for social stressors but only in those who already have a genetic predisposition (Read et al. 2001b; Read 2005). In this model, life events became mere 'triggers' of an underlying genetic time-bomb. This apparent integration is more a colonisation of the psychological and social by the biological, resulting in increased bio-genetic research and decreased psychosocial research (Read et al. 2001b). The colonisation even went so far as to invent the euphemism 'psycho-education' for programmes promulgating the illness ideology to families (Aderhold and Gottwalz 2004; Read et al. 2004b; Read et al. 2004c). Dr Sharfstein (2005: 3) has urged his colleagues to 'examine the fact that as a profession, we have allowed the bio-psychosocial model to become the bio-bio-bio model'.

Public opinion

Despite the dominance of the bio-genetic paradigm among some 'experts', the public continues its longstanding belief that the bad things that happen to us, especially when we are little and defenceless, can cause serious problems later in life.

Surveys have consistently found that while most people understand that both nature and nurture influence our mental health, we place much more emphasis on adverse life events than on biology or genetics (Read and Haslam 2004; Read et al. 2006). In a 1987 US survey the two most frequently cited causes of schizophrenia were 'Environmental stress' and 'Major unpleasant emotional experiences'. Furthermore 'Poor parenting, bad upbringing' was cited by the public more often than by mental health professionals (Wahl 1987). One survey of US citizens found that 91 per cent cited 'Stressful circumstances' as a cause of schizophrenia (Link et al. 1999).

When Londoners were asked about schizophrenia, 'Overall subjects seemed to prefer environmental explanations – e.g. "being mercilessly persecuted by family and friends" and "having come from backgrounds that promote stress" ' (Furnham and Rees 1988: 218). Another London study found that the most endorsed causal model of schizophrenia was 'Unusual or traumatic experiences or the failure to negotiate some critical stage of emotional development' (Furnham and Bower 1992). 'It seems that lay people have not been converted to the medical view and prefer psychosocial explanations' (p. 207). 'Subjects agreed that schizophrenic behaviour had some meaning and was neither random nor simply a symptom of an illness' (p. 206).

Two New Zealand studies replicated a US finding (Hill and Bale 1981) that young adults endorse the 'Interactional' (psychosocial) items of the Mental Health Locus of Origin scale more frequently than the 'Endogenous' (bio-genetic) items (Read and Harre 2001; Read and Law 1999). In both studies the item most strongly endorsed was 'The mental illness of some people is caused by abuse or neglect in childhood.'

An Australian survey found that for schizophrenia, 'Problems from child-hood such as being badly treated or abused, losing one or both parents when young or coming from a broken home' was rated as a likely cause by 88 per cent, whereas only 59 per cent endorsed 'inherited or genetic' (Jorm et al. 1997). This same understanding, that psychosocial factors are more important than bio-genetic, has been replicated in Germany (Angermeyer and Matschinger 1999), Ireland (Barry and Greene 1992), India (Srinivasan and Thara 2001), Mongolia and Russia (Dietrich et al. 2004).

The reaction of biological psychiatrists, eagerly supported by the drug industry (Mosher et al. 2004), has been to bemoan the public's lack of 'mental health literacy' (Jorm 2000), while redoubling efforts to persuade us to think more like themselves (Jorm et al. 1997; Wahl 1999). One of the first research papers (Thompson et al. 2002) emanating from the current World Psychiatric Association campaign to improve attitudes about schizophrenia portrays the belief that schizophrenia is a 'debilitating disease', caused pre-dominantly by biochemical imbalance, as 'sophisticated' and 'knowledgeable'. The study was funded by the drug company Eli Lilly.

Destigmatisation programmes designed to educate us to think more like biological psychiatry and the drug companies, ignore the fact that study after study has demonstrated that bio-genetic causal beliefs are correlated with increased fear and prejudice (Dietrich et al. 2004; Mehta and Farina 1997; Read and Haslam 2004; Read et al. 2006; Walker and Read 2002).

So who is right, the majority of people around the world or one branch of one profession (biological psychiatry) and the drug companies?

The evidence of a relationship between childhood abuse and psychosis

Child abuse or neglect and becoming a psychiatric patient

Physical and sexual abuse

It has been demonstrated that child abuse can play a causal role in PTSD, dissociative disorders, depression, suicidality, eating disorders, anxiety dis-orders, sexual dysfunction, drug and alcohol abuse and personality disorders (Boney-McCoy and Finkelhor 1996; Fergusson et al. 1996; Kendler et al. 2000; Mullen et al. 1993; Swanston et al. 2003).

Nevertheless some psychiatrists still believe that the more severe diagnostic categories, such as schizophrenia, are less related, or unrelated, to child abuse (Read 1997) despite all the research showing that child abuse is related to severity of disturbance, whichever way you measure severity. Psychiatric patients subjected to child sexual abuse (CSA) or child physical abuse (CPA) have earlier first admissions, longer and more frequent hospitalisations, spend longer in seclusion, receive more medication, are more likely to try to kill themselves and to self-mutilate, and have higher global symptom severity (Beck and van der Kolk 1987; Briere et al. 1997; Goff et al. 1991a; Lipschitz et al. 1999b; Pettigrew and Burcham 1997; Read 1998; Read et al. 2001a; Read et al. 2005; Sansonnet-Hayden et al. 1987).

A review has summarised 40 studies of inpatients, and outpatients where the sample contained 50 per cent or more people diagnosed psychotic (Read et al. 2004a). Half of the 2396 women had suffered CSA. The majority of both the women (69 per cent) and the men (60 per cent) had experienced either CSA or CPA. Many of these studies provided details of the abuse. In a study of child and adolescent inpatients (Lipschitz et al. 1999a) the CSA began on average at 8 years of age and lasted on average 2.1 years. Most of the CSA was intrafamilial and involved penetration or oral sex. The CPA started on average at 4.4 years of age, lasted an average of 6.4 years, and involved physical injury in most cases (Lipschitz et al. 1999b).

The same review compared general population studies and samples of psychiatric patients that employed very similar methodology and found CPA to be four to six times more common in psychiatric patients, with CSA seven to ten times more common. The proportion of CSA that was perpetrated by family members (incest) was calculated to be twice as high (62 per cent) among psychiatric patients as in the general population (29 per cent) (Read et al. 2004a).

These comparisons with general populations may underestimate the differences. People tend to underreport abuse while in hospital (Dill et al. 1991; Read 1997; see also Chapter 9). When researchers surveyed female inpatients *after* they returned to the community, 85 per cent disclosed CSA (Mullen et al. 1993).

The notion that psychiatric patients cannot be believed when they disclose abuse is not supported by the relevant research. Studies have shown that disclosures by patients have high reliability and high levels of corroborating evidence (Read et al. 2005; see also Chapter 9). One study, for instance, found that 'The problem of incorrect allegations of sexual assaults was no different for schizophrenics than the general population' (Darves-Bornoz et al. 1995: 82).

Psychological abuse and neglect

Adult inpatient studies report rates of childhood neglect ranging from 22 per cent to 62 per cent (Heads et al. 1997; Muenzenmaier et al. 1993; Saxe et al. 1993). In a study of adult outpatient 'schizophrenics' 35 per cent had suffered emotional abuse as children, 42 per cent physical neglect, and 73 per cent emotional neglect (Holowka et al. 2003). A study of adolescent inpatients found that 52 per cent had experienced emotional abuse, 61 per cent physical neglect and 31 per cent emotional neglect (Lipschitz et al. 1999b). Two studies allow comparison with a community survey using identical methods. Thus 2 per cent of women in general reported being 'seriously neglected as a child' (Kessler et al. 1995), compared to between 4 per cent and 36 per cent of women psychiatric patients (Neria et al. 2002; Switzer et al. 1999). The male figures are: general population 3 per cent, patients between 8 per cent and 35 per cent. In a New Zealand community survey, women emotionally abused as children were five times more likely to have had a psychiatric admission (Mullen et al. 1996).

Child abuse and psychosis

Contrary to current bio-genetic ideology, but consistent with public opinion, psychosis is at least as related to child abuse as are other diagnoses such as PTSD and depression (Read et al. 2005). In fact there is evidence, presented next, that the relationship with psychosis may be even stronger than the relationship with many of the other diagnostic categories (Read et al. 2004a).

Clinical research scales

The 'Psychoticism' scale of the *Symptom Checklist 90-Revised* has been found to be more related to child abuse than the other nine clinical scales (Bryer et al. 1987; Ellason and Ross 1997; Lundberg-Love et al. 1992; Swett et al. 1990). The Schizophrenia scale of the *Minnesota Multiphasic Personality Inventory* (MMPI) is significantly elevated in adults who suffered CPA (Cairns 1998), CSA (Hunter 1991; Tsai et al. 1979) and incest (Scott and Stone 1986). Medical patients who had suffered CSA scored significantly higher on the Schizophrenia and Paranoia scales, but not on the Depression scale (Belkin et al. 1994).

Clinical diagnoses

The same pattern emerges from studies using actual diagnoses in clinical practice (Read et al. 2005). Adults diagnosed 'schizophrenic' are more likely than the general population to have run away from home as children (Malmberg et al. 1998), to have attended child guidance centres (Ambelas 1992) and to have been placed in children's homes (Cannon et al. 2001). Of 5362 children, those whose mothers had poor parenting skills when they were 4 years old were significantly more likely to be schizophrenic as adults (Jones et al. 1994). In a sample of adult outpatients diagnosed 'schizophrenic' 85 per cent had suffered some form of childhood abuse or neglect (73 per cent emotional neglect, 50 per cent sexual abuse) (Holowka et al. 2003). A chart review found that 52 per cent of female inpatients diagnosed schizophrenic had suffered 'parental violence' (Heads et al. 1997). In a study of 426 inpatients diagnosed psychotic, the CPA rate for the women was 29 per cent (Neria et al. 2002), compared to 5 per cent in the general population using identical methods (Kessler et al. 1995). The rates for men were: patients 17 per cent, general population 3 per cent.

Some studies find that diagnoses of psychosis and schizophrenia are about as strongly related to child abuse as other diagnoses (e.g. Neria et al. 2002; Ritsher et al. 1997; Wurr and Partridge 1996). Many studies, however, provide further evidence that child abuse and neglect may be even more strongly related to diagnoses of schizophrenia than to diagnoses indicating less severe disturbance.

In a 30-year study of over 500 child guidance clinic attenders, 35 per cent of those who later became 'schizophrenic' had been removed from home because of neglect, a rate double that of any other diagnosis (Robins 1966). In another study, of over 1000 people, those who at age 3 had mother–child interactions characterised by 'harshness towards the child; no effort to help the child' were, at age 26, significantly more likely than others to be diagnosed with 'schizophreniform disorder', but not mania, anxiety or depression (Cannon et al. 2002).

From a study of 93 women attending a psychiatric emergency room (Briere et al. 1997), it can be calculated that CSA was more common in psychosis (70 per cent) and depression (74 per cent), than in anxiety (27 per cent) or mania (43 per cent). Among 139 female outpatients 78 per cent of those diagnosed 'schizophrenic' had suffered CSA; the percentages for other diagnoses were: panic disorder 26 per cent, anxiety disorders 30 per cent, major depressive disorder 42 per cent (Friedman et al. 2002). Among children admitted to a psychiatric hospital, 77 per cent of those who had been sexually abused were diagnosed psychotic, compared to 10 per cent of the other children (Livingston 1987).

The symptoms that lead to diagnoses such as 'schizophrenia' are also more common in those who have been abused (Read et al. 2005). In a study of 'chronically mentally ill women' those who had been abused or neglected experienced more psychotic symptoms than other patients (Muenzenmaier et al. 1993). The same is repeatedly found in the general population (Berenbaum 1999; Janssen et al. 2004; Ross and Joshi 1992; Startup 1999).

The five DSM-IV 'characteristic symptoms' of schizophrenia are: hallucinations, delusions, disorganised thinking ('thought disorder'), grossly disorganised or catatonic behaviour, and negative symptoms (APA 1994: 285). In one community survey 46 per cent of people with three or more of these symptoms had suffered CPA or CSA, compared to 8 per cent of those with none of the symptoms (Ross and Joshi 1992). An inpatient study found one or more of these symptoms in 75 per cent of those who had suffered

CPA, in 76 per cent of those who had suffered CSA, and in 100 per cent of those subjected to incest (Read and Argyle 1999). A study of 200 adult out-patients found that 35 per cent of those abused as children had two or more symptoms compared to 19 per cent of the non-abused patients (Read et al. 2003). Not only are abused patients more likely to have psychotic symptoms, but they also manifest those symptoms at an earlier age than non-abused patients (Goff et al. 1991a).

Specific symptoms

Researchers from the British school of cognitive behaviour therapy (e.g. Bentall 2003), have argued that it is more productive, theoretically and clinic-ally, to research specific behaviours and cognitions than the heterogenous and disjunctive construct of schizophrenia, which has poor reliability and validity (Bentall 2004; Read 2004c).

In a study of inpatient 'schizophrenics' those who had suffered CSA or CPA had significantly more of the 'positive' symptoms of schizophrenia, but slightly fewer 'negative' symptoms, than those not abused. The symptoms significantly related to abuse were, in order of the strength of the relationship: Voices Commenting, Ideas of Reference, Thought Insertion, Paranoid Idea-tion, Reading Others' Minds and Visual Hallucinations (Ross et al. 1994).

HALLUCINATIONS

The onset of most auditory hallucinations has been found to be preceded by either a traumatic event or an event triggering memories of an earlier trauma (Honig et al. 1998). An inpatient study in New Zealand found some form of hallucination in 53 per cent of those subjected to CSA, 58 per cent of those subjected to CPA, and 71 per cent of those who suffered both forms of abuse (Read and Argyle 1999). This 'dose effect' was replicated in another New Zealand study, of 200 outpatients, which found hallucinations in 19 per cent of the non-abused patients, 47 per cent of those subjected to CPA, 55 per cent of those subjected to CSA and 71 per cent of those subjected to both CPA and CSA (Read et al. 2003). The figures for 'command hallucinations' to harm self or others were: non-abused 2 per cent, CPA 18 per cent, CSA 15 per cent, CSA+CPA 29 per cent. The figures for voices commenting were: non-abused 5 per cent, CPA 21 per cent, CSA 27 per cent, CSA+CPA 36 per cent. As previously noted, the study by Ross et al. (1994) found that voices com-menting was the most strongly related of all psychotic symptoms to child abuse.

A study of adult bipolar affective disorder patients found that those subjected to CPA were no more likely than other patients to experience hal-lucinations (or delusions). Those subjected to CSA were no more likely to have visual hallucinations. However, they were twice as likely to have auditory hallucinations and six times as likely to hear voices commenting (Hammersley et al. 2003).

These findings that abused adult inpatients are more likely to hallucinate, has been replicated with adolescent and child inpatients (Famularo et al. 1992; Sansonnet-Hayden et al. 1987). Hallucinations are particularly common in incest survivors (Ellenson 1985; Ensink 1992; Heins et al. 1990; Read and Argyle 1999). Among non-patients, predisposition to auditory, but not visual, hallucinations was significantly higher in those who reported multiple trauma (Morrison and Petersen 2003).

An outpatient study found tactile hallucinations *only* in those who had suffered CSA or CPA. The figures for olfactory hallucinations were: non-abused 1 per cent, CPA 9 per cent, CSA 10 per cent, CSA+CPA 21 per cent (Read et al. 2003).

DELUSIONS

The New Zealand outpatient study (Read et al. 2003) produced weaker support for a relationship between child abuse and delusions. Although 40 per cent of the CSA patients experienced some form of delusion, compared to 27 per cent of the non-abused, this was not statistically significant. Furthermore the study did not replicate the relationships between child abuse and Ideas of Reference or Mind Reading (Ross et al. 1994). It did, however, provide a degree of support for their finding of a relationship between child abuse and Paranoid Ideation. Paranoid delusions were present for 40 per cent of the CSA outpatients, compared to 23 per cent of the non-abused patients. An outpatient study found paranoid delusions in 36 per cent of incest survivors but none of the non-familial cases of CSA (Read et al. 2003).

THOUGHT DISORDER

Bryer et al. (1987) found a significant relationship between 'psychotic thinking' and CSA. However, in 2004 a review of the sparse literature concerning thought disorder found that most studies have not found a relationship with either CSA or CPA (Read et al. 2004a).

CATATONIA

In his original 1874 conception of catatonia, Kahlbaum (1973: 4) believed it was usually precipitated by 'very severe physical or mental stress . . . [such as] a very terrifying experience'. More recent commentators still see catatonia as an extreme fear response (Moskowitz 2004; Perkins 1982). There is, however, no research at all examining the relationship between childhood trauma and the DSM schizophrenia symptom of 'grossly disorganised or catatonic behaviour'.

NEGATIVE SYMPTOMS

Studies of adult (Lysaker et al. 2001; Read et al. 2003; Resnick et al. 2003) and child (Famularo et al. 1992) inpatients have found no differences in rates of negative symptoms between abused and non-abused. Two adult inpatient studies even found slightly fewer such symptoms in abused patients (Goff et al. 1991a; Ross et al. 1994).

SUMMARY

From the small, but growing, body of literature on the relationship between child abuse and specific 'schizophrenic' symptoms, we might reasonably conclude the following:

- Hallucinations – almost definitely related (especially auditory hallucinations, including voices commenting and command hallucinations, and probably also visual, olfactory and tactile)
- Delusions – probably (more likely paranoid than grandiose)
- Thought disorder – probably not (unless the trauma is 'retriggered' by subsequent repeat trauma – see below)
- Negative symptoms – probably not
- Catatonia – no data.

In terms of types of child abuse there is, thus far, a small amount of evidence suggesting that 'schizophrenic' symptoms may be more powerfully related to CSA than to CPA, with the most consistently evidenced specific relationship being that between CSA and auditory hallucinations, especially voices commenting (Read et al. 2004a). However, it is likely that psychotic symptoms are related more to the severity rather than the type of abuse, with the more severe forms of abuse – incest and being subjected to both CSA and CPA – being related to particularly high rates of hallucinations (i.e., a 'dose effect') (Read and Argyle 1999; Read et al. 2003). In a study of 100 incest survivors, a cumulative trauma-score (multiple types of abuse and multiple abusers) was significantly higher in those who later experienced auditory or visual hallucinations (Ensink 1992: 109–138).

Symptom content

The actual content of psychotic symptoms has historically been under-emphasised. The prevailing bio-genetic climate dictated that it was adequate merely to know if someone heard voices. However, researchers have recently begun to document that the content of hallucinations and delusions can tell us heaps about current and past events in someone's life, providing further support for the public's impressions (Read et al. 2005).

One study found that in severely maltreated children 'the content of the reported visual and/or auditory hallucinations or illusions tended to be strongly reminiscent of concrete details of episodes of traumatic victimization' (Famularo et al. 1992: 866). The same has been found to be true for many adolescents (Sansonnet-Hayden et al. 1987) and adults who suffered CSA (Heins et al. 1990). This is also consistent with the finding that the characteristics of stressful events prior to onset of hallucinations and delusions are often evident in the content of those symptoms (Raune et al. 1999). Ensink found that the content of hallucinations of adult CSA survivors contain both 'flash-back elements and more symbolic representations' of traumatic experiences (1992: 126). Her many examples include visual hallucinations, e.g. 'I saw sperm in my food and in my drinks' (p. 124).

High rates of sexual delusions have been found in incest survivors diagnosed psychotic: 'One believed that her body was covered with ejaculate and another that she had had sexual relations with public figures' (Beck and Van der Kolk 1987: 1475). In the New Zealand study of 200 outpatients the percentages who experienced 'schizophrenic' symptoms (of any kind) with sexual content were: non-abused 2 per cent, CSA 7 per cent, CPA 7 per cent (not statistically significant). There was, however, a significant relationship between child abuse and symptom content pertaining to evil or the devil: non-abused 3 per cent, CSA 15 per cent, CPA 12 per cent. Among those who had suffered both CSA and sexual assault as an adult, 28 per cent experienced symptoms about evil or the devil (Read et al. 2003).

Examples from the New Zealand outpatient study included

> One person, whose chart included a forensic report stating that 'was abused over many years through anal penetration with the use of violence', hears the perpetrator's voice telling the patient to touch 'children' ... Another's chart read 'Sexual abuse: abused from an early age ... Raped several times by strangers and violent partners'. This person believes that they are 'being tortured by people getting into body for example the Devil and the Beast and 'At one stage had bleeding secondary to inserting a bathroom hose into self, stating "wanting to wash" self as "people are trying to put aliens into my body"' ... Another, who suffered 'ongoing sexual abuse by relative', hears the voice of the relative telling 'to jump from bridge and kill self. Has already tried to commit suicide several times'.
>
> (Read et al. 2003: 12)

Heins et al. (1990) documented more examples. A man who had been raped several times by an uncle at age 7, heard voices telling him he was 'sleazy' and should kill himself. A woman who had been sexually assaulted by her father from a very young age, and raped as a teenager, had the delusion that 'people were watching her as they thought she was a sexual pervert and auditory hallucinations accusing her of doing "dirty sexy things"'. Another woman, whose father had raped her monthly from age 8 and who was raped several times by a cousin at age 11, heard voices calling her a 'slut'. Read and Argyle (1999) found that the content of just over half (54 per cent) of the 'schizophrenic' symptoms of abused adult inpatients were obviously related to the abuse. A woman who had been sexually abused by her father from age 5 heard 'male voices outside her head and screaming children's voices inside her head'. In another example a man who had been sexually abused from age 4 believed his body was asymmetrical and that women only wanted sex with him because of the thrill of being with a freak.

Coincidental, contributory, or causal?

Most of the studies cited thus far are correlational. They do not, therefore, prove that the relationship is a causal one. It would be surprising, however, if it was not. Just about every other mental health problem studied has been found to have a relationship with child abuse even after controlling for probable intervening variables (Boney-McCoy and Finkelhor 1996; Fergusson et al. 1996; Kendler et al. 2000; Pettigrew and Burcham 1997; Swanston et al. 2003). After controlling for other childhood disruptions and disadvantages, women whose CSA involved intercourse were 12 times more likely than non-abused females to have had psychiatric admissions and 26 times more likely to have tried to kill themselves (Mullen et al. 1993).

Six studies *have* controlled for other factors that might explain the relationship between child abuse and psychosis. In one study, of 93 female psychiatric patients, 53 per cent of those who had suffered CSA had 'nonmanic psychotic disorders (e.g., schizophrenia, psychosis not otherwise specified)' compared to 25 per cent of those who were not victims of CSA. After controlling for 'the potential effects of demographic variables, most of which also predict victimization and/or psychiatric outcome' CSA was still strongly related to psychotic disorders ($p = 0.001$) (Briere et al. 1997).

Another study controlled for subsequent retraumatisation in the form of rapes or attempted rapes (ASA) and serious physical assaults (APA) after age 16 (Read et al. 2003). Patients who had experienced both CSA and ASA had particularly high rates of psychotic symptoms: hallucinations – non-abused 18.5 per cent, CSA+ASA 86 per cent; delusions – non-abused 27 per cent, CSA+ASA 71 per cent; thought disorder – non-abused 13 per cent, CSA+ASA 71 per cent. In a regression analysis, childhood abuse (CSA or CPA) was a significant predictor of hallucinations even after taking into account (i.e. without) APA and ASA. This was the case for auditory hallucinations in general and voices commenting in particular, and also for tactile hallucinations. However, for command, visual and olfactory hallucinations, the relationships with child abuse were, in the absence of later retraumatisation, no longer significant. Similarly, while delusions (both paranoid and grandiose) and thought disorder were predicted by childhood and adulthood abuse in combination, childhood abuse was not significantly related to these symptoms in the absence of later retraumatisation (Read et al. 2003).

The third study, of 1612 documented cases of CSA in Australia, recorded subsequent rates of treatment for a range of diagnoses in the public mental health system and compared these to rates of treatment in the general population (Spataro et al. 2004). The abused males were 1.3 times more likely, and the abused females 1.5 times more likely, to have been treated for a 'schizophrenic disorder' than the general population. These differences 'did not reach significance'. The researchers list numerous limitations, in their otherwise sophisticated and rigorous prospective study, all of which 'reduce the probability of finding a positive association between CSA and mental disorders'. These included: the presence of people in the general population sample who had suffered CSA, the inclusion of only severe forms of CSA, and the fact that 'the average age of our subjects was in their early 20's thus many have yet to pass the peak years for developing schizophrenic and related disorders'. Furthermore the general population were significantly older than the subjects and had, therefore, a greater chance of developing schizophrenia. One final and particularly crucial bias weakening the strength of the relationships in this study between CSA and schizophrenia or any other mental health problem was *not* identified by the researchers. All the abuse cases had been identified and verified by the relevant authorities (Read and Hammersley 2005). This means that many or most will have been removed from the abusive situation and that some will have received support or therapy. Such situations are rare and are powerful predictors of long-term outcomes, not least via their influence on attributions about blame for the abuse (Barker-Collo and Read 2001; Morrison et al. 2003). We therefore agree with the authors when they point out, in relation to their schizophrenia findings, that 'Care must be taken in interpreting this and other negative findings'. Perhaps 'extreme care' would be more accurate. Within days of its publication colleagues in New Zealand were sending us copies of this paper to prove to us that we were wrong about child abuse and schizophrenia. Interestingly, they didn't send us a copy of the paper we summarise next.

The fourth study, employing data from the second British National Survey of Psychiatric Morbidity, involved interviews of 8580 British people. Those with psychotic disorders were 15.5 times more likely to have suffered CSA than those with no psychiatric disorder. The odds ratios for other disorders were: 'non-psychotic disorder' 6.9; alcohol dependence 2.4; drug dependence 1.8 (Bebbington et al. 2004). This confirms, again, that far from CSA being unrelated to psychosis, it is actually more related to psychosis than other disorders (Read 1997; Read et al. 2004a).

This study addressed the causation issue by controlling not only for a long list of other adverse events, including bullying, violence in the home, running away from home, being in a children's institution and so on (all of which were significantly related to psychosis in their own right), but also for current level of depression. After doing so CSA was still 2.9 times more prevalent in psychotic people than in those with no psychiatric disorder ($p = 0.008$). The researchers concluded, rather cautiously, that 'This is suggestive of a social contribution to aetiology' (Bebbington et al. 2004: 220).

The fifth study was a retrospective survey of 17,337 Californians (Whitfield et al. 2005). It found, for both men and women, that CPA, CSA, childhood emotional abuse, and several other adverse childhood events, all significantly increased the risk of hallucinations. After controlling for substance abuse, gender, race and education, those who had experienced the greatest number of types of adverse events in childhood were 4.7 times more likely to have experienced hallucinations. The researchers concluded:

> Our data and those of others suggest that a history of child maltreatment should be obtained by health care providers with patients who have a current or past history of hallucinations. This is important because the effects of childhood and adulthood trauma are treatable and prevent-able. . . . Finding such a trauma-symptom or trauma-illness association may be an important factor in making a diagnosis, treatment plan, and referral and may help patients by lessening their fear, guilt or shame about their possibly having a mental illness.
>
> (Whitfield et al. 2005: 806)

The sixth study involved a general population sample of 4045. This was a prospective study. Psychosis-free adults were interviewed three years later. The study controlled for age, sex, level of education, unemployment, urbanicity, ethnicity, discrimination, marital status, presence of any psychiatric diag-nosis, positive psychotic symptoms or mental health care in first-degree rela-tives, and lifetime drug use. On three separate measures of psychosis, the people who had been abused before age 16 were 2.5, 7.3 and 9.3 times more likely to be psychotic. Furthermore there was, again, a 'dose–response' rela-tionship. For example, those who had experienced child abuse of mild sever-ity were 2.0 times more likely than non-abuse participants to have 'pathology level' psychosis, compared to 10.6 and 48.4 times more likely for those who had suffered moderate and high severity of abuse respectively (Janssen et al. 2004).

Can trauma lead to psychosis without a genetic predisposition?

Because Janssen and colleagues controlled for psychosis in relatives, their study adds to the growing body of literature showing that you do not have to have a genetic predisposition to develop psychosis. This has also been established in research demonstrating the relationship between urban living and schizophrenia (Lewis et al. 1992; Mortensen et al. 1999). Children growing up in deprived economic conditions but who have no family history of psychosis are seven times more likely to develop schizophrenia than non-deprived children (Harrison et al. 2001). When all the methodological flaws in the studies that have sustained the notion of a genetic predisposition are taken into consideration, there is no robust evidence of its existence (Joseph 2004). Bad things happening, often enough, early enough or sufficiently severely, can drive us mad with or without a genetic predisposition (Read et al. 2005).

Possible pathways from abuse to psychosis

Requirements for investigating how childhood trauma leads to psychotic symptoms

The assumption of a genetic basis for psychosis has not led to an intense exploration of the processes by which trauma as a child can lead to 'psychotic symptoms' later in life. Equally important is the question of why some abused children grow up with other sets of 'symptoms' – from depression and anxiety to posttraumatic stress disorder and dissociation – while others seem to do relatively well. Research into the mechanisms by which childhood trauma leads to differential outcomes, including psychosis, is finally underway. Some guiding principles might help us avoid resource-wasting dead ends:

- Brain differences do not imply biological aetiology: the environment affects the brain.
- Psychological phenomena are more reliable entities for study than diagnostic categories.
- Individual 'psychotic symptoms' are situated on dimensions of understandable, ordinary psychological processes which are reactive to past and present life events and circumstances.
- 'Symptoms of psychosis' have psychological meaning, and they can serve a function, such as defending against intolerable feelings and memories.
- Diagnoses are descriptive, not explanatory constructs.
- The relationship between childhood events and adult outcomes involves a complex set of (often reciprocal) interactions between a large number of personal and social mediating variables.

With these guiding principles in mind we can review just some of the progress already made in our efforts to understand just *how* childhood trauma can contribute to the development of psychotic symptoms.

Heightened sensitivity to stressors: the traumagenic neurodevelopmental model

Heightened reactivity to stressors has long been accepted as a cardinal feature of 'schizophrenia' (Walker and DiForio 1997) and is thought to be at the core of the 'constitutional vulnerability' that forms the diathesis in the stress-diathesis model.

Unfortunately, most brain researchers investigating the causes of 'schizophrenia' operate as if the brain exists in a social vacuum and that any brain dysfunction they unearth is proof of a biological aetiology, usually genetic or perinatal (e.g. Crow 2004). Nevertheless, brain research can help us understand what is going on in the brains of traumatised children who later develop the heightened sensitivity so characteristic of people labelled 'schizophrenic'.

Activation of the hypothalamic-pituitary-adrenal (HPA) axis is one of the primary manifestations of the stress response. Walker and DiForio (1997: 672) identified 'a unique neural response to HPA activation' in schizophrenia. The adrenal cortex, stimulated by adrenocortropic hormone (ACTH) from the pituitary, releases glucocorticoids (including cortisol in humans). The hippocampus contains a high density of glucocorticoid receptors and plays a vital role in the feedback system that modulates the activation of the HPA axis. 'When exposure to stressors persists and heightened glucocorticoid release is chronic, there can be permanent changes in the HPA axis. Most notably, the negative feedback system that serves to dampen HPA activation is impaired' (Waller and DiForio 1997: 670).

Studies of the role of dopamine in producing increased sensitivity following prolonged or severe exposure to stress has led to the realisation that 'experience-dependent effects may be an important ontogenetic mechanism in the formation, and even stability, of individual differences in dopamine system reactivity' (Depue and Collins 1999: 507; Walker and DiForio 1997: 323–324). Thus stress exposure elevates the release of not only cortisol but also dopamine, a neurotransmitter consistently claimed to be linked to 'schizophrenia'.

Walker and DiForio (1997: 679) stressed the importance, for understanding the causes of 'schizophrenia', of 'identifying the patient characteristics that predict sensitivity to stressors'. One response to this was an article entitled 'The contribution of early traumatic events to schizophrenia in some patients: A traumagenic neurodevelopmental model' (Read et al. 2001b). This article documents the research showing that over-reactivity and dysregulation of the HPA axis is found in abused children. It also presented the research showing that the dopamine irregularities so frequently cited as evidence that schizophrenia is a predominantly or purely bio-genetically based phenomenon are found in traumatised children. Of crucial importance were findings that these brain 'abnormalities' caused by childhood trauma can persist into adulthood. Heim et al. (2000) had concluded:

Our findings suggest that HPA and autonomic nervous system hyper reactivity, presumably due to cortisol releasing factor hypersecretion, is a persistent consequence of childhood abuse that may contribute to the diathesis for adulthood psychopathological conditions.

(Heim et al. 2000: 592)

The traumagenic neurodevelopmental model is an example of a more genuine integration of the reciprocal, complex interactions between social, psychological and biological factors than the 'bio-psychosocial' / 'stress-diathesis' model which has for decades underemphasised the fact that our brains are affected by our environment throughout life. This is especially true – due to high plasticity – during childhood. The article further documented that the neurological abnormalities that have also been cited as evidence that schizophrenia is a 'brain disease' are found in the brains of traumatised children, including structural changes such as hippocampal damage, cerebral atrophy, ventricular enlargement, and reversed cerebral asymmetry. The deficits in cognitive functioning that occur in association with these structural brain abnormalities can also be the result of child abuse (Read et al. 2001b: 332).

Since that 2001 article, the evidence that child abuse causes long-lasting adverse changes in the HPA axis, hippocampus and dopamine system has continued to accumulate (e.g. Bremner et al. 2003; Cichetti and Walker 2001; Nemeroff 2004; Penza et al. 2003). These long-term changes can even be caused by prenatal stress on the mother (Huiznick et al. 2004), showing that even brain 'abnormalities' that exist from birth need not be genetically based. The question *Does Stress Damage the Brain?* (Bremner 2002) is finally and firmly on the global research agenda. The focus, however, continues to be on PTSD, depression or anxiety and the implications for psychosis and schizophrenia are still undervalued. There are some exceptions (e.g. Huiznick et al. 2004; Teicher et al. 2003). One article, which discusses the role of N-methyl-D-aspartate (NMDA) receptors in the apparent lack of coordination between locally specialised brain functions in 'schizophrenia', has argued:

Physical and sexual abuse in childhood has been linked to an increased risk of schizophrenia. While there is not enough evidence at this point to determine whether adverse environmental experiences during development are associated with the development of impaired NMDA receptor expression and cognitive coordination in humans, we suggest that this may be as fruitful an area to explore as that of behaviour genetics of cognitive coordination in schizophrenia.

(Phillips and Silverstein 2003: 117)

The traumagenic neurodevelopmental model proposes that trauma, if sufficiently prolonged, severe or early, can actually create the vulnerability in the vulnerability–stress equation. It can contribute to the oversensitivity to later stress, without any genetic implications. Some studies have confirmed that adverse life events can render individuals more vulnerable to the onset of psychotic experiences via increasing their emotional reactivity to subsequent stressors (Myin-Germeys et al. 2003) and that the consequent emotional reactivity to daily stress can contribute to the underlying vulnerability for psychotic disorders (Myin-Germeys et al. 2001).

Hallucinations: decontextualised trauma flashbacks?

We have seen earlier that the psychotic symptom most strongly and consistently related to child abuse is the experiencing of hallucinations. When trauma is identified in psychotic people (i.e., when we understand the origin of the phenomenology) hallucinations are frequently reclassified as 'pseudo-hallucinations', 'psychotic-like hallucinations', 'dissociative hallucinations' or 'trauma-based flashbacks' (Read 1997). A diagnosis of 'schizophrenia' – made on the basis of precisely the same hallucinations – is then changed, to PTSD, Dissociative Disorder etc. even though, as discussed earlier, some psychotic hallucinations are nothing more or less than memories of traumatic events identical to the split-off flashbacks considered indicative of PTSD (Read et al. 2005).

Other 'psychotic hallucinations' are also trauma based but involve confusion between inner and outer experience. Some intrusive, flashback memories of child abuse occur with awareness that the experience is indeed an internal event relating to the past, i.e. a memory of the trauma. Others occur without this awareness and are experienced as external events in the present. This misattributing of an internal event to an external source (faulty 'source monitoring') has become a central tenet of many – but not all – of the recent, impressive advances made by British cognitive psychologists in our understanding of psychotic phenomena (e.g. Bentall 2003, 2004; Birchwood et al. 2000; Freeman et al. 2002; Kingdon and Turkington 1994; Morrison 2002, 2004). For example, after reviewing the research demonstrating the relationship between auditory hallucinations and inner speech, Bentall (2004) concludes:

> The various theories that try to account for this relationship all amount to the proposition that people hear hallucinated voices when they misattribute their own inner speech to a source that is external or alien to themselves. Hallucinations in other modalities can presumably be explained in the same way. Visual hallucinations, for example, may be the result of failing to discriminate between mental imagery and visual perceptions.
>
> (Bentall 2004: 198)

To experience the memory of the perpetrator's voice calling you a 'slut', or the memory of the smell of semen, as external events in the present can serve as a defence against remembering what actually happened as a child. Although the consequence of this misattribution may lead to delusional explanations of the experience (see below) at least one does not have to relive the actual trauma and the associated feelings.

From a less psychodynamic perspective Bentall (2003) offers the following additional explanation:

> Source-monitoring failures tend to occur when we experience intrusive or automatic thoughts . . . It follows that a person who has poor source-monitoring skills will be most vulnerable to hallucinations when experiencing a flood of intrusive thoughts and images. Trauma (we know from the research literature on post-traumatic stress disorder) often has exactly this effect.
>
> (Bentall 2003: 483)

This notion of faulty source-monitoring (or projection, as psychodynamic folk might call it) might seem to apply more readily to visual, tactile and olfactory hallucinations than to voices. Flashbacks of the sounds, sights, touch sensations and smells involved in the abuse can be experienced, piecemeal as it were, as hallucinations occurring in the external present. Sensory and perceptual components of traumatic events can be re-experienced without any awareness of their relatedness to past events (van der Kolk and Fisler 1995). Nadel and Jacobs (1996) offer an elegant explanation in their discussion of trauma-induced inactivation of the hippocampus – the brain region responsible for the contextualisation of memories.

Many trauma-related voices, however, are not the actual words said at the time of the abuse and cannot really, therefore, be characterised as flashbacks. Some of the examples of symptom content offered earlier, including command hallucinations to harm oneself, are clearly negative self-statements developed during or since the abuse. The same externalising/projecting outwards into the present may nevertheless serve the defensive function of not having to acknowledge the awful origins of the self-statements.

Conceptualising hallucinations as dissociative events offers a potentially powerful perspective. The failure to integrate traumatic events at the time of their occurrence can result in the persistence of disaggregated stimuli which, compartmentalised and independent of context, emerge later in life (Moskowitz et al., in press). Voices commenting, a common hallucination in schizophrenia, is also very common in patients with Dissociative Identity Disorder (DID) (Ross et al. 1990). The most common voices in both schizophrenia and DID are punitive and hostile (Honig et al. 1998; Putnam 1989). Such powerfully negative internal self-statements are precisely the kind of inner speech that we might be better off, in the short term at least, experiencing as located outside ourselves and as unrelated to anything real in our past.

Finally, in keeping with the principle that psychotic symptoms are understandable psychological processes, we should remember that the self trauma model (not usually applied to psychosis) posits that flashbacks and intrusive trauma memories (whether called hallucinations or pseudo-hallucinations) are the mind/brain's natural attempt to process and thereby integrate trauma memories (Briere 2002). For some trauma survivors the mind/brain 'heals' itself. For others the memories remain fragmented and terrifying. Some of the factors that might contribute to these two quite different outcomes are identified in the Complex Pathways section below.

Paranoid delusions: faulty attempts to explain trauma-based hallucinations?

British cognitive psychologists have advanced our understanding of paranoid delusions (e.g. Trower and Chadwick 1995; Bentall et al. 1994). The Manchester-based group has focused on faulty attributions for negative events. Most of us tend to have a 'self-serving' bias. We tend to blame circumstances or other people when bad things happen but assume that we are responsible when good things happen. The opposite is true if we are depressed. People who experience paranoid delusions have an exaggerated 'self-serving' bias. More importantly, they are particularly prone to blaming other people, rather than general impersonal circumstances. It is thought, therefore, that although paranoid delusions can involve living in fear of harm from others' delusions, they can be a defence against low self-esteem (Bentall 2004: 201–202).

Nadel and Jacobs's (1996) work on the inhibitory impact of prolonged stress on hippocampal functioning (while sparing the amygdala's assignment of emotional valence) provides a physiological underpinning for decontextualised fear. Garety's London-based group focus on the role of anxiety and conceptualise persecutory delusions as threat beliefs. 'The beliefs are hypothesized to arise from a search for meaning for internal or external experiences that are unusual, anomalous, or emotionally significant for the individual' (Freeman et al. 2002: 331).

Attention has also been drawn to ways in which information confirming false beliefs is sought out or privileged and information disconfirming the belief is avoided. Paranoid people selectively attend to and recall threat-related information (Bentall et al. 1995). Potential disconfirming evidence is avoided by the use of 'safety behaviours' used to avoid the imagined threat (Freeman et al. 2001; Morrison 1998). Studies have also shown that people with paranoid delusions tend to jump to conclusions quickly when coming up with causal explanations for unusual or negative events (Garety et al. 1991) and, importantly for our current topic, that this is particularly the case when the content of the task is emotionally charged (Young and Bentall 1997).

In essence then what has been discovered is that some people, when faced with negative, emotionally loaded, or unusual or anomalous experiences quickly jump to the suspicion of external threat, i.e. they become paranoid. Hearing voices when there is nobody there is often (but not always) a negative experience, and is often experienced as unusual or anomalous. Paranoid delusions are sometimes, therefore, understandable attempts to make sense of hallucinations (across sense modalities).

Paranoid delusions can, of course, develop in the absence of hallucinations. There would seem to be some similarity between the hypervigilance to threat (acknowledged, in PTSD patients, to be the outcome of trauma), and the supposedly delusional belief that people are out to get you in traumatised people who are diagnosed psychotic. With or without the need to explain trauma flashbacks/hallucinations, having been severely or repeatedly sexually abused as a young child is likely to render other people a serious potential threat, a threat that can easily be generalised to anyone or anything that is reminiscent of the perpetrator or the circumstances surrounding the abuse. Again, Nadel and Jacob's (1996) work on the impact of trauma on the brain is salient. Whether we label this PTSD, DID or schizophrenia, the resulting fear, distortions and impoverishment of lives remain.

Clearly, a growing number of researchers now include childhood trauma in their theorising or research. Researchers and theorists from psychological frameworks beyond a cognitive paradigm also have much to contribute to the understanding of delusions and hallucinations. These include attachment theory (Shapiro and Levondosky 1999; Trower and Chadwick 1995), including a developmental and family perspective (Harrop and Trower 2003), dissociation (Moskowitz et al., in press; Ross 2004) and psychodynamics (Heilbrun et al. 1986; Silver et al. 2004).

Rudegeair and Farrelly (2003) offer an evolutionary perspective on dissociation and its relationship to psychosis. They argue that the human phylogeny has seen the proliferation of pre-frontal cortex for assessing and manipulating an increasingly complex social context through the orchestration of social memories, appreciation for the meaning of the immediate 'social moment', and the selection of a socially effective response. The resulting ontogenetic challenge for the developing individual is the integration of initially separate ego states in the service of social efficiency. In this model, intrapsychic integration is seen as a developmentally vulnerable goal easily disrupted by childhood trauma and attachment failures resulting in the persistence of separate 'dissociated' states and a susceptibility to errors in contextualisation, manifesting as errors of perception and interpretation of social meaning.

Complex pathways

The relationships between childhood trauma and psychotic experiences in adulthood are mediated by a myriad of intervening and interacting factors, in the psychological, social and biological domains (Read et al. 2005). We already know, for instance, that the more severe the abuse, the greater the probability of severe mental health problems in adulthood, including suicidality and admission to psychiatric hospital (Fergusson et al. 1996; Mullen et al. 1993). This same 'dose effect' has now been established, in large-scale prospective studies, for psychosis (Janssen et al. 2004; Whitfield et al. 2005).

An article has summarised the progress made thus far examining multifactor models of response to CSA and its impact on mental health using pathway analysis methodologies (Barker-Collo and Read 2003). For instance, abuse severity factors include early age of abuse onset, use of violence, presence of other forms of abuse/neglect and intrafamilial abuse (e.g. incest) versus abuse by a stranger. Another crucial factor is whether the abused person tells anyone and how that person responds. In a New Zealand survey of 191 women who were sexually abused as children, the average time it took to tell anyone was 16 years (McGregor 2003). Another important mediator is whether the abuse survivor blames herself or the perpetrator for the abuse. This would appear to be of obvious relevance to the later development of the sorts of attributions that underlie paranoid delusions. One of the complex models has focused on attachment and coping styles (Shapiro and Levendosky 1999) as mediators of the effects of CSA on later psychological and interpersonal functioning.

Retraumatisation

It will be imperative that future studies seeking to track the complex pathways from child abuse to adult psychosis (and other mental health problems) include revictimisation. People who have been abused as children are more likely to be abused as adults (Cloitre et al. 1996; Muenzenmaier et al. 1993). Most psychiatric patients, male and female, suffer serious physical assaults as adults. One study found that in the year before admission to hospital 63 per cent of patients had suffered physical violence by their partners and 46 per cent of those who lived at home had been assaulted by family members, predominantly parents (Cascardi et al. 1996). Most female psychiatric patients suffer sexual assaults (Goodman et al. 2001; Mueser et al. 1998; Switzer et al. 1999), with about a third being raped (Briere et al. 1997; Cloitre et al. 2001; Craine et al. 2001; Neria et al. 2002; Switzer et al. 1999), frequently by spouses (Chandra et al. 2003). A study of women inpatients predominantly diagnosed psychotic found that 'two-thirds of the sexually coercive experiences occurred prior to the onset of the mental disorder' (Chandra et al. 2003: 332). About a quarter of male patients are sexually assaulted as adults (Goodman et al. 2001; Mueser et al. 1998).

A study of 409 female inpatients found that sexual assault was significantly related to a diagnosis of schizophrenia but, at least in this sample, not to mania, depression, substance abuse or borderline personality disorder (Cloitre et al. 1996). Among female psychiatric patients, physical assault (by non-partners) was significantly related to only one diagnostic group: 'nonmanic psychotic disorders (e.g. schizophrenia, psychosis not otherwise specified)'. Overall 37 per cent had been raped, but this was the case for 51 per cent of those with a diagnosis of 'nonmanic psychotic disorder' (Briere et al. 1997).

A Dutch study of people diagnosed with schizophrenia or dissociative disorder found that 'In most patients, the onset of auditory hallucinations was preceded by either a traumatic event or an event that activated the memory of earlier trauma' (Honig et al. 1998: 646).

As we have seen earlier, when the ability of child abuse and adulthood abuse to predict schizophrenic symptoms were analysed in relation to each other (by logistic regression) only voices commenting and tactile hallucinations were predicted by child abuse if no adult abuse followed. However, both hallucinations and delusions were predicted by child abuse if that child abuse *is* followed by abuse in adulthood. Even thought disorder and grandiose delusions were predicted by child and adult abuse together (Read et al. 2003).

Conclusions and implications

A recent chapter elsewhere has delineated no fewer than 37 'Unanswered Questions and Next Steps' that emanate from the data linking childhood trauma and psychosis (Read et al. 2004a). Many of the research questions could be easily and economically addressed if trauma researchers would include psychosis in their list of outcome measures, and if psychosis researchers would start asking questions about the lives of the people they are trying to understand.

Diagnosis

The relationship between childhood trauma and psychosis raises major issues for our diagnostic system that should be addressed by the authors of DSM-V. The relationships among trauma, psychosis and dissociation are complex, and are only beginning to be unravelled (Moskowitz et al., in press; Ross 2004). The same is true of the relationships among trauma, psychosis and PTSD (Seedat et al. 2003). Some leading researchers, who have done more than most to highlight the importance of trauma in 'serious mental illness' (SMI), proposed a model 'in which PTSD is hypothesized to mediate the negative effects of trauma on the course of SMI' (Mueser et al. 2002: 123). Such an approach begs the question of whether trauma has a causal role in psychosis, and would seem to require no changes to our diagnostic system. This has been the downside to the introduction of PTSD. It seems to have created a sort of blind spot to the massive overlap among the symptoms on different pages of DSM-IV, and to the similarity of mechanisms underlying them (Seedat et al. 2003). We too often assume that if trauma is identified the diagnosis must be PTSD, because we *know* that trauma can't cause psychosis.

It is revealing to remember that before PTSD, the symptoms that are now considered indicative of the new diagnosis were frequently considered evidence of schizophrenia (Seedat et al. 2003). It is obviously better for people to be labelled with PTSD than schizophrenia, because they have a better chance of getting to talk to someone about what has happened to them, and a lower chance of being exposed to a lifetime of anti-psychotic medications and their various adverse effects (Ross and Read 2004). However, this rediagnosing serves to maintain the illusion that trauma cannot cause psychosis (Read 1997). Therefore we would prefer that most DSM categories, and certainly schizophrenia, schizophreniform disorder, schizoaffective disorder, dissociative disorders, substance abuse, depression, anxiety disorders, eating disorders, personality disorders and sexual dysfunctions, have a 'posttraumatic' or 'with trauma history' subcategory. Failing this unlikely outcome we can live with the analysis provided, after thoughtful consideration of the relevant research, by Morrison et al. (2003):

> Some psychotic patients will develop PTSD in response to their psychosis, some people will develop psychosis in the first place as a result of traumatic experiences, some may develop both, and for some people a vicious circle may develop between their psychotic experiences and their PTSD symptoms. It is also possible that some shared mechanism (such as dissociation, attributional style or interpretations of intrusions) may be responsible for mediating the development or maintenance of the disorders. The possibility that psychosis and PTSD are part of a spectrum of reactions to trauma is, in fact, similar to proposals that suggest there is a distinct subtype of psychotic disorders that is trauma-induced.
>
> (Morrison et al. 2003: 345)

Treatment

Chapter 9 in this book covers perhaps the most immediate clinical implication – the need for mental health staff to ask people with psychotic symptoms what has happened in their lives. Beyond this are the treatment implications (Read and Ross 2003). The whole range of psychological treatments now known to be effective with the symptoms of psychosis (Cullberg 2006; Johannessen et al. 2006; Martindale et al. 2001; Read et al. 2004d; Ross and Read 2003) must be offered to more clients, traumatised or otherwise. These include cognitive-behavioural (Gould et al. 2001; Haddock et al. 2003; Kingdon and Turkington 1994; Morrison 2002, 2004; Morrison et al. 2004; Wiersma et al. 2004), psychodynamic (Gottdiener 2004; Karon and vanden Bos 1981; Silver et al. 2004), family therapy (real family therapy, not ideologically driven 'psycho-education' packages) (Aderhold and Gottwalz 2004), non-medical residential-based services (Mosher 2004), the psychosocial components of early intervention services (Johannessen 2004) and user-run services (Chamberlin 2004). Whether we can accomplish an effective integration of these approaches with the approaches currently used for non-psychotic traumatised people (Briere 2002; Courtois 1999; McGregor 2003) remains to be seen. The potential retraumatising impact of hospitalisation must temper our use of this intervention (Morrison et al. 2003).

Some will interpret the neurological and biochemical concomitants of the psychological effects of trauma as an argument for yet more chemical solutions. Arguing against this, however, is a study showing that for patients suffering from chronic depression, psychotherapy is significantly more effective than medication for the patients who had experienced childhood trauma (Nemeroff et al. 2003). Also, older studies have shown that 'schizophrenia' is more effectively treated by ordinary human beings in ordinary homes than by medications in hospitals (Mosher 2004). These findings, that human interventions can be more effective than chemical ones, have recently been replicated in the domain of preventive interventions for youth considered at risk for psychosis. A randomised, controlled trial has demonstrated that people from such a high-risk population are significantly less likely to develop psychosis if they receive cognitive therapy, with or without anti-psychotic medication (Morrison et al. 2004). Human treatments carry none of the diverse dangers of medication including those of the new 'atypical' anti-psychotics (Bentall and Morrison 2002; Mosher et al. 2004; Ross and Read 2004).

Prevention

Finally, if we look up for a moment from our research and our clinical practice, there are some rather important broader implications. One study has shown that an environmental enrichment programme at age 3 to 5 can reduce 'schizotypal personality' and antisocial scores in early adulthood (Raine et al. 2003).

> The belief that because 'schizophrenia' is an illness and therefore life events and circumstances can play no role in its causation has led to the awful conclusion that nothing can be done to prevent it. Rather than lobby governments to fund primary prevention programmes that could improve the quality of life for children, adolescents, and their families, biological psychiatry gives politicians a perfect excuse for doing nothing.
>
> (Read et al. 2004b: 4)

Many mental health professionals see more human pain in a week than most of us see in a lifetime. Paradoxically, these societally-ordained witnesses seem paralysed into silence about the source of the pain flowing over them. To ask a human being to sit day after day with often frightened and sometimes frightening survivors of the worst that life can throw at people, *and* to find the energy, and hope, to simultaneously try to plug the source, seems unfair. On the other hand, an exclusive focus on the distressed individual may be stopping us focusing on what we mean by mental health, healthy families, healthy communities and just societies. If we focus more of our debate here, we might learn more about how to enhance their development.

(Davies and Burdett 2004: 279)

References

Aderhold, V., and Gottwalz, E. (2004) Family therapy and schizophrenia: Replacing ideology with openness. In J. Read, L. Mosher and R. Bentall (eds) *Models of madness* (pp. 335–348). Hove: Brunner-Routledge.

Ambelas, A. (1992) Preschizophrenics: Adding to the evidence, sharpening the focus. *British Journal of Psychiatry, 31*, 401–444.

American Psychiatric Association (APA) (1994) *Diagnostic and statistical manual of mental disorders* (4th edn). Washington, DC: APA.

Angermeyer, M., and Matschinger, H. (1999) Lay beliefs about mental disorders: A comparison between the western and eastern parts of Germany. *Social Psychiatry and Psychiatric Epidemiology, 34*, 275–281.

Barker-Collo, S., and Read, J. (2003) Models of response to childhood sexual abuse: Their implications for treatment. *Trauma, Violence and Abuse, 4*, 95–111.

Barry, M., and Greene, S. (1992) Implicit models of mental disorder: A qualitative approach to the delineation of public attitudes. *Irish Journal of Psychology, 13*, 141–160.

Bebbington, P., Bhugra, D., Brugha, T., Singleton, N., Farrell, M., Jenkins, R., et al. (2004) Psychosis, victimisation and childhood disadvantage: Evidence from the second British National Survey of Psychiatric Morbidity. *British Journal of Psychiatry, 185*, 220–226.

Beck, J., and van der Kolk, B. (1987) Reports of childhood incest and current behaviour of chronically hospitalized psychotic women. *American Journal of Psychiatry, 144*, 1474–1476.

Belkin, D., Greene, A., Rodrigue, J., and Boggs, S. (1994) Psychopathology and history of sexual abuse. *Journal of Interpersonal Violence, 9*, 535–547.

Bentall, R. (2003) *Madness explained: Psychosis and human nature.* London: Penguin.

Bentall, R. (2004) Abandoning the concept of schizophrenia: The cognitive psychology of hallucinations and delusions. In J. Read, L. Mosher and R. Bentall (eds) *Models of madness* (pp. 195–208). Hove: Brunner-Routledge.

Bentall, R., and Morrison, A. (2002) More harm than good: The case against using anti-psychotic drugs to prevent severe mental illness. *Journal of Mental Health, 11*, 351–356.

Bentall, R., Kaney, S., and Bowen-Jones, K. (1995) Persecutory delusions and recall of threat-related, depression-related and neutral words. *Cognitive Therapy and Research, 19*, 331–43.

Bentall, R. P., Kinderman, P., and Kaney, S. (1994) The self, attributional processes and abnormal beliefs: Towards a model of persecutery delusions. *Behaviour Research and Therapy, 32*, 331–341.

Berenbaum, H. (1999) Peculiarity and reported child maltreatment. *Psychiatry, 62*, 21–35.

Birchwood, M., Meaden, A., Trower, P., Gilbert, P., and Plaistow, J. (2000) The power and omnipotence of voices: Subordination and entrapment by voices and significant others. *Psychological Medicine, 30*, 337–44.

Boney-McCoy, S., and Finkelhor, D. (1996) Is youth victimization related to trauma symptoms and depression after controlling for prior symptoms and family relationships? *Journal of Consulting and Clinical Psychology, 64*, 1406–1416.

Bremner, J. (2002) *Does Stress Damage the Brain?* London: W. W. Norton.

Bremner, J., Vythilingam, M., Vermetten, E., Southwick, S., McGlashan, T., Nazeer, A., et al. (2003) MRI and PET study of deficits in hippocampal structure and function in women with childhood sexual abuse and PTSD. *American Journal of Psychiatry, 160*, 924–932.

Briere, J. (2002) Treating adult survivors of severe childhood abuse and neglect. In J. Myers et al. (eds) *ASPAC Handbook on Child Maltreatment*, 2nd edn, Newbury Park, CA: Sage.

Briere, J., Woo, R., McRae, B., Foltz, J., and Sitzman, R. (1997) Lifetime victimization history, demographics and clinical status in female psychiatric emergency room patients. *Journal of Nervous and Mental Disease, 185*, 95–101.

Bryer, J., Nelson, B., Miller, J., and Krol, P. (1987) Childhood sexual and physical abuse as factors in psychiatric illness. *American Journal Psychiatry, 144*, 1426–1430.

Cairns, S. (1998) MMPI–2 and Rorschach assessments of adults physically abused as children. Unpublished doctoral dissertation. University of Manitoba.

Cannon, M., Walsh, E., Hollis, C., Maresc, K., Taylor, E., Murray, M., and Jones, P. (2001) Predictors of later schizophrenia and affective psychoses among attendees at a child psychiatry department. *British Journal of Psychiatry, 178*, 420–426.

Cannon, M., Caspi, A., Moffitt, T., Harrington, H., Taylor, A., Murray, R., and Poulton, R. (2002) Evidence for early-childhood, pan-developmental impairment specific to schizophreniform disorder. *Archives of General Psychiatry, 59*, 449–456.

Cascardi, M., Mueser, K., Degiralomo, J., and Murrin, M. (1996) Physical aggression against psychiatric inpatients by family members and partners. *Psychiatric Services, 47*, 531–533.

Chamberlin, J. (2004) User-run services. In J. Read, L. Mosher, and R. Bentall (eds) *Models of madness* (pp. 283–290). Hove: Brunner-Routledge.

Chandra, P., Deepthivarma, S., Carey, M., Carey, K., and Shalinianant, M. (2003) A cry from the wilderness: Women with severe mental illness in India reveal their experiences with sexual coercion. *Psychiatry: Interpersonal and Biological Processes, 66*, 323–334.

Cichetti, D., and Walker, E. (2001) Editorial. Stress and development: Biological and psychological consequences. *Development and Psychopathology, 13*, 413–418.

Cloitre, M., Tardiff, K., Marzuk, P., Leon, A., and Portera, L. (1996) Childhood abuse and subsequent sexual assault among female inpatients. *Journal of Traumatic Stress, 9*, 473–482.

Cloitre, M., Tardiff, K., Marzuk, P., Leon, A., and Portera, L. (2001) Consequences of childhood abuse among male psychiatric inpatients: Dual roles as victims and perpetrators. *Journal of Traumatic Stress, 14*, 47–60.

Courtois, C. (1999) *Recollections of Sexual Abuse: Treatment Principles and Guidelines*. New York: W. W. Norton.

Craine, L., Henson, C., Colliver, J., and MacLean, D. (1988) Prevalence of a history of sexual abuse among female psychiatric patients in a state hospital system. *Hospital and Community Psychiatry, 39*, 300–304.

Crow, T. (2004) Cerebral asymmetry and the lateralization of language: Core deficits in schizophrenia as pointers to the gene. *Current Opinion in Psychiatry, 17*, 97–106.

Cullberg, J. (2006) *Psychoses: An integrative perspective*. London: Routledge.

Darves-Bornoz, J.-M., Lempérière, T., Degiovanni, A., and Gaillard, P. (1995) Sexual victimization in women with schizophrenia and bipolar disorder. *Social Psychiatry and Psychiatric Epidemiology, 30*, 78–84.

Davies, E., and Burdett, J. (2004) Preventing 'schizophrenia': Creating the conditions for saner societies. In J. Read, L. Mosher and R. Bentall (eds) *Models of Madness* (pp. 271–282). Hove: Brunner-Routledge.

Depue, R., and Collins, P. (1999) Neurobiology of the structure of personality: Dopamine, facilitation of incentive motivation, and extraversion. *Behavioural and Brain Sciences, 22*, 491–569.

Dietrich, S., Beck, M., Bugantugs, B., Kenzine, D., Matschinger, H., and Angermeyer, M. (2004) The relationships between public causal beliefs and social distance toward mentally ill people. *Australian and New Zealand Journal of Psychiatry, 38*, 348–354.

Dill, D., Chu, J., Grob, M., and Eisen, S. (1991) The reliability of abuse history reports: A comparison of two inquiry formats. *Comprehensive Psychiatry, 32*, 166–169.

Ellason, J., and Ross, C. (1997) Childhood trauma and psychiatric symptoms. *Psychological Reports, 80*, 447–50.

Ellenson, G. (1985) Detecting a history of incest. *Social Casework*, November, 525–32.

Ensink, B. (1992) *Confusing Realities*. Amsterdam: Vu University.

Famularo, R., Kinscherff, R., and Fenton, T. (1992) Psychiatric diagnoses of maltreated children: Preliminary findings. *Journal of the American Academy of Child and Adolescent Psychiatry, 31*, 863–867.

Fergusson, D., Horwood, J., and Lynskey, M. (1996) Childhood sexual abuse and psychiatric disorder in young adulthood: II. Psychiatric outcomes of childhood sexual abuse. *Journal of the American Academy of Child and Adolescent Psychiatry, 34*, 1365–1374.

Freeman, D., Garety, P., and Kuipers, E. (2001) Persecutory delusions: Developing the understanding of belief maintenance and emotional distress. *Psychological Medicine, 31*, 1293–1306.

Freeman, D., Garety, P., Kuipers, E., Fowler, D., and Bebbington, P. (2002) A cognitive model of persecutory delusions: A cognitive model of persecutory delusions. *British Journal of Clinical Psychology, 41*, 331–347.

Friedman, S., Smith, L., Fogel, D., Paradis, C., Viswnathan, R., Ackerman, R., and Trappler, B. (2002) The incidence and influence of early traumatic life events in patients with panic disorder: A comparison with other psychiatric outpatients. *Anxiety Disorders, 16*, 259–72.

Furnham, A., and Bower, P. (1992) A comparison of academic and lay theories of schizophrenia. *British Journal of Psychiatry, 62*, 201–210.

Furnham, A., and Rees, J. (1988) Lay theories of schizophrenia. *International Journal of Social Psychiatry, 34*, 212–220.

Garety, P., Hemsley, D., and Wessely, S. (1991) Reasoning in deluded schizophrenic and paranoid patients: Biases in performance on a probabilistic inference task. *Journal of Nervous and Mental Disease, 179*, 194–201.

Goff, D., Brotman, A., Kindlon, D., Waites, M., and Amico, E. (1991a) Self-reports of child abuse in chronically psychotic patients. *Psychiatry Research, 37*, 73–80.

Goff, D., Brotman, A., Kindlon, D., Waites, M., and Amico, E. (1991b) The delusion of possession in chronically psychotic patients. *Journal of Nervous and Mental Disease, 179*, 567–571.

Goodman, L., Salyers, M., Mueser, K., Rosenberg, S., Swartz, M., Essock, S., et al. (2001) Recent victimization in women and men with severe mental illness. *Journal of Traumatic Stress, 14*, 615–632.

Gottdiener, W. (2004) Psychodynamic psychotherapy for schizophrenia: Empirical support. In J. Read, L. Mosher and R. Bentall (eds) *Models of madness* (pp. 307–318). Hove: Brunner-Routledge.

Gould, R., Mueser, K., Bolton, E., Mays, V., and Goff, D. (2001) Cognitive therapy for psychosis in schizophrenia: An effect size analysis. *Schizophrenia Research, 48*, 335–342.

Haddock, G., Barrowclough, C., Tarrier, N., Morning, J., O'Brien, R., Schofield, N., et al. (2003) Cognitive-behavioural therapy and motivational intervention for schizophrenia and substance misuse: 18-month outcomes of a randomised controlled trial. *British Journal of Psychiatry, 183*, 418–426.

Hammersley, P., Dias, A., Todd, G., Bowen-Jones, K., Reilly, B., and Bentall, R. (2003) Childhood traumas and hallucinations in bipolar affective disorder. *British Journal of Psychiatry, 182*, 543–547.

Harrison, G., Gunnell, D., Glazebrook, C., Page, K., and Kwiecinski, R. (2001) Association between schizophrenia and social inequality at birth. *British Journal of Psychiatry, 179*, 346–350.

Harrop, P., and Trower, C. (2003) *Why does schizophrenia develop at late adolescence?* London: John Wiley and Sons.

Heads, T., Taylor, P., and Lease, M. (1997) Childhood experiences of patients with schizophrenia and a history of violence: A special hospital sample. *Criminal Behaviour and Mental Health, 7*, 117–130.

Heilbrun, A., Diller, R., and Dodson, V. (1986) Defensive projection and paranoid delusions. *Journal of Psychiatric Research, 20*, 161–173.

Heim, C., Newport, D. J., Heit, S., Graham, Y., Wilcox, M., Bonsall, R., et al. (2000) Pituitary-adrenal and autonomic responses to stress in women after sexual and physical abuse in childhood. *Journal of the American Medical Association, 284*, 592–597.

Heins, T., Gray, A., and Tennant, M. (1990) Persisting hallucinations following childhood sexual abuse. *Australian and New Zealand Journal of Psychiatry, 24*, 561–565.

Hill, D., and Bale, R. (1981) Measuring beliefs about where psychological distress originates and who is responsible for its alleviation: Two new scales for clinical researchers. In H. Lefcourt.(ed.) *Research with the locus of control construct* (Vol. 2, pp. 122–139). New York: Academic Press.

Holowka, D., King, S., Saheb, D., Pukall, M., and Brunet, A. (2003) Childhood abuse and dissociative symptoms in adult schizophrenia. *Schizophrenia Research, 60*, 87–90.

Honig, A., Romme, M., Ensink, B., Escher, S., Pennings, M., and de Vries, M. (1998)

Auditory hallucinations: A comparison between patients and nonpatients. *Journal of Nervous and Mental Disease, 186*, 646–651.

Huiznick, A., Mulder, E., and Buitelaar, J. (2004) Prenatal stress and risk for psychopathology: Specific effects or induction of general susceptibility. *Psychological Bulletin, 130*, 115–142.

Hunter, J. (1991) A comparison of psychosocial maladjustment of adult males and females sexually molested as children. *Journal of Interpersonal Violence, 6*, 205–217.

Janssen, I., Krabbendam, L., Bak, M., Hanssen, M., Vollebergh, W., de Graaf, R., and van Os, J. (2004) Childhood abuse as a risk factor for psychotic experiences. *Acta Psychiatrica Scandinavica, 109*, 38–45.

Johannessen, J.-O. (2004) The development of early intervention services. In J. Read, L. Mosher and R. Bentall (eds) *Models of madness* (pp. 319–333). Hove: Brunner-Routledge.

Johannessen, J.-O., Martindale, B., and Cullberg, J. (eds) (2006) *Evolving psychosis: Different stages, different treatments*. London: Routledge.

Jones, P., Rodgers, B., Murray, R., and Marmont, M. (1994) Child developmental risk factors for adult schizophrenia in the British 1946 birth cohort. *Lancet, 344*, 1398–1402.

Jorm, A. (2000) Mental health literacy: Public knowledge and beliefs about mental disorders. *British Journal of Psychiatry, 177*, 396–401.

Jorm, A., Korten, A., Jacomb, P., Christensen, H., Rodgers, B., and Pollitt, P. (1997) Public beliefs about causes and risk factors for depression and schizophrenia. *Social Psychiatry and Psychiatric Epidemiology, 32*, 143–148.

Joseph, J. (2004) Schizophrenia and heredity: Why the emperor has no genes. In J. Read, L. Mosher and R. Bentall (eds) *Models of Madness* (pp. 67–84). Hove: Brunner-Routledge.

Kahlbaum, K. (1973) *Catatonia*. Baltimore, MD: Johns Hopkins University Press.

Karon, B., and vanden Bos, G. (1981) *Psychotherapy of schizophrenia: The treatment of choice*. New York: Aronson.

Kendler, K., Bulik, S., Silberg, J., Hettema, J., Myers, J., and Prescott, C. (2000) Childhood sexual abuse and adult psychiatric and substance use disorders in women. *Archives of General Psychiatry, 57*, 953–959.

Kessler, R., Sonnega, A., Bromet, E., Hughes, M., and Nelson, C. (1995) PTSD in the National Comorbidity Survey. *Archives of General Psychiatry, 52*, 1048–1060.

Kingdon, D., and Turkington, D. (1994) *Cognitive-behavioural therapy of schizophrenia*. Hove: Lawrence Erlbaum.

Lewis, G., David, A., Andreasson, S., and Allebeck, P. (1992) Schizophrenia and city life. *Lancet, 340*, 137–140.

Link, B., Phelan, J., Bresnahan, M., Stueve, A., and Pescosolido, B. (1999) Public conceptions of mental illness. *American Journal of Public Health, 89*, 1328–1333.

Lipschitz, D., Winegar, R., Hartnick, E., Foote, B., and Southwick, S. (1999a) PTSD in hospitalized adolescents: Diagnostic comorbidity and clinical correlates. *Journal of the American Academy of Child and Adolescent Psychiatry, 38*, 385–392.

Lipschitz, D., Winegar, R., Nicolau, A., Hartnick, E., Wolfson, M., and Southwick, S. (1999b) Perceived abuse and neglect as risk factors for suicidal behaviour in adolescent inpatients. *Journal of Nervous and Mental Disease, 187*, 32–39.

Livingston, R. (1987) Sexually and physically abused children. *Journal of the American Academy of Child and Adolescent Psychiatry, 26*, 413–415.

Lundberg-Love, P., Marmion, S., Ford, K., Geffner, R., and Peacock, L. (1992) The long-term consequences of childhood incestuous victimization upon adult women's psychological symptomatology. *Journal of Child Sexual Abuse, 1*, 81–102.

Lysaker, P., Meyer, P., Evans, J., Clements, C., and Marks, K. (2001) Childhood sexual trauma and psychosocial functioning in adults with schizophrenia. *Psychiatric Services, 52*, 1485–1488.

McGregor, K. (2003) Therapy – It's a two-way thing: Women survivors of child sexual abuse describe their therapy experiences. Unpublished doctoral dissertation. University of Auckland, New Zealand.

Malmberg, A., Lewis, G., and Allebeck, P. (1998) Premorbid adjustment and personality in people with schizophrenia. *British Journal of Psychiatry, 172*, 308–313.

Martindale, B., Bateman, A., Crowe, M., and Margison, F. (eds) (2000) *Psychosis: Psychological approaches and their effectiveness*. London: Gaskell.

Mehta, S., and Farina, A. (1997) Is being 'sick' really better? Effect of the disease view of mental disorder on stigma. *Journal of Social and Clinical Psychology, 16*, 405–419.

Morrison, A. (1998) A cognitive analysis of the maintenance of auditory hallucinations. *Behavioural and Cognitive Psychotherapy, 26*, 289–302.

Morrison, A. (ed.) (2002) *A casebook of cognitive therapy for psychosis*. Hove: Brunner-Routledge.

Morrison, A. (2004) Cognitive therapy for people with psychosis. In J. Read, L. Mosher and R. Bentall (eds) *Models of madness* (pp. 291–306). Hove: Brunner-Routledge.

Morrison, A., and Petersen, T. (2003) Trauma and metacognition as predictors of predisposition to hallucinations. *Behavioural and Cognitive Psychotherapy, 31*, 235–246.

Morrison, A., Frame, A., and Larkin, W. (2003) Relationships between trauma and psychosis: A review and integration. *British Journal of Clinical Psychology, 42*, 331–353.

Morrison, A. P., French, P., Walford, L., Lewis, S. W., Green, J. M., Kilcommons, A., et al. (2004) A randomised controlled trial of cognitive therapy for the prevention of psychosis in people at ultra-high risk. *British Journal of Psychiatry, 185*, 291–297.

Mortensen, P., Pedersen, C., Westergaard, T., Wohlfahrt, J., Ewald, H., Mors, O., Andersen, P. K., and Melbye, M. (1999) Effects of family history and place of season of birth on the risk of schizophrenia. *New England Journal of Medicine, 340*, 603–608.

Mosher, L. (2004) Non-hospital, non-drug intervention with first-episode psychosis. In J. Read, L. Mosher and R. Bentall (eds) *Models of madness* (pp. 349–364). Hove: Brunner-Routledge.

Mosher, L., Gosden, R., and Beder, S. (2004) Drug companies and schizophrenia: Unbridled capitalism meets madness. In J. Read, L. Mosher and R. Bentall (eds) *Models of madness* (pp. 115–130). Hove: Brunner-Routledge.

Moskowitz, A. (2004) 'Scared stiff': Catatonia as an evolutionary-based fear response. *Psychological Review, 111*, 984–1002.

Moskowitz, A., Read, J., Farrelly, S., Rudegeair, T., and Williams, O. (in press) Are all psychotic symptoms dissociative? In P. Dell and J. O'Neil (eds) *Dissociation and the dissociative disorders: DSM-IV and beyond*. McLean, VA: International Society for the Study of Dissociation.

Muenzenmaier, K., Meyer, I., Struening, E., and Ferber, J. (1993) Childhood abuse and neglect among women outpatients with chronic mental illness. *Hospital and Community Psychiatry, 44*, 666–670.

Mueser, K., Trumbetta, S., Rosenberg, S., Vidaver, R., Goodman, L., Osher, F., and Foy, D. (1998) Trauma and PTSD in severe mental illness. *Journal of Consulting and Clinical Psychology, 66*, 493–499.

Mueser, K. T., Rosenburg, S. D., Goodman, L. A., and Trumbetta, S. L. (2002) Trauma, PTSD and the course of severe mental illness: an interactive model. *Schizophrenia Research, 53*, 123–143.

Mullen, P., Martin, J., Anderson, J., Romans, S., and Herbison, G. (1993) Childhood sexual abuse and mental health in adult life. *British Journal of Psychiatry, 163*, 721–32.

Mullen, P., Martin, J., Anderson, J., Romans, S., and Herbison, G. (1996) The long-term impact of the physical, emotional, and sexual abuse of children: A community study. *Child Abuse and Neglect, 20*, 7–21.

Myin-Germeys, L., van Os, J., Schwartz, J., Stone, A., and Delespaul, P. (2001) Emotional reactivity to daily life stress in psychosis. *Archives of General Psychiatry, 58*, 1137–1144.

Myin-Germeys, L., Krabbendam, P., Delespaul, P., and van Os, J. (2003) Do life events have their effect on psychosis by influencing the emotional reactivity to daily life stress? *Psychological Medicine, 33*, 327–333.

Nadel, L., and Jacobs, W. (1996) The role of the hippocampus in PTSD, panic and phobia. In N. Kato (ed.) *The Hippocampus: Functions and clinical relevance* (pp. 455–463). Amsterdam: Elsevier Science.

Nemeroff, C. (2004) Neuobiological consequences of childhood trauma. *Journal of Clinical Psychiatry, 65* (suppl. 1), 18–28.

Nemeroff, C., Heim, C., Thase, M., Klein, D., Rush, A., Schatzberg, A., et al. (2003) Differential responses to psychotherapy versus pharmacotherapy in patients with chronic forms of major depression and childhood trauma. *Proceedings of the National Academy of Sciences of the U.S.A., 100*, 14293–14296.

Neria, Y., Bromet, E., Sievers, S., Lavelle, J., and Fochtman, L. (2002) Trauma exposure and PTSD in psychosis: Findings from a first-admission cohort. *Journal of Consulting and Clinical Psychology, 70*, 246–251.

Penza, K., Heim, C., and Nemeroff, C. (2003) Neurobiological effects of childhood abuse: Implications of the pathophysiology of depression and anxiety. *Archives of Women's Mental Health, 6*, 15–22.

Perkins, R. (1982) Catatonia: The ultimate response to fear? *Australian and New Zealand Journal of Psychiatry, 16*, 282–287.

Pettigrew, J., and Burcham, J. (1997) Effects of childhood sexual abuse in adult female psychiatric patients. *Australian and New Zealand Journal of Psychiatry, 31*, 208–213.

Phillips, W., and Silverstein, S. (2003) Convergence of biological and psychological perspectives on cognitive coordination in schizophrenia. *Behavioral and Brain Sciences, 26*, 65–138.

Putnam, F. (1989) *Diagnosis and Treatment of Multiple Personality Disorder*. New York: Guilford Press.

Raine, A., Mellingen, K., Liu, J., Venables, P., and Mednick, S. (2003) Effects of environmental enrichment at ages 3–5 years on schizotypal personality and antisocial behavior at ages 17 and 23 years. *American Journal of Psychiatry, 160*, 1627–1635.

Raune, D., Kuipers, E., and Bebbington, P. (1999) Psychosocial stress and delusional and verbal auditory hallucination themes in first episode psychosis: Implications for early intervention. Paper presented at Psychological Treatments of Schizophrenia, Oxford, 23–24 September 1999.

Read, J. (1997) Child abuse and psychosis: A literature review and implications for professional practice. *Professional Psychology: Research and Practice, 28*, 448–56.

Read, J. (1998) Child abuse and severity of disturbance among adult psychiatric inpatients. *Child Abuse and Neglect, 22*, 359–368.

Read, J. (2004a) A history of madness. In J. Read, L. Mosher and R. Bentall (eds) *Models of madness* (pp. 9–20). Hove: Brunner-Routledge.

Read, J. (2004b) The invention of 'schizophrenia'. In J. Read, L. Mosher and R. Bentall (eds) *Models of madness* (pp. 21–34). Hove: Brunner-Routledge.

Read, J. (2004c) Does 'schizophrenia' exist? Reliability and validity. In J. Read, L. Mosher and R. Bentall (eds) *Models of madness* (pp. 43–56). Hove: Brunner-Routledge.

Read, J. (2005) The bio-bio-bio model of madness. *The Psychologist, 18*, 196–197.

Read, J., and Argyle, N. (1999) Hallucinations, delusions and thought disorders among adult psychiatric inpatients with a history of child abuse. *Psychiatric Services, 50*, 1467–1472.

Read, J., and Hammersley, P. (2005) Child sexual abuse and schizophrenia. Correspondence. *British Journal of Psychiatry, 186*, 76.

Read, J., and Hammersley, P. (2006) Can very bad childhoods drive us crazy? Science, ideology and taboo. In J. Johannessen, B. Martindale and J. Cullberg (eds) *Evolving psychosis: Different stages, different treatments* (pp. 270–292). Hove: Brunner-Routledge.

Read, J., and Harre, N. (2001) The role of biological and genetic causal beliefs in the stigmatisation of 'mental patients'. *Journal of Mental Health, 10*, 223–235.

Read, J., and Haslam, N. (2004) Public opinion: Bad things happen and can drive you crazy. In J. Read, L. Mosher and R. Bentall (eds) *Models of madness* (pp. 133–146). Hove: Brunner-Routledge.

Read, J., and Law, A. (1999) The relationship of causal beliefs and contact with users of mental health services to attitudes to the 'mentally ill'. *International Journal of Social Psychiatry, 45*, 216–229.

Read, J., and Ross, C. (2003) Psychological trauma and psychosis: Another reason why people diagnosed schizophrenic must be offered psychological therapies. *Journal of the American Academy of Psychoanalysis and Dynamic Psychiatry, 31*, 247–267.

Read, J., Agar, K., Barker-Collo, S., Davies, E., and Moskowitz, A. (2001a) Assessing suicidality in adults: Integrating childhood trauma as a major risk factor. *Professional Psychology: Research and Practice, 32*, 367–372.

Read, J., Perry, B., Moskowitz, A., and Connolly, J. (2001b) The contribution of early traumatic events to schizophrenia in some patients: A traumagenic neurodevelopmental model. *Psychiatry: Interpersonal and Biological Processes, 64*, 319–345.

Read, J., Agar, K., Argyle, N., and Aderhold, V. (2003) Sexual and physical abuse during childhood and adulthood as predictors of hallucinations, delusions and thought disorder. *Psychology and Psychotherapy: Theory, Research and Practice, 76*, 1–22.

Read, J., Goodman, L., Morrison, A., Ross, C., and Aderhold, V. (2004a) Childhood trauma, loss and stress. In J. Read, L. Mosher and R. Bentall (eds) *Models of madness* (pp. 223–252). Hove: Brunner-Routledge.

Read, J., Mosher, L., and Bentall, R. (2004b) 'Schizophrenia' is not an illness. In J. Read, L. Mosher and R. Bentall (eds) *Models of madness* (pp. 3–7). Hove: Brunner-Routledge.

Read, J., Seymour, F., and Mosher, L. (2004c) Unhappy families. In J. Read, L. Mosher and R. Bentall (eds) *Models of madness* (pp. 253–268). Hove: Brunner-Routledge.

Read, J., Mosher, L., and Bentall, R. (eds) (2004d) *Models of madness: Psychological, social and biological approaches to schizophrenia.* Hove: Brunner-Routledge.

Read, J., van Os, J., Morrison, A. P., and Ross, C. A. (2005) Childhood trauma, psychosis, and schizophrenia: A literature review with theoretical and clinical implications. *Acta Psychiatrica Scandinavica, 112*, 330–350.

Read, J., Haslam, N., Sayce, L., and Davies, E. (2006) Prejudice and schizophrenia A review of the 'Mental Illness is an Illness Like any Other' approach. *Acta Psychiatrica Scandinavica* (in press).

Resnick, S., Bond, G., and Mueser, K. (2003) Trauma and PTSD in people with schizophrenia. *Journal of Abnormal Psychology, 112*, 415–423.

Ritsher, J., Coursey, R., and Farrell, E. (1997) A survey on issues in the lives of women with severe mental illness. *Psychiatric Services, 48*, 1273–1282.

Robins, L. (1966) *Deviant children grown up.* Baltimore, MD: Williams & Wickins.

Ross, C. (2004) *Schizophrenia: Innovations in diagnosis and treatment.* New York: Howarth Press.

Ross, C., and Joshi, S. (1992) Schneiderian symptoms and childhood trauma in the general population. *Comprehensive Psychiatry, 33*, 269–273.

Ross, C., and Read, J. (2004) Antipsychotic medication: Myths and facts. In J. Read, L. Mosher and R. Bentall (eds), *Models of madness* (pp. 115–130). Hove: Brunner-Routledge.

Ross, C., Miller, S., Reagor, P., Bjornson, L., Fraser, G., and Anderson, G. (1990) Schneiderian symptoms in multiple personality disorder and schizophrenia. *Comprehensive Psychiatry, 31*, 111–118.

Ross, C., Anderson, G., and Clark, P. (1994) Childhood abuse and positive symptoms of schizophrenia. *Hospital and Community Psychiatry, 45*, 489–491.

Rudegeair, T., and Farrelly, S. (2003) Is all psychosis dissociative? Paper presented at Annual Conference of the International Society for the Study of Dissociation, Chicago, IL, November.

Sansonnet-Hayden, H., Haley, G., Marriage, K., and Fine, S. (1987) Sexual abuse and psychopathology in hospitalized adolescents. *Journal of the American Academy of Child and Adolescent Psychiatry, 26*, 753–757.

Saxe, G., van der Kolk, B., Berkowitz, R., Chinman, G., Hall, K., Lieberg, G., and Schwartz, J. (1993) Dissociative disorders in psychiatric inpatients. *American Journal of Psychiatry, 150*, 1037–1042.

Scott, R., and Stone, D. (1986) MMPI profile constellations in incest families. *Journal of Consulting and Clinical Psychology, 54*, 364–368.

Seedat, S., Stein, M., Oosthuizen, P., Emsley, R., and Stein, D. (2003) Linking PTSD and psychosis: A look at epidemiology, phenomenology, and treatment. *Journal of Nervous and Mental Disease, 191*, 675–81.

Shapiro, D., and Levendosky, A. (1999) Adolescent survivors of childhood sexual abuse: The mediating role of attachment style and coping in psychological and interpersonal functioning. *Child Abuse and Neglect, 23*, 1175–1191.

Sharfstein, S. (2005) Big Pharma and American psychiatry: The good, the bad, and the ugly. *Psychiatric News, 40*, 3–4.

Silver, A., Koehler, B., and Karon, B. (2004) Psychodynamic psychotherapy of schizophrenia: Its history and development. In J. Read, L. Mosher and R. Bentall (eds) *Models of madness* (pp. 209–222). Hove: Brunner-Routledge.

Spataro, J., Mullen, P., Burgess, P., Wells, D., and Moss, A. (2004) A prospective study in males and females of the impact of child sexual abuse on mental health. *British Journal of Psychiatry, 184*, 416–421.

Srinivasan, T., and Thara, R. (2001) Beliefs about causation of schizophrenia: Do Indian families believe in supernatural causes? *Social Psychiatry and Psychiatric Epidemiology, 36*, 134–140.

Startup, M. (1999) Schizotypy, dissociative experiences and childhood abuse. *British Journal of Clinical Psychology, 38*, 333–344.

Swanston, H., Plunkett, A., O'Toole, B., Shrimpton, S., Parkinson, P., and Oates, R. (2003) Nine years after child sexual abuse. *Child Abuse and Neglect, 27*, 967–984.

Swett, C., Surrey, J., and Cohen, C. (1990) Sexual and physical abuse histories and psychiatric symptoms among male psychiatric outpatients. *American Journal of Psychiatry, 147*, 632–636.

Switzer, G., Dew, M., Thompson, K., Goycoolea, J., Derricott, T., and Mullins, S. (1999) PTSD and service utilization among urban mental health centre clients. *Journal of Traumatic Stress, 12*, 25–39.

Teicher, M., Andersen, S., Polcari, A., Anderson, C., Navalta, C., and Kim, N. (2003) The neurobiological consequences of early stress and childhood maltreatment. *Neuroscience and Biobehavioral Reviews, 27*, 33–44.

Thompson, A., Stuart, H., Bland, R., Arboleda-Florez, J., Warner, R., and Dickson, R. (2002) Attitudes about schizophrenia from the pilot site of the WPA worldwide campaign against the stigma of schizophrenia. *Social Psychiatry and Psychiatric Epidemiology, 37*, 475–482.

Trower, P., and Chadwick, P. (1995) Pathways to defence of the self: A theory of two types of paranoia. *Clinical Psychology: Science and Practice, 2*, 263–278.

Tsai, M., Feldman-Summers, S., and Edgar, M. (1979) Childhood molestation: Variables related to differential impacts on psychosexual functioning in adult women. *Journal of Abnormal Psychology, 88*, 407–417.

van der Kolk, B., and Fisler, R. (1995) Dissociation and the fragmentary nature of traumatic memories: Overview and exploratory study. *Journal of Traumatic Stress, 8*, 23–43.

Wahl, O. (1987) Public versus professional conceptions of schizophrenia. *Journal of Community Psychology, 15*, 285–291.

Wahl, O. (1999) Mental health consumers' experience of stigma. *Schizophrenia Bulletin, 25*, 467–478.

Walker, E., and DiForio, D. (1997) Schizophrenia: A neural diathesis-stress model. *Psychological Review, 104*, 667–685.

Walker, I., and Read, J. (2002) The differential effectiveness of psychosocial and bio-genetic causal explanations in reducing negative attitudes towards 'mental illness'. *Psychiatry: Interpersonal and Biological Processes, 65*, 313–325.

Whitfield, C., Dube, S., Felitti, V., and Anda, R. (2005) Adverse childhood experiences and hallucinations. *Child Abuse and Neglect, 29*, 797–810.

Wiersma, D., Jenner, A., Nienhuis, F., and van de Willige, D. (2004) Hallucination focused integrative treatment improves quality of life in schizophrenia patients. *Acta Psychiatrica Scandinavica, 109*, 194–201.

Wurr, C., and Partridge, I. (1996) The prevalence of a history of childhood sexual abuse in an acute adult inpatient population. *Child Abuse and Neglect, 20*, 867–872.

Young, H., and Bentall, R. (1997) Probabilistic reasoning in deluded, depressed and normal subjects. *Psychological Medicine, 27*, 455–465.

Zubin, J., and Spring, B. (1997) Vulnerability: A new view of schizophrenia. *Journal of Abnormal Psychology, 86*, 103–126.

Chapter 3

The trauma of being psychotic

An analysis of posttraumatic stress disorder in response to acute psychosis

Sarah Bendall, Patrick McGorry and Helen Krstev

Psychosis can be a terrifying experience. One young woman described hearing her mother's screams in her head and believing that her mother, who was overseas at the time, was being tortured and her screams were being telepathically communicated to her. If this were actually happening, logic and knowledge of the world aside, this young woman's situation would be a horrific one to be in. While the potentially terrifying nature of psychosis is clear to those who have experienced it and the people who care for them, both personally and professionally, it has received very little attention by either psychosis or trauma researchers. This chapter presents case studies, reviews the literature on posttraumatic stress disorder (PTSD) as a result of psychotic experience and hospitalisation, integrates it with current understandings of PTSD, and raises some conceptual issues that make understanding the trauma of psychosis unique.

Personal accounts of psychosis

The following personal accounts attest to the traumatic nature of psychotic experiences and events. The trauma may be as a result of the nature of the symptoms themselves and the consequent threat to physical and/or psychical integrity or as a result of the restrictive and at times forceful nature of hospitalisation.

A common psychotic experience is one of being controlled and punished . . .

> I had one particular friend. I called him the 'Controller.' He was my secret friend. He took on all of my bad feelings. He was the sum total of my negative feelings and my paranoia. I could see him and hear him, but no one else could.
>
> The problems were compounded when I went off to college. Suddenly, the Controller started demanding all my time and energy. He would punish me if I did something he didn't like. He spent a lot of time yelling at me and making me feel wicked. I didn't know how to stop him from

screaming at me and ruling my existence. It got to the point where I couldn't decipher reality from what the controller was screaming. So I withdrew from society and reality. I couldn't tell anyone what was happening because I was so afraid of being labelled 'crazy'. I didn't understand what was going on in my head. I really thought that other 'normal' people had Controllers too.

(Jordan 1995: 501–502)

shortly after I was taken to hospital for the first time in a rigid catatonic condition, I was plunged up in a cataclysm and totally dislocated. I myself had been responsible for setting the destructive forces into motion, although I had acted with no intent to harm, and defended myself with healthy indignation against the accusations of others. If I had done something wrong, I certainly was suffering the consequences along with everyone else. Part of the time I was exploring a new planet (a marvellous and breathtaking adventure) but it was too lonely, I could persuade no one to settle there, and I had to get back to the earth somehow. The earth, however, had been devastated by atomic bombs and most of its inhabitants killed. Only a few people – myself and the dimly perceiving nursing staff – had escaped. At other times, I felt totally alone on the new planet. The issue of world salvation was of predominant importance and I was trying to tell people how to go back to the abandoned earth. All personal matters relating to my family were forgotten. At times when the universe was collapsing, I was not sure that things would turn out all right. I thought I might have to stay in the endless hell-fire of atomic destruction. The chief horror consisted in the fact that I would never be able to die. I thought I would either have to figure out some form of suicide or else get a lobotomy.

(Anonymous 1964: 95)

Fears of being annihilated are also some of the shared experiences of people experiencing psychosis.

Going to work was pure hell. I continued to hear voices. One day while sitting at my desk I saw a fly I had never seen. It could not have been real, not in February. One of my duties was to read information intended for military personnel. I remember reading about Hellfire missiles. I imagined the manmade hellfire killing people. I became convinced that I was reading top secret information and that someone would try to have me killed so that I couldn't talk.

(Herrig 1995: 340)

For many the experience of hospitalisation is incredibly traumatic which at first may be met with resistance and rebellion but eventually is met with helplessness and despair, shattering one's sense of self, as Esso Lette describes:

> when I was first hospitalised, I was young, passive, extremely dependent, and naïve. I did not understand what was happening, and I was not sufficiently in touch with the world to care. I was so regressed that I hardly spoke and stayed in bed as much as possible, eagerly seizing my voices as companions. I believed I was living on Venus and, according to hospital charts, I stood on chairs and tables speaking in an incomprehensible language . . . One private hospital in Denver was particularly destructive. I was banned from group therapy sessions, my food was monitored, my time was regulated, and my roommates were removed from my room and thus from my negative influence.
>
> Toward the end of my hospitalisation, I was placed in seclusion and restraints everyday. I was forbidden to cross a red line painted on the floor, much less leave the unit. Not surprisingly, I did not improve, as such power struggles and automatic limit setting are rarely therapeutic. The more I was ostracized and punished, the angrier I became and the more I rebelled. Slowly, however, my desperation turned to resignation and hopelessness.
>
> (Lette 1987: 487)

Christina, a young person experiencing her first episode of psychosis, described her harrowing experience of hospitalisation as follows:

> as I run my hands along the smooth surface around me I feel the small wooden pricks of the surface which I touch. It is a wooden box which surrounds me and I feel trapped, I have nowhere to move, my body aches with pain from this cramped position . . .
>
> I am my own prisoner, entrapped in both body and mind, locked in this tiny box. There is no way to control the situation and I am physically unable to be freed from the corners surrounding me, crying out, sobbing like a newborn baby; oh why, oh why did I place myself here!
>
> It's a delusion and I don't know what reality is any more. The only reality I have is my nightmare, which is real as hell. Will I never, ever be allowed to see my family again?
>
> (Early Psychosis Prevention and Intervention
> Centre (EPPIC) 2000: 13)

Experiences of psychosis as criterion A

There has been debate as to whether the experience of psychosis can be considered a traumatic event (Shaw et al. 1997). This is an interesting nosological issue since the criterion for the trauma in PTSD (criterion A) has changed in different editions of the *Diagnostic and Statistical Manual of Mental Disorders* (APA 1980, 1987, 1994), showing that trauma is difficult to define in itself. How the experience of psychosis fits the definition or not, is dependent on the criteria of the DSM at the time.

Researchers agree that experiences of hospitalisation in the midst of a psychotic episode can meet criterion A for PTSD in both the DSM-III-R (McGorry et al. 1991; Priebe et al. 1998) and the DSM-IV (Priebe et al. 1998). These experiences include forced medication and seclusion and thus can be considered both outside of normal experience and to involve threat to the physical integrity of the self.

There is contention, however, with regard to the experience of the symptoms of psychosis and their eligibility for criterion A. The DSM-IV (APA 1994) requires that the trauma that can elicit PTSD have the following elements:

1   The person experienced, witnessed, or was confronted with an event or events that involved actual or threatened death or serious injury, or a threat to the physical integrity of self or other, and
2   The person's response involved intense fear, helplessness, or horror.

(APA 1994: 428)

People with psychosis often respond to their symptoms with fear, helplessness and horror (Morrison et al. 2003). It is more contentious, however, whether people with psychosis have experienced an event that involves actual or threatened death, injury or threat to the physical integrity of the self. Many researchers in the area have suggested that the subjective experience of sufferers from psychosis should be taken at face value and accepted as traumatic as if their hallucinations and delusions were happening in the real world (Lundy 1992; Morrison et al. 2003; Mueser and Rosenburg 2003; Shaner and Eth 1989; Williams-Keeler et al. 1994). This means, for example, that the young woman described in the first paragraph would be considered to have experienced a trauma because she *believed* her mother was being tortured. Studies into PTSD resulting from experiences other than psychosis have found that the subjective experience of threat is a better predictor of distress than the objective experience (Alvarez-Conrad et al. 2001; Bernat et al. 1998; Girelli et al. 1986) supporting the idea that it is the subjective experience of psychosis that should be considered.

Alternatively, Shaw suggested that the criterion for a traumatic event should extend from threat to physical integrity to threat to psychological integrity (Shaw et al. 1997) and thus a wider experience of psychosis would meet criteria. Psychotic experiences that are more diffuse and confusing and are associated with changes to the self and the world would be incorporated. The personal account by the anonymous author above gives a graphic account of the traumatic nature of this kind of experience. The suggestion is supported by evidence that 'mental defeat' is associated with longer duration of PTSD in torture survivors (Ehlers et al. 2000). Mental defeat is defined as 'the perceived loss of all autonomy, a state of giving up in one's own mind all efforts to retain one's identity as a human being with a will of one's own' (Ehlers et al. 2000: 45). This definition has resonance with the state of being of a person with acute psychosis in relation to their symptoms, even if their symptoms are not about specific traumatic beliefs.

While the DSM's focus is on the nature of the trauma, the empirical evidence suggests that there are, in fact, other factors that predict the development of PTSD including the response of others to the victim (Briere 1997). This supports the suggestion that it may be the experience of social extrusion and stigma that is experienced as traumatic as the real world interfaces with the person with psychosis (Mueser and Rosenburg 2003).

The conceptualisation of the traumatic nature of psychotic experience is complex and multifaceted, and will be discussed in detail later in this chapter. It will be argued throughout this chapter that psychosis is highly traumatic for some people and thus, for the purposes of this review, it will be assumed that psychosis can be the traumatic trigger for PTSD.

Rates of PTSD in people with psychosis

A series of studies have investigated the incidence of PTSD in people with psychosis. These have found rates varying from 11 to 67 per cent (Frame and Morrison 2001; McGorry et al. 1991; Meyer et al. 1999; Priebe et al. 1998; Shaw et al. 1997; Shaw et al. 2002). These studies have used a variety of methodologies and measures and have measured symptoms at various times in the process of psychosis, which may account for the varying rates of PTSD found in the samples.

The first of these studies was conducted by McGorry and his colleagues in 1991. They assessed thirty-six people with psychosis over a period of twelve months, recruiting and assessing them as psychiatric inpatients and then assessing them again four and eleven months after discharge from hospital. They were assessed using the PTSD scale (Friedman et al. 1986) and the Impact of Events Scale (IES: Horowitz et al. 1979). They found that 46 per cent of people met criteria for PTSD at the four-month follow-up and 35 per cent did so at the eleven-month follow-up.

A study of forty-five people with psychosis was conducted with people recruited during an inpatient admission at either a general hospital psychiatric unit or an acute ward in a large psychiatric hospital (Shaw et al. 1997). Participants were assessed in hospital shortly before discharge and then again within approximately one week of discharge. Psychotic symptomatology was measured using the Factor Construct Rating Scale (FCRS: Overall 1968), a modified version of the Brief Psychiatric Rating Scale, and PTSD symptoms were measured using the Clinician Administered PTSD Scale (CAPS: Blake et al. 1990) and the IES (Horowitz et al. 1979). Results showed that 49 per cent of people met criteria for PTSD.

Another study recruited forty-six people who had been admitted to the Turku City Hospital (Meyer et al. 1999). Participants were interviewed one and nine weeks after admission to the inpatient ward. Half had been discharged by the time the second interview took place. Severity and quality of psychotic symptoms were assessed at weeks one and nine using the Positive and Negative Symptom Scale (PANSS: Kay et al. 1987). Traumatic symptomatology was assessed at week one with the Impact of Events Scale-Revised (IES-R: Marmar et al. 1996) and at week nine with the CAPS (Blake et al. 1990); 11 per cent of the sample met criteria for PTSD. This study also found that PANSS score was associated with PTSD at week eight.

A larger study included 105 people (Priebe et al. 1998). It is unclear when the patients were assessed in relation to an acute episode. Psychopathology was assessed using the Brief Psychiatric Rating Scale (BPRS: Overall and Gorham 1962) and the Present State Examination (PSE: Wing et al. 1974) and traumatic symptoms were measured using the PTSD Interview (Watson et al. 1991); 51 per cent of people in the sample met criteria for PTSD. They were significantly more likely to be unemployed.

A more recent study measured PTSD in a group admitted to hospital with acute psychosis (Frame and Morrison 2001). Sixty people were recruited and 67 per cent of them had PTSD at discharge and 50 per cent at four- to six-month follow-up.

Shaw and her colleagues conducted another study that was similar to their 1997 study (Shaw et al. 2002). The forty-five participants with psychosis were assessed when they had reached a level of recovery that enabled them to participate in the research. This was usually around the time of discharge although no figures are given as to mean length of admission in this group. The schizophrenia and mania sections of the World Health Organization's (WHO 1993) Composite International Diagnostic Interview (CIDI), the FCRS and a modified BPRS (Overall and Gorham 1962) were used to measure psychotic symptoms. PTSD and acute stress were measured by the CAPS-1 (Blake et al. 1995), the IES and the Stanford Acute Stress Reaction Questionnaire (SARQ: Koopman et al. 1994); 52 per cent of participants met criteria for PTSD. They were significantly more likely to have suicidal thoughts.

These studies use a variety of methods to measure PTSD, both self-report and clinician administered measures, and the majority found rates of approximately 50 per cent. Meyer et al.'s (1999) results are strikingly different, with a rate of 11 per cent. Meyer et al. (1999) suggested that people with affective psychosis may be more prone to PTSD than people with schizophrenia as people with depression have been shown to be more prone to PTSD than others (Chubb and Bisson 1996; Mueser et al. 1998). However, other studies did not find different rates of PTSD in different diagnostic categories (McGorry et al. 1991; Shaw et al. 1997).

What is it about psychosis that is traumatic?

It is clear then, that many people experience the symptoms of PTSD in the immediate aftermath of an acute episode of psychosis. What is less clear is what it is about the psychotic experience that is traumatic.

Psychotic symptoms

Many of the studies that have researched the prevalence rates of PTSD in psychosis have also investigated more specifically the relationship between psychotic symptoms and PTSD. Some studies found that more psychotic symptoms correlated with higher levels of PTSD symptomatology (Meyer et al. 1999; Shaw et al. 2002) although another found only weak evidence for this (Priebe et al. 1998). Meyer et al. (1999) investigated correlations over two time points and found that a higher level of positive symptoms at both week one and eight was correlated with higher traumatisation at week eight. They suggested two possible explanations for this: that ongoing positive symptoms are more traumatic than quickly resolving ones or that presence of PTSD symptoms delays recovery from psychosis.

Studies have also investigated how much of PTSD symptomatology is attributable to psychotic symptoms rather than other experiences of psychosis such as hospitalisation or other traumas. Meyer and colleagues (1999) categorised posttraumatic symptoms by their cause in their study. They asked general trauma questions to elucidate the origin of the traumatic experience 'e.g., whether the PTSD symptoms had been present during the last week/ month in relation to any traumatic experience' (Meyer et al. 1999: 345). They specified whether traumatic symptoms were due to psychotic symptoms or other experiences. They found that psychotic symptoms caused post-traumatic symptoms in 69 per cent of cases (Meyer et al. 1999). Frame and Morrison (2001) used multiple regression to analyse their results and found that psychotic symptoms explained 52 per cent of the variance in PTSD symptoms, more than both hospitalisation and other traumas.

Which particular psychotic symptoms are traumatic has also been an area of inquiry. In the Shaw et al. (1997) study, the distress and intrusion caused by specific psychotic symptoms was measured using the schizophrenia and mania section of the CIDI (WHO 1993) with additional subscales to measure the posttraumatic symptoms associated with each psychotic or manic symptom. Psychotic symptoms were generally reported as more distressing than manic symptoms. Specific positive symptoms were found to be related to higher levels of distress and intrusion in relation to that symptom. Persecutory delusions, passivity phenomena, and visual hallucinations were the psychotic symptoms rated as most distressing. Shaw et al. (2002) then used this 1997 data to look specifically at which psychotic symptoms were associated with PTSD and found that people who experienced being controlled, visual hallucinations, being followed, believing others were hearing their thoughts, and having their mind read were all associated with post-psychotic PTSD. In another study, unusual thought content and suspiciousness/ persecution were the psychotic symptoms most associated with PTSD symptoms (Meyer et al. 1999).

These data suggest that the positive symptoms of psychosis are the experiences that contribute the most to the development of post-psychotic PTSD (Frame and Morrison 2001; Meyer et al. 1999) and a range of positive symptoms have been found to be the most traumatic. These include persecutory delusions, passivity phenomena, visual hallucinations, and unusual thought content (Meyer et al. 1999; Shaw et al. 1997, 2002).

Hospitalisation

Understanding the nature of the traumatic impact of hospitalisation on people with psychosis is central to any attempt to reduce the trauma of hospitalisation, and has received research attention. McGorry and his colleagues asked for qualitative information regarding the source of post-traumatic symptoms and concluded that symptoms 'seemed to be linked especially to the experience of hospitalisation and less so to the psychotic experience per se, for example, recurrent nightmares involving forced sedation or seclusion' (McGorry et al. 1991: 256).

Shaw et al. (1997) investigated participants' experiences of hospitalisation using the Hospital Experiences Questionnaire (HECS) which they designed for the study. Fifty-seven hospital experiences (e.g., being in seclusion, being physically abused, being away from family and friends) were rated by each person on a four-point Likert scale (1 = not at all; 4 = very much/often) for distress engendered and for intrusive thoughts or memories (Shaw et al. 1997, 2002). Hospitalisation experiences were found to be distressing (Shaw et al. 1997). For example, the 36 per cent of participants who were placed in seclusion at some time in their hospitalisation, scored a mean distress level of 3.63 and mean intrusion level of 2.5 for this item. Other hospitalisation experiences that caused high distress were being physically abused (n = 7 of 45; distress rating = 3.43; intrusion rating = 2.14), being on a closed ward (n = 24; distress rating = 3.38; intrusion rating = 2.71) and being detained (n = 38; distress rating = 3.37; intrusion rating = 3.71). No association was found between a greater number of negative hospitalisation experiences and PTSD, however (Shaw et al. 2002).

Meyer and colleagues (1999) found that 25 per cent of posttraumatic symptoms were related to the hospitalisation experience. However, no hospitalisation experience, including voluntary versus involuntary admission, was associated with overall traumatisation scores at either one or nine weeks' post admission.

Another traumatic experience associated with hospitalisation is verbal, physical and sexual abuse from inpatients and/or staff of the unit. This is an issue that has been inadequately studied (Frueh et al. 2000). Violence was reported by participants in some of the studies under discussion (Priebe et al. 1998; Shaw et al. 1997). Shaw and colleagues found that 67 per cent of their participants had been harassed by other patients for money or cigarettes or had witnessed verbal abuse; 25 per cent had witnessed physical abuse or experienced sexual or verbal abuse; 15 per cent had experienced physical abuse; 9 per cent reported physical or sexual abuse by staff. It was noted, however, that it was difficult to clarify whether these memories were real or delusional. In the Meyer et al. (1999) study, 5 per cent of traumatic experiences recorded were not due to hospitalisation experiences (such as seclusion or restraint) or positive symptoms. It is not clear whether these experiences occurred during hospitalisation and thus may have included abuse from inside the hospital.

Several studies have investigated the relationship between involuntary admission status and level of PTSD and found no relationship between the two (Frame and Morrison 2001; Meyer et al. 1999; Priebe et al. 1998). This suggests that it is not the involuntary nature of the admission that makes it traumatic for people with psychosis. This is supported by studies that have found that people recovered from acute psychosis did not object to the idea of involuntary admission (Adams and Hafner 1991; Hammill et al. 1989).

The relationship between hospitalisation and psychotic symptoms

There is evidence that hospitalisation contributes less to the development of post-psychotic PTSD than do the psychotic symptoms themselves (Frame and Morrison 2001; Meyer et al. 1999). However, when asked qualitatively, patients highlighted the traumatic nature of hospitalisation (McGorry et al. 1991). This could reflect the complex relationship that must exist between psychotic symptoms and hospitalisation. Coercive measures in hospital often occur due to the acute positive symptoms of psychosis and the objective coercive measure will be subjectively experienced differently depending on the nature of the positive symptoms the person is experiencing. There are several lines of evidence to support this: Shaw and colleagues (1997) found it impossible to differentiate between PTSD as a result of psychotic or hospitalisation experiences in their study. There is also evidence from an innovative study into the pastel drawings of inpatients with psychosis drawn in art therapy groups on a unit where seclusion was extensively used (Wadeson and Carpenter 1976). Although not asked to draw about the seclusion room specifically, many pictures were in fact about this. Qualitative results showed that pictures of the seclusion room could be divided into (a) strong feelings about the experience of seclusion and (b) frightening delusions connected with the experience of seclusion. This study shows that negative hospitalisation experiences can become enmeshed with psychotic symptomatology. It also shows the utility of qualitative research into the meaning that people apply to coercive measures in order to understand this relationship better. It is also possible that the opposite interaction occurs in some people and that hospitalisation helps people feel safe and therefore ameliorates the traumatic nature of positive symptoms, although this has not been investigated to the authors' knowledge.

Phase of illness and PTSD

Several researchers have suggested that the first episode of psychosis and its treatment may be a particularly traumatic experience (McGorry et al. 1991; Mueser and Rosenburg 2003; Shaner and Eth 1989; Williams-Keeler et al. 1994). It is also possible that the converse is true, that multiple episodes or persistent positive symptoms are more traumatic due to the longer duration of the traumatic stressor. Longer duration of trauma has been associated with higher rates of PTSD in people who have experienced traumas other than psychosis (Horowitz et al. 1995). While several studies report the number of people experiencing their first episode within their sample, they do not report whether they have differing rates of PTSD (Meyer et al. 1999; Shaw et al. 1997). McGorry et al.'s (1991) participants were in the early phase of their illness. They found no relationship between number of admissions and level of PTSD. Meyer et al. (1999) found no significant differences in level of PTSD between those experiencing their first involuntary admission and those with more than one involuntary admission.

The complex relationship between psychotic and PTSD symptoms: conceptual issues

Psychosis and PTSD are both complex disorders. Any attempt to understand the nature of post-psychotic PTSD requires an understanding of the nature, phenomenology and course of both disorders. An exploration of these issues gives some insight into this complex relationship.

The early course of post-psychotic PTSD

Studies have shown that rates of PTSD immediately after any trauma are startlingly high. Studies of PTSD symptoms in people who had been assaulted found rates of between 30 per cent (Patterson et al. 1990) and 94 per cent (Rothbaum et al. 1992) (within a month of the assault). Rates of PTSD are known to diminish substantially over the course of the first year after the traumatic event. In Rothbaum et al.'s (1992) study, 94 per cent met PTSD criteria thirteen days after the assault, 65 per cent met criteria thirty-five days after the assault and 47 per cent did so ninety-four days after the assault. In a study of survivors of a plane crash, 54 per cent had PTSD shortly after the event and 10–15 per cent did so one year later (Sloane 1988). This shows that a significant number of the people who endure a traumatic experience, develop the symptoms of PTSD immediately after their experience but symptoms abate in the normal course of their lives. This data has led some trauma theorists to suggest that PTSD symptoms may be a normal and adaptive response to overwhelming trauma that aids psychological adaptation to the experience of the trauma (Briere 1992; Jackson and Iqbal 2000). Studies into post-psychotic PTSD have found a similar pattern. People with psychosis show a high rate of PTSD shortly after hospitalisation for acute psychosis (67 per cent in Frame and Morrison 2001; 52 per cent in Shaw et al. 1997). Studies examining rates of PTSD symptoms in the year after acute psychosis have found that rates diminish over this time. In one study, rates of PTSD dropped from 67 per cent post-discharge to 50 per cent four to six months post-discharge (Frame and Morrison 2001). Another study found that 46 per cent of people were experiencing PTSD four months after discharge from hospital, and 35 per cent eleven months post-discharge (McGorry et al. 1991). Post-psychotic PTSD seems to follow the same general course as PTSD from other traumas. This provides support for the idea that the PTSD seen in psychosis is analogous to that from other traumas and that psychosis should be a criterion A event.

Psychosis as ongoing trauma

A major problem with comparing post-psychotic PTSD rates with PTSD rates from other traumas, however, is that the psychotic symptoms (the traumatic stressor) had not entirely resolved when PTSD was measured in the studies reviewed in this chapter. The traumatic stressors in the comparison studies (plane crash and assault) were discrete and had occurred at a certain point in the past. PTSD, by definition, occurs after the end or resolution of a trauma and PTSD is usually studied after the trauma has abated for ethical and practical reasons. Thus, our understanding of PTSD is based around the idea that trauma is discrete and PTSD occurs in the aftermath. However, in many situations trauma and posttraumatic symptoms are less discrete and may be experienced simultaneously for many months or years. Child sexual or physical abuse and domestic violence are examples of ongoing abuse where traumatic experiences and symptoms can co-occur. Experts in the field have suggested new, more complex conceptualisations for the symptoms that occur in these situations such as child sexual abuse accommodation syndrome (Summit 1983) and complex PTSD (Herman 1992a). The uncontrollable nature of these ongoing traumatic experiences has been conceptualised as a condition that makes the experience more traumatic (Herman 1992b). It has also been found that longer duration of trauma leads to an increased risk for PTSD (Horowitz et al. 1995). Psychosis is more likely to fit into the ongoing trauma conceptualisation since there is often a long duration of untreated psychosis, especially in the first episode (Harrigan et al. 2003). Even when treatment has started, symptoms can take some time to resolve (Lieberman et al. 1993) and, at times, do not resolve even after treatment (Edwards et al. 1998).

Studying PTSD in people who may still be experiencing trauma is problematic since we know very little about the nature of symptoms of trauma in people who are experiencing ongoing trauma. Research and theoretical emphasis may need to be shifted to conceptualisations of the ongoing traumatic nature of psychosis.

The relationship between self, beliefs and psychotic trauma

The trauma of psychosis is unique because it often stems from the fundamentally mistaken beliefs associated with hallucinations and delusions rather than an objective trauma. Hallucinations and delusions often change through the course of psychosis. The dynamic nature of the traumatic stressor means that the process of recovery from psychosis will have a profound impact on the beliefs associated with the positive psychotic symptoms. For example, the young woman in the first paragraph may gain insight into her positive symptoms and understand that the screams she is hearing are not her mother's but a manifestation of a psychotic illness. Her symptoms may or may not alter, but her understanding of those symptoms will change and thus change the traumatic impact of the symptoms. However, the realisation of the seriousness of her illness may also be traumatic. The fundamental adjustment that has to be made from the belief that the psychotic symptoms are real, to the psychotic symptoms as coming from within presents great challenges to the concept of the self (Jackson and Iqbal 2000).

The beliefs that people generate in response to their traumatic experience have been widely studied in the PTSD field and have a large impact on recovery from PTSD (Brewin and Holmes 2003). A striking example is that tortured political activists are less likely to develop PTSD from their torture experiences than tortured non-activists (Basoglu et al. 1997). The activists' beliefs that their experiences were in some way understandable in the context of their political fight provided some protection against PTSD. The important role of beliefs has also been found in people with psychosis: the distress caused by auditory hallucinations is contingent on whether the voices are evaluated as benevolent or malevolent, an evaluation that is only partially contingent on the content of the voices (Chadwick and Birchwood 1995). Belief formation in psychosis is therefore particularly important due to the fluidity of psychotic experiences as a traumatic stressor throughout the recovery process.

People with psychosis do not form their beliefs about their psychotic experiences in a social vacuum. Issues such as social stigma, the recovery environment, and access to appropriate treatment all contribute to the way in which individuals will form their beliefs about their psychotic experiences. In a meta-analysis of fourteen separate risk factors for PTSD, social support was found to have the largest effect size (Brewin et al. 2000). This is a very complex issue in PTSD since social attitudes to different kinds of traumas are very different. Survivors of spousal violence, road traffic accidents and psychosis, for example, may experience a different quality of social support. This evidence suggests that issues such as social stigma may have an effect on the development of post-psychotic PTSD.

Phenomenological overlap

Positive symptoms

Research studies have highlighted the difficulty of differentiating between delusions and hallucinations and intrusive memories of delusions and hallucinations (Meyer et al. 1999; Shaw et al. 1997). Indeed, it has been found that paranoid delusions were particularly related to intrusive thoughts (Shaw et al. 1997). Since the intrusive symptoms of PTSD are 'sudden sensory memories that seem immediately real' (APA 1987: 250), and since delusions are firmly held beliefs that are not real, an intrusive thought of a delusion will be phenomenologically very similar to a delusion. This is equally so of hallucinations. Researchers have pointed out the difficulty of separating these issues in research studies (e.g., Meyer et al. 1999), which must lead to consideration of the difficulties encountered by patients, many of whom do not know of the existence of posttraumatic intrusive symptoms. An intrusive thought of a psychotic symptom could be interpreted as the beginning of a relapse and trigger anxiety and distress in the patient. In fact, in some people, a relapse may be diagnosed when a person may be experiencing posttraumatic intrusive activity rather than a recurrence of illness.

Negative symptoms

Negative symptoms have many similarities to the avoidance and numbing symptoms of PTSD (Lundy 1992; McGorry et al. 1991; Stampfer 1990). Stampfer (1990) presents a comprehensive theoretical argument that negative symptoms are inseparable from avoidance and numbing in PTSD. He suggests that negative symptoms are not specific to psychosis, that they are not invariably present in psychosis and that there are many phenomenological similarities between the two including flattened affect, social withdrawal, feeling disconnected from others and diminished interest in life. The little published research in this area does not provide support for Stampfer's theory. McGorry et al. (1991) investigated the relationship between negative symptoms and PTSD and found no correlations between negative symptoms and the avoidance symptoms of PTSD (as measured by the IES) but did find that people with higher levels of PTSD symptoms were more depressed at both four and eleven months. Priebe et al. (1998) also found that there was no correlation between negative symptoms and level of traumatic symptoms. As yet unpublished data from EPPIC has found a relationship between negative and PTSD symptoms and case study evidence has shown the relationship between negative symptoms and PTSD in some people (Lundy 1992). More published research is needed to draw firm conclusions in this area.

Conclusion

Compelling descriptions of personal experiences of psychosis and empirical evidence that approximately half of those in the immediate aftermath of an acute psychotic episode will meet criteria for PTSD provide evidence that acute psychosis can be a highly traumatic experience. It is therefore suggested that the subjective experience of psychosis should be viewed as a trauma that can cause PTSD.

While the negative experience of hospitalisation contributes to PTSD in people with psychosis and must continue to be addressed in psychiatric settings, it is the positive symptoms of psychosis that have been found to be the most traumatic part of the experience of psychosis. The qualitative and phenomenological experience of the traumatic nature of psychosis is yet to be clearly understood. A more sophisticated understanding of the nature of psychosis as a traumatic stressor must be developed. The trauma of psychosis is a uniquely subjective experience that changes over the course of illness and has a major impact on beliefs about the self and the world.

The provision of high quality, comprehensive treatment of people with psychosis must include evidence-based trauma therapy for the trauma associated with psychosis (as well as other traumas patients may have experienced). Adaptations of traditional PTSD treatment are necessary to address the unique nature of the trauma of psychosis.

References

Adams, N. H. S., and Hafner, R. J. (1991) Attitudes of psychiatric patients and their relatives to involuntary treatment. *Australian and New Zealand Journal of Psychiatry, 25*, 231–237.

Alvarez-Conrad, J., Zoellner, L. A., and Foa, E. B. (2001) Linguistic predictors of trauma pathology and physical health. *Applied Cognitive Psychology, 15*, 159–170.

American Psychiatric Association (1980) *Diagnostic and statistical manual of mental disorders* (3rd edn). Washington, DC: APA.

American Psychiatric Association (1987) *Diagnostic and statistical manual of mental disorders* (3rd revised edn). Washington, DC: APA.

American Psychiatric Association (1994) *Diagnosis and statistical manual of mental disorders* (4th edn). Washington, DC: APA.

Anonymous (1964) An autobiography of a schizophrenic experience. In B. Kaplan (ed.) *The inner world of mental illness: A series of first person accounts of what it was like* (pp. 89–115). New York: Harper Row.

Basoglu, M., Mineka, S., Paker, M., Aker, T., Livanou, M., and Gok, S. (1997) Psychological preparedness for trauma as a protective factor in survivors of torture. *Psychological Medicine, 27*, 1421–1433.

Bernat, J. A., Ronfeldt, H. M., Calhoun, K. S., and Arias, I. (1998) Prevalence of traumatic events and peritraumatic predictors of posttraumatic stress symptoms in a nonclinical sample of college students. *Journal of Traumatic Stress, 11*, 645–664.

Blake, D., Weathers, F., Nagy, L., Kaloupek, D., Klauminzer, G., Charney, D., et al. (1990) *Clinician-administered PTSD scale (CAPS)*. Boston, MA: National Center for Posttraumatic Stress Disorder, Behavioral Science Division.

Blake, D., Weathers, F., Nagy, L., Kaloupek, D., Gusman, F., Charney, D., et al. (1995) The development of a clinician-administered PTSD scale. *Journal of Traumatic Stress, 8*, 75–90.

Brewin, C. R., and Holmes, E. A. (2003) Psychological theories of posttraumatic stress disorder. *Clinical Psychology Review, 23*, 339–376.

Brewin, C. R., Andrews, B., and Valentine, J. D. (2000) Meta-analysis of risk factors for post-traumatic stress disorder in trauma-exposed adults. *Journal of Consulting and Clinical Psychology, 68*, 748–766.

Briere, J. (1992) *Child abuse trauma: Theory and treatment of the lasting effects.* Newbury Park, CA: Sage.

Briere, J. (1997) *Psychological assessment of adult posttraumatic states.* Washington, DC: APA.

Chadwick, P. D. J., and Birchwood, M. J. (1995) The omnipotence of voices II: The Beliefs About Voices Questionnaire (BAVQ). *British Journal of Psychiatry, 166*, 11–19.

Chubb, H. L., and Bisson, J. I. (1996) Early psychological reactions in a group of individuals with pre-existing and enduring mental health difficulties following a major coach accident. *British Journal of Psychiatry, 169*, 430–433.

Early Psychosis Prevention and Intervention Centre (EPPIC) (2000) *Trips and journeys: Personal accounts of early psychosis.* Melbourne: EPPIC.

Edwards, J., Maude, D., McGorry, P. D., Harrigan, S., and Cocks, J. (1998) Prolonged recovery in first-episode psychosis. *British Journal of Psychiatry, 172 (suppl. 33)*, 107–116.

Ehlers, A., Maercker, A., and Boos, A. (2000) Posttraumatic stress disorder following political imprisonment: The role of mental defeat, alienation, and perceived permanent change. *Journal of Abnormal Psychology, 107*, 508–519.

Frame, L., and Morrison, A. P. (2001) Causes of posttraumatic stress disorder in psychotic patients. *Archives of General Psychiatry, 58*, 305–306.

Friedman, M. J., Schneiderman, C. K., West, A. N., and Corson, J. A. (1986) Measurement of combat exposure, posttraumatic stress disorder, and life stress among Vietnam combat veterans. *American Journal of Psychiatry, 143*, 537–539.

Frueh, B. C., Dalton, M. E., Johnson, M. R., Hiers, T. G., Gold, P. B., Magruder, K. M., et al. (2000) Trauma within the psychiatric setting: Conceptual framework, research directions, and policy implications. *Administration and Policy in Mental Health, 28*, 147–154.

Girelli, S. A., Resick, P. A., Marhoefer-Dvorak, S., and Hutter, C. K. (1986) Subjective distress and violence during rape: Their effects on long-term fear. *Victims and Violence, 1*, 35–46.

Hammill, K., McEvoy, J. P., Koral, H., and Schneider, N. J. (1989) Hospitalised schizophrenic patient views about seclusion. *Journal of Clinical Psychiatry, 50*, 174–177.

Harrigan, S. M., McGorry, P. D., and Krstev, H. (2003) Does treatment delay in first-episode psychosis really matter? *Psychological Medicine, 33*, 97–110.

Herman, J. L. (1992a) Complex PTSD: A syndrome in survivors of prolonged and repeated trauma. *Journal of Traumatic Stress, 5*, 377–391.

Herman, J. L. (1992b) *Trauma and recovery: The aftermath of violence – from domestic abuse to political terror*. New York: Basic Books.

Herrig, E. (1995) First person account: A personal experience. *Schizophrenia Bulletin, 21*, 339–342.

Horowitz, A. V., Wilner, N., and Alvarz, N. (1979) Impact of events scale: A measure of subjective distress. *Psychosomatic Medicine, 41*, 209–218.

Horowitz, K., Weine, S., and Jekel, J. (1995) PTSD symptoms in urban adolescent girls: Compounded community trauma. *Journal of the American Academy of Child and Adolescent Psychiatry, 34*, 1353–1361.

Jackson, C., and Iqbal, Z. (2000) Psychological adjustment to early psychosis. In M. Birchwood, D. Fowler and C. Jackson (eds) *Early intervention in psychosis* (pp. 64–100). Chichester: John Wiley.

Jordan, J. C. (1995) First person account: Schizophrenia – adrift in an anchorless reality. *Schizophrenia Bulletin, 21*, 501–503.

Kay, S. R., Fiszbein, A., and Opler, L. A. (1987) The positive and negative syndrome scale (PANSS) for schizophrenia. *Schizophrenia Bulletin, 13*, 261–276.

Koopman, C., Classen, C., and Spiegel, D. (1994) Predictors of posttraumatic stress symptoms among survivors of the Oakland/Berkeley, Calif., firestorm. *American Journal of Psychiatry, 151*, 888–894.

Lette, E. (1987) The treatment of schizophrenia: A patient's perspective. *Hospital and Community Psychiatry, 38*, 486–491.

Lieberman, J., Jody, D., Giesler, S., Alvir, J., Loebel, A., Szymanski, S., et al. (1993) Time course and biologic correlates of treatment responses in first-episode schizophrenia. *Archives of General Psychiatry, 50*, 369–376.

Lundy, M. S. (1992) Psychosis-induced posttraumatic stress disorder. *American Journal of Psychotherapy, 46*, 485–491.

McGorry, P. D., Chanen, A., McCarthy, E., Van Riel, R., McKenzie, D., and Singh, B. S. (1991) Posttraumatic stress disorder following recent-onset psychosis: An unrecognized postpsychotic syndrome. *Journal of Nervous and Mental Disease, 179*, 253–258.

Marmar, C. R., Weiss, D. S., Metzler, T. J., and Delucchi, K. (1996) Characteristics of emergency services personnel related to peritraumatic dissociation during critical incident exposure. *American Journal of Psychiatry, 153*, 94–102.

Meyer, H., Taiminen, T., Vuori, T., Aeijaelae, A., and Helenius, H. (1999) Post-traumatic stress disorder symptoms related to psychosis and acute involuntary hospitalization in schizophrenic and delusional patients. *Journal of Nervous and Mental Disease, 187*, 343–352.

Morrison, A. P., Frame, L., and Larkin, W. (2003) Relationships between trauma and psychosis: A review and integration. *British Journal of Clinical Psychology, 42*, 331–353.

Mueser, K. T., and Rosenburg, S. D. (2003) Treating the trauma of first episode psychosis: A PTSD perspective. *Journal of Mental Health, 12*, 103–108.

Mueser, K. T., Goodman, L. A., Trumbetta, S. L., Rosenberg, S. D., Osher, F. C., Vidaver, R., et al. (1998) Trauma and posttraumatic stress disorder in severe mental illness. *Journal of Consulting and Clinical Psychology, 66*, 493–499.

Overall, J. E. (1968) Standard psychiatric description: The factor construct rating scale (FCRS). *Triangle, 8*, 178–184.

Overall, J. E., and Gorham, D. R. (1962) The brief psychiatric rating scale. *Psychological Reports, 10*, 799–812.

Patterson, D. R., Carrigan, L., Questad, K. A., and Robinson, R. S. (1990) Post-traumatic stress disorder in hospitalised patients with burn injuries. *Journal of Burn Care Rehabilitation, 11*, 181–184.

Priebe, S., Broker, M., and Gunkel, S. (1998) Involuntary admission and post-traumatic stress disorder symptoms in schizophrenia patients. *Comprehensive Psychiatry, 39*, 220–224.

Rothbaum, B. O., Foa, E. B., Riggs, D. S., Murdock, T., and Walsh, W. (1992) A prospective examination of post-traumatic stress disorder in rape victims. *Journal of Traumatic Stress, 5*, 455–475.

Shaner, A., and Eth, S. (1989) Can schizophrenia cause post-traumatic stress disorder? *American Journal of Psychotherapy, 43*, 588–597.

Shaw, K., McFarlane, A., and Bookless, C. (1997) The phenomenology of traumatic reactions to psychotic illness. *Journal of Nervous and Mental Disease, 185*, 434–441.

Shaw, K., McFarlane, A. C., Bookless, C., and Air, T. (2002) The aetiology of postpsychotic posttraumatic stress disorder following a psychotic episode. *Journal of Traumatic Stress, 15*, 39–47.

Sloane, P. (1988) Post-traumatic stress in survivors of an airplane crash-landing: A clinical and exploratory research intervention. *Journal of Traumatic Stress, 1*, 211–229.

Stampfer, H. G. (1990) 'Negative symptoms': A cumulative trauma stress disorder? *Australian and New Zealand Journal of Psychiatry, 24*, 516–528.

Summit, R. C. (1983) The child sexual abuse accommodation syndrome. *Child Abuse and Neglect, 7*, 177–193.

Wadeson, H., and Carpenter, W. T. (1976) Impact of the seclusion room experience. *Journal of Nervous and Mental Disease, 163*, 318–328.

Watson, C. G., Juba, M. P., Manifold, V., Kucala, T., and Anderson, P. E. D. (1991) The PTSD interview: Rationale, description, reliability, and concurrent validity of a DSM-III-based technique. *Journal of Clinical Psychology, 47*, 179–188.

Williams-Keeler, L., Milliken, H., and Jones, B. (1994) Psychosis as precipitating trauma for PTSD: A treatment strategy. *American Journal of Orthopsychiatry, 64*, 493–498.

Wing, J. K., Cooper, J. E., and Sartorius, N. (1974) *The measurement and classification of psychiatric symptoms*. London: Cambridge University Press.

World Health Organization (1993) *Composite International Diagnostic Interview (CIDI)*. Geneva: WHO.

Chapter 4

Psychosis with comorbid PTSD

M. Kay Jankowski, Kim T. Mueser and
Stanley D. Rosenberg

Multiple studies of people with severe mental illness (SMI) have found elevated levels of trauma exposure, and of problems related to being traumatized. Several models have been put forth to account for these observed relationships. First, because there is abundant evidence that stress can precipitate psychotic episodes, negative life events have long been thought to act as stressors that contribute to an underlying vulnerability to psychosis. Second, SMI may increase the likelihood of trauma exposure through associated correlates like homelessness and substance abuse. Third, a pre-existing psychiatric condition may increase vulnerability to the emergence or chronicity of posttraumatic symptoms following exposure. Research to date supports the likely contribution of these, and other possible mechanisms, linking trauma exposure, SMI and PTSD.

For example, psychosis may itself represent a criterion A trauma. Or the potential symptom overlap between depression and PTSD, or schizophrenia and PTSD, may conflate the apparent rates of PTSD in those diagnostic groups (Franklin and Zimmerman 2001; Priebe et al. 1998). Alternatively, PTSD associated with psychotic experiences may be misdiagnosed as primary psychosis (Hamner et al. 2000). There is growing evidence showing that PTSD, a common consequence of trauma exposure, is sometimes associated with psychotic experiences that do not appear to be due to other major psychiatric disorders. Therefore, any consideration of the relationship between trauma and psychosis must consider both the extent to which traumatic experiences contribute to or exacerbate pre-existing psychosis, as well as the extent to which psychosis may represent an associated symptom of posttraumatic stress disorder rather than reflect a separate condition.

This chapter addresses the complex relationships between trauma and psychosis. We begin with a review of the research on rates of trauma in persons with SMI, followed by consideration of the clinical correlates of trauma exposure in this population. We next consider rates of PTSD in persons with SMI, and briefly address the clinical correlates of PTSD in this population. We then present a model in which we hypothesize that PTSD mediates the course of SMI, contributing to a worse outcome through both direct and indirect mechanisms. The implications of this model for understanding the relationship between trauma and psychosis are considered, as well as implications for the treatment of PTSD in these clients. We next briefly review evidence showing that psychosis can occur secondary to PTSD, but, if unrecognized, may lead to the incorrect diagnosis of psychotic disorders such as schizophrenia. Last, we consider the question of whether the experience of a psychotic episode and its treatment may in itself be conceptualized as a traumatic event, which in turn could lead to the development of a PTSD-like syndrome.

Throughout this chapter, we use terms such as severe mental illness because of their widespread utilization within the public mental health system in the United States. SMI (also called serious mental illness, severe and persistent mental illness, psychiatric disability) is defined in terms of a diagnosable mental illness according to the DSM-IV, with associated persistent impairment in role functioning (i.e., work), social relationships, or ability to care for oneself. Although there are slight differences among states in their definition of SMI, in general they are quite similar and such definitions are used in determining criteria for disability income.

Trauma in the general population versus people with severe mental illness

Abundant evidence documents that rates of lifetime trauma in the general population are high. In the National Comorbidity Study, 56 per cent of respondents reported exposure to at least one traumatic event during their lives, with one as the modal number of exposures (Kessler et al. 1995). In general, men are more likely to experience or witness physical assault, whereas women are more likely to be sexually victimized (Breslau et al. 1997; Kessler et al. 1995). Within the general population, trauma exposure has been associated with a wide range of negative effects, including increased use of medical and mental health services (Drossman et al. 1990; Freedy et al. 1994; Golding et al. 1988; Moeller et al. 1993; Rapkin et al. 1990; Rosenberg et al. 2000a; Rosenberg et al. 2000b; Zayfert et al. 2002), substance use disorders (Brown et al. 1998; Jacobson et al. 2001; Keane and Wolfe 1990; Stewart et al. 1998), and psychological distress, including PTSD (Beitchman et al. 1992; Polusny and Follette 1995; Widom 1999).

While trauma is common in the general population, persons with SMI are even more likely to be traumatized. Between 34 per cent and 53 per cent of clients with SMI report childhood sexual or physical abuse (Darves-Bornoz et al. 1995; Greenfield et al. 1994; Jacobson and Herald 1990; Rose et al. 1991; Ross et al. 1994), and 43 per cent to 81 per cent report some type of victimization over their lives (Carmen et al. 1984; Goodman et al. 2001; Hutchings and Dutton 1993; Jacobson 1989; Jacobson and Richardson 1987; Lipschitz et al. 1996). Studies of the prevalence of interpersonal trauma in women with SMI indicate especially high victimization, with rates ranging as high as 77 per cent to 97 per cent for episodically homeless women (Davies-Netzley et al. 1996; Goodman et al. 1995). Thus, interpersonal violence is so common in the SMI population that it can be considered to be a normative experience (Goodman et al. 1997b).

Traumatic experiences in clients with SMI are related to both the severity of psychiatric problems and increased use of acute care services. In particular, clients with SMI who have a history of trauma report more severe symptoms, such as hallucinations, depression, and anxiety (Briere et al. 1997; Craine et al. 1988; Figueroa et al. 1997; Goodman et al. 1997a). Consistent with the relationship between trauma and symptom severity in clients with SMI, exposure to interpersonal violence is correlated with worse psychosocial functioning (Lysaker et al. 2001), more time in the hospital, and more emergency room calls (Briere et al. 1997; Carmen et al. 1984; Goodman et al. 2001).

There appear to be multiple factors contributing to the high rates of trauma exposure in people with SMI. First, people exposed to abuse in childhood are more likely to develop schizophrenia, suggesting that such abuse represents a risk factor for increased vulnerability to development of the illness. For example, Read et al. (2001) have proposed a traumagenic neurodevelopmental model of schizophrenia in which they posit that the effects of stress on the developing brain contribute to the development of the disorder.

Second, after a SMI has developed, people are at elevated risk for victimization because their psychiatric problems may increase their potential exposure to violence. Common consequences or correlates of SMI include poverty (Aro et al. 1995), housing instability and homelessness (Drake et al. 1989b), substance use disorders (Mueser et al. 2003), and engaging in other risky behaviors such as sex trading. Psychopathology itself is also a risk factor for violent victimization in this population, which may be related in part to impairments in social judgment (Penn et al. 1997) and the effects of stigma (Farina 1998). The available evidence also suggests that a sub-set of people with SMI are caught up, at least episodically, in a 'cycle of violence,' in which they alternately play the role of victim and perpetrator (Cascardi et al. 1996; Hiday et al. 1999). Furthermore, as reviewed below, the available research on the SMI population reveals high rates of PTSD.

PTSD in clients with SMI

Various estimates of lifetime prevalence of PTSD in the general population range between 8 per cent and 12 per cent (Breslau et al. 1991; Kessler et al. 1995; Resnick et al. 1993). The little available research on point-prevalence of PTSD indicates rates of 2.7 per cent for women and 1.2 per cent for men (Stein et al. 1997). The most common psychiatric comorbidities associated with PTSD are depression and substance use disorder.

Studies of PTSD in clients with SMI indicate higher rates of PTSD. Eight studies have examined the prevalence of PTSD in the SMI population. One study of first admissions for psychosis reported a rate of 14 per cent (Neria et al. 2002), and the remaining seven studies reported rates ranging between 28 per cent and 43 per cent (Cascardi et al. 1996; Craine et al. 1988; McFarlane et al. 2001; Mueser et al. 1998; Mueser et al. 2001; Mueser et al. 2004b; Switzer et al. 1999). As in the general population (Saunders et al. 1992), PTSD severity in clients with SMI is related to the severity of trauma exposure, the number of traumatic events, and childhood victimization (Cascardi et al. 1996; Mueser et al. 1998; Neria et al. 2002).

Early traumatic life events appear to be risk factors for the development of major depressive disorder (MDD), psychotic disorders, and PTSD. In addition, the existence of another major mental illness may increase vulnerability, neurobiologically or psychologically, to the development of PTSD at any given level of trauma exposure. In a sample of clients drawn from a large health maintenance organization, for example, Breslau et al. (1991) reported that the prevalence of PTSD among those exposed to trauma was 24 per cent. This rate of PTSD following trauma exposure is approximately half the average rate of PTSD found in the studies of trauma and PTSD in clients with SMI (reviewed in previous paragraph), and is consistent with other research showing that the presence of a mental illness increases a person's chance of developing PTSD following exposure to a traumatic event (North et al. 1997).

Several other contributory factors, both real and artifactual, have also been suggested. For example, the potential symptom overlap between depression and PTSD, or schizophrenia and PTSD, may conflate the apparent rates of PTSD in those diagnostic groups. Alternatively, PTSD associated with psychotic symptoms may be misdiagnosed as a primary psychotic disorder (discussed later in this chapter). Finally, since almost all of the studies on this topic have looked at populations in treatment, it is reasonable to hypothesize that the high rates of PTSD in those seeking psychiatric care for other disorders are partially due to 'Berkson's fallacy,' or the tendency of people with multiple disorders to seek care more than those with a single diagnosis, resulting in higher rates of comorbidity in treatment samples than in population samples (Berkson 1949).

PTSD also is related to worse functioning in clients with SMI, including more severe psychiatric problems, worse health, and higher rates of psychiatric and medical hospitalization (Mueser et al. 2004b; Resnick et al. 2003; Switzer et al. 1999). The high rate of PTSD and its correlation with worse functioning suggest the need for a comprehensive, explanatory model to better understand, and guide treatment for, this comorbid condition. However, prior to that, we consider measurement issues in the assessment of trauma and PTSD in clients with SMI.

Reliability and validity of trauma and PTSD assessments in clients with SMI

The validity of people's accounts of traumatic events has been a topic of much controversy, especially concerning reports by adults of childhood sexual abuse (Brandon et al. 1998; Herman 1992; Loftus and Ketcham 1994; Pope and Hudson 1995). Even greater concern pertains to the reports of persons with SMI, whose disorder may result in psychotic distortions or delusions with themes involving sexual or physical abuse (Coverdale and Grunebaum 1998). Given the very private nature of most interpersonal traumatic experiences, external verification of trauma reports is not possible for most people, either with or without a psychiatric disorder.

While the accuracy of reports of victimization is difficult to ascertain, the reliability (or consistency) of reports over time can be more easily determined. Temporal reliability of trauma reports is a necessary, but not sufficient condition to establish validity. The few studies of the temporal stability of trauma exposure measures in non-SMI individuals report fair to moderate test-retest reliability (Goodman et al. 1999; Green 1996; Lauterbach and Vrana 1996; Norris and Kaniasty 1996). Less research has addressed the stability of trauma reports in clients with SMI, but some studies have demonstrated comparable levels of test-retest reliability (Goodman et al. 1999; Mueser et al. 2001). Goodman et al. (1999) showed that the internal reliability and the test-retest reliability of client self-reports of PTSD symptom severity over two weeks was high (r and coefficient alphas ≥ 0.80). Another study of structured clinical interviews for the diagnosis of PTSD (the Clinician Administered PTSD Scale: CAPS) (Blake et al. 1995) in clients with SMI demonstrated high internal reliability and inter-rater reliability, moderate test-retest reliability over two weeks, and moderate convergent validity with the PTSD Checklist (PCL: Blanchard et al. 1996), a self-report measure of PTSD (Mueser et al. 2001). In addition, when more stringent PTSD severity criteria for the CAPS were employed to define a PTSD case, the test-retest reliability increased substantially. Finally, in a larger study of computerized versus interviewer-based assessment of clients with SMI (Wolford 1999), PCL scores showed high test-retest and internal reliability, and correlated highly (>0.75) with structured interviews based on the CAPS. Depending on cut-off scores used, diagnostic agreement between CAPS and PCL were in the range of 0.80 (Rosenberg et al. 2002). These studies indicate that reliable and valid assessments of PTSD can be conducted in clients with SMI.

We have reviewed research documenting that trauma exposure and PTSD can be measured reliably in the SMI population, and studies showing that the prevalence of PTSD in clients with SMI exceeds that in the general population. Furthermore, trauma and PTSD are correlated with worse functioning and higher service utilization among clients with SMI. In the next section we present a model whereby we hypothesize that PTSD worsens the course of SMI.

Trauma, PTSD and SMI: an interactive model

There are both empirical and theoretical reasons for hypothesizing that PTSD mediates the impact of trauma on worsening the course of SMI (Mueser et al. 2002). In our model, we suggest that PTSD is chiefly responsible for the frequently observed relationships between trauma and more severe symptoms and higher use of acute care services in clients with SMI, both directly (via PTSD symptoms) and indirectly (via common correlates of PTSD such as substance abuse and retraumatization). We describe the hypothesized interactions in our model below.

Based on factors known to influence the course of schizophrenia and other types of SMI, specific symptoms of PTSD, and associated conditions (e.g., substance abuse) are expected to exacerbate the psychiatric disorder, leading to a worse outcome and use of higher cost psychiatric services. We recognize that trauma may play a role in the development of SMI (Read et al. 2001), and that PTSD and its associated problems is not the only mediator of the negative effects of trauma on SMI. For example, Morrison et al. (2003) have argued that trauma plays a direct role in the etiology of some types of psychosis, and depression is a well-established consequence of trauma (Duncan et al. 1996). Nevertheless, we believe that PTSD is an important, parsimonious, but hitherto neglected factor in understanding how trauma influences SMI: if PTSD does in fact mediate the course of SMI, then effective treatment of PTSD could improve the course of disorders such as schizophrenia, bipolar disorder, or severe treatment refractory depression.

Our model has been developed with particular reference to schizophrenia, and the majority of evidence we draw upon to support it is from research on this disorder. However, the high rates of trauma across a variety of other SMIs such as bipolar disorder and severe major depression, coupled with similarities in factors affecting their course, suggest that the impact of trauma and its interactions with other factors are common across these disorders. Although it is likely that diagnostic-specific interactions exist between trauma and different types of SMI, we suggest that the importance of their similarities outweighs these differences.

In our model, illustrated in Figure 4.1, we hypothesize that PTSD is a comorbid disorder which mediates the relationships between trauma, increased symptom severity, and higher use of acute care services in persons with a SMI. We hypothesize that PTSD can both directly and indirectly increase symptom severity, risk of relapse, and use of acute care services in patients with a SMI. PTSD symptoms can directly affect SMI through the avoidance of trauma-related stimuli, distress related to re-experiencing the trauma, and overarousal. Common correlates of PTSD can also indirectly

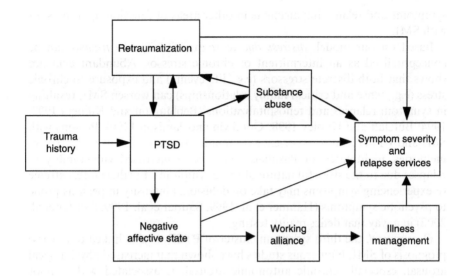

influence SMI, including substance abuse, retraumatization, negative feeling states, and a poor working alliance with treatment providers. In the next section we elaborate on the direct effects of PTSD on SMI posited by our model, followed by the indirect effects.

Direct effects of PTSD on SMI

We hypothesize that each of the three symptom clusters that define PTSD according to DSM-IV, avoidance of stimuli related to the trauma, distress related to re-experiencing the trauma, and overarousal, affect SMI. Based on factors known or believed to influence SMI, each of these PTSD symptom clusters may be expected to directly affect the comorbid psychiatric disorder.

Because most violence in the lives of persons with SMI is interpersonal in nature (Mueser et al. 1998), *avoidance of trauma-related stimuli* often extends to close relationships, leading to reduced social contacts and social isolation (Allen 1995; American Psychiatric Association 1994; Jordan et al. 1992). Multiple studies have shown that lack of social contacts is a strong predictor of symptom relapses and rehospitalizations in persons with SMI (Avison and Speechley 1987; Harrison et al. 1996; Rajkumar and Thara 1989; Strauss and Carpenter 1972). It has been hypothesized that social isolation may increase vulnerability to psychotic symptoms because of the lack of opportunities for reality testing with others, the absence of meaningful stimulation such as work, or the failure to experience the buffering effects of a supportive social network (Bell et al. 1996; Cresswell et al. 1992; Wing and Brown 1970). Thus, severe avoidance and social isolation due to PTSD are expected to worsen symptoms and related impairments in other areas of functioning in persons with SMI.

Based on our model, *distress due to re-experiencing the trauma* can be conceptualized as an intermittent or chronic stressor. Abundant evidence shows that both discrete stressors (e.g., life events) and exposure to chronic stress (e.g., tense and critical family relationships) can worsen SMI, resulting in symptom relapses and rehospitalizations (Bebbington and Kuipers 1992, 1994; Butzlaff and Hooley 1998; Goodwin and Jamison 1990). Persons with SMI and PTSD who re-experience traumatic events in the form of intrusive memories, nightmares, or flashbacks may be at increased vulnerability to relapses due to the stressful nature of these symptoms. Furthermore, extreme re-experiencing symptoms may take on delusional intensity in persons prone to psychotic symptoms (Hamner et al. 1999; Sautter et al. 1999; Sautter et al. 2002) in a way that defies reality testing.

Overarousal, the third symptom cluster of PTSD, is also linked to a worse prognosis of SMI. Numerous studies have shown that increased physiological arousal, especially chronic autonomic arousal, is associated with a poor prognosis in persons with SMI (Dawson and Nuechterlein 1984; Straube and Öhman 1990; Zahn 1986). Primary PTSD is associated with chronic over-arousal reflected across a wide range of different measures, such as heart rate, skin conductance, and catecholamine excretion, especially in response to stimuli reminiscent of the traumatic event (Orr and Kaloupek 1997; Southwick et al. 1997). Therefore, comorbid PTSD may worsen the course of SMI by further increasing arousal in persons who are already physiologically compromised and who often, even in the absence of trauma, experience high levels of activation. In addition, overgeneralization of vigilance may be to the detriment of the person's ability to assess actual probabilities of threat, increasing vulnerability to retraumatization (see below).

Little research has evaluated the relationship between specific PTSD symptoms or PTSD diagnosis and symptom severity or course of SMI. However, as previously reviewed, the suggested associations between symptoms and trauma exposure in persons with SMI, coupled with the evidence of high rates of trauma and PTSD in this population, are consistent with the hypothesis that PTSD symptoms directly affect other psychiatric symptoms.

Indirect effects of PTSD on SMI

In addition to the direct effects of PTSD on SMI, our model posits that common clinical or behavioral correlates of PTSD indirectly affect psychiatric problems. Four common correlates of PTSD are hypothesized to worsen SMI, which are *substance abuse, retraumatization, strong negative affective states*, and interpersonal difficulties (e.g., establishing trust) leading to a *poor working alliance*. We discuss each of these indirect effects in turn below.

Substance abuse

Persons with PTSD often abuse alcohol and drugs in order to avoid or minimize unpleasant, intrusive memories of traumas, to decrease arousal, or to improve sleep (Breslau et al. 2003; Stewart et al. 1998), and there is evidence that PTSD tends to precede the development of substance use disorders in the general population (Chilcoat and Breslau 1998a, 1998b; McFarlane 1998). There is also a high prevalence of substance use disorders in the SMI population (Mueser et al. 2003; Regier et al. 1990), and such substance abuse has been linked with higher lifetime exposure to trauma, especially in childhood (Briere et al. 1997; Carmen et al. 1984; Craine et al. 1988; Goodman et al. 1999; Rose et al. 1991).

Prospective research has shown that substance abuse in people with SMI contributes to a wide range of negative outcomes, including worse symptoms and relapses (Drake et al. 1989a; Drake et al. 1996; Kozaric-Kovacic et al. 1995; Linszen et al. 1994), as well as more hospitalizations and higher use of other acute care services (Bartels et al. 1993; Dickey and Azeni 1996; Haywood et al. 1995; Swartz et al. 1998). PTSD, therefore, may indirectly worsen the course of SMI via its effects on increased substance abuse.

In addition to the direct effects of substance abuse on course of SMI, our model hypothesizes that substance abuse also increases vulnerability to trauma (or retraumatization), which (as discussed below) can also lead to a worse course of illness. Several studies indicate that within the SMI population substance use disorders are associated with violent victimization (Hiday et al. 1999; Lam and Rosenheck 1998).

Retraumatization

Research on trauma has shown that earlier victimization, especially childhood sexual abuse, increases risk of later victimization and PTSD over the lifetime (Burnam et al. 1988; Nishith et al. 2000; Polusny and Follette 1995), and the high number of traumas experienced by persons with SMI has been noted by many (Goodman et al. 1995; Lipschitz et al. 1996; Muenzenmaier et al. 1993; Mueser et al. 1998). Furthermore, the number of traumas experienced is a strong predictor of PTSD in both the general population (Astin et al. 1995; King et al. 1996; Resnick and Kilpatrick 1994) and among persons with SMI (Mueser et al. 1998).

Several analogue studies of ambiguous situations involving potential interpersonal threat show that women with a history of sexual victimization have poorer recognition of risk and indicate they would leave a threatening situation later than women with no history of sexual victimization (Meadows et al. 1995; Meadows et al. 1997; Wilson et al. 1999). PTSD may further interfere with such skills to prevent exposure to additional interpersonal violence. Although PTSD may cause greater vigilance and attention to potential danger, high levels of anxiety associated with the disorder may hinder the ability of individuals with PTSD to protect themselves and avert dangerous situations altogether. Moreover, the types of cognitive distortions commonly associated with PTSD related to interpersonal violence (for example, 'I don't deserve to be treated well'; 'Men will only like me if I have sex with them') may put individuals at increased risk for revictimization as well. Skills for averting exposure to traumatic events may be further hampered by the general deficits in social skills prominent in persons with SMI (Bellack et al. 1990; Bellack et al. 1992; Bellack et al. 1994). Regardless of the precise pathways, PTSD is related to revictimization and this association may be even stronger among persons with SMI.

The experience of recent life events, including traumas, has been repeatedly linked to an increased risk of relapse and rehospitalization in persons with SMI (Bebbington and Kuipers 1992; Briere et al. 1997; Carmen et al. 1984). Revictimization therefore, either in the form of exposure to recent traumas or ongoing interpersonal victimization in patients with SMI and PTSD, can have a deleterious effect on the psychiatric disorder, similar to other types of life stress. To the extent that PTSD contributes to such revictimization, it will indirectly worsen the course of SMI.

Strong negative affective states

Strong negative emotions, such as fear and anxiety, sadness and depressed mood, shame, and anger, are also commonly associated with PTSD. These negative feeling states may contribute to a worsening course of SMI in a number of ways. It is common for people with PTSD to feel anxious and afraid in situations that are not objectively dangerous. Fear and anxiety may have a negative effect on SMI insofar as these emotions are associated with heightened autonomic arousal and may also lead to avoidance behaviors, which have been shown earlier in this chapter to be associated with a worse course of illness. Feelings of sadness and depressed mood, shame and guilt, and anger also frequently co-occur with PTSD and might negatively affect a person's SMI by interfering in important activities such as self-care, managing their illness, work, recreation and establishing and maintaining meaningful interpersonal relationships. For example, strong and frequent feelings of sadness and depression might cause people to lose motivation to care for themselves, manage their illness and engage in pleasurable, recreational activities. Anger, on the other hand, frequently causes problems in interpersonal relationships, and shame often negatively affects self-esteem and exacerbates feelings of being stigmatized.

Poor working alliance

Because of the interpersonal nature of most traumas, PTSD and social dysfunction, including pervasive feelings of mistrust, are closely linked (American Psychiatric Association 1994; Carmen et al. 1984; Figley 1985). Problems related to hypervigilance, recurrent disturbing memories, efforts to avoid trauma-related stimuli, anger, and mistrust can have an impact on the ability to form and maintain close relationships (Browne and Finkelhor 1986; Roesler and McKenzie 1994). Efforts to keep secrets or avoid topics related to traumatic events can further interfere with close relationships, and ultimately exacerbate anxiety about the experiences themselves (Kelly and McKillop 1996).

Based on our model, we hypothesize that interpersonal problems related to PTSD may interfere with the ability of clients with SMI to establish a working alliance (or therapeutic alliance) with clinicians. The concept of working alliance has been defined by Bordin (1976) as including: (1) the perceived relevance of the *tasks* involved in treatment, (2) agreement as to the *goals* of the intervention, and (3) the strength of the interpersonal *bonds* between the clinician and individual (e.g., mutual trust and acceptance). To the extent that a therapeutic relationship includes these three components, a good working alliance will exist that can serve as a vehicle for change towards desired outcomes.

For clients with a SMI, poor relationships with clinicians can result in their receiving fewer illness management services than necessary for the optimal management of their disorder (e.g., medication, case management), thereby increasing their risk of relapses and rehospitalizations. Evidence supporting this is found in several studies indicating that the quality of the therapeutic alliance with the case manager is related to symptom severity and hospitalizations in clients with SMI (Gehrs and Goering 1994; Neale and Rosenheck 1995; Priebe and Gruyters 1993; Solomon et al. 1995). Thus, PTSD may worsen the course of SMI by interfering with clients' ability to form a good working relationship with their treatment providers.

Treatment of PTSD in people with SMI

The proposed model has clinical implications for developing interventions to lessen the hypothesized effect of trauma on these disorders. Given the central role of PTSD posited by this model, we believe treatment efforts should be focused on PTSD, rather than attempting to address the broader range of effects associated with trauma exposure in the SMI population. In this section, we briefly discuss treatment of PTSD in the general population and potential modifications for treating PTSD in clients with SMI.

There is growing evidence from studies of the general population that well-delineated, theoretically based treatment models are effective in the treatment of PTSD. In 1997, the International Society for Traumatic Stress Studies (ISTSS) established a Treatment Guidelines Task Force, and this group has published PTSD treatment guidelines (Foa et al. 2000a, 2000b). Employing the coding system developed by the Agency for Health Care Policy and Research (AHCPR: US Department of Health and Human Services), the best supported interventions for PTSD symptoms were cognitive-behavioral treatment approaches.

Within this class of interventions, *exposure therapy* had the most studies supporting its efficacy. Exposure therapy involves helping clients decrease avoidance of trauma-related stimuli by encouraging them to directly confront feared thoughts, feelings, memories, and situations (Foa and Rothbaum 1998). Prolonged *imaginal exposure*, in which clients talk at length in sessions about specific traumatic events while conjuring up vivid memories of those experiences, leading to habituation of anxiety to those feared memories, is the mainstay of exposure therapy. Imaginal exposure is typically combined with *in vivo* exposure, in which clients approach and remain in situations that remind them of traumatic events but which are objectively safe.

Following exposure, *cognitive restructuring* (also called *cognitive therapy*), had the second strongest empirical support. Cognitive restructuring for PTSD is aimed at helping clients identify distorted or self-defeating thoughts, often related to traumatic experiences (e.g., 'no one can be trusted'), evaluating whether evidence supports these beliefs, and (if not) altering them accordingly. Three studies have compared exposure therapy with cognitive restructuring for PTSD, with none of them reporting significant differences in outcomes (Marks et al. 1998; Resick et al. 2002; Tarrier et al. 1999). Some studies have also evaluated the effects of combined exposure and cognitive restructuring treatment, and found the two to be superior to waitlist controls or non-exposure/cognitive restructuring comparison treatments (McDonagh-Coyle et al. 2005; Marks et al. 1998), but not to either exposure therapy or cognitive restructuring alone (Marks et al. 1998). Thus, research on cognitive-behavioral treatment of PTSD in the general population suggests that exposure and cognitive restructuring are effective, but does not suggest one is more effective than the other.

Several factors require consideration in attempting to modify cognitive-behavioral interventions for PTSD in clients with SMI. First, clients with SMI are exquisitely sensitive to the effects of stress (Bebbington and Kuipers 1992; Butzlaff and Hooley 1998), and treatment strategies must therefore be selected to minimize any unnecessary stress. Exposure therapy has been reported to be both stressful and difficult to successfully implement in persons with PTSD in the general population (McDonagh-Coyle et al. 2005; Tarrier et al. 1999; Zayfert and Becker 2000), and therefore it is reasonable to speculate that exposure therapy would be even more difficult to tolerate in this population. Cognitive restructuring, on the other hand, is not considered a particularly stressful treatment strategy. It is a technique used in the treatment of a wide range of disorders in the general population (e.g., depression, anxiety, anger management), and there is extensive evidence documenting that cognitive restructuring can be effectively implemented in clients with SMI, with multiple randomized controlled trials showing that it is effective at reducing persistent psychotic experiences (Drury et al. 1996; Durham et al. 2003; Rector et al. 2000; Sensky et al. 2000; Tarrier et al. 2000). Thus, cognitive restructuring may have higher potential for implementation and transportability in clients with SMI than exposure therapy.

Several other issues unique to a SMI population also need to be considered in developing a CBT programme to treat PTSD in this population. Because cognitive deficits are often present in clients with SMI (Dickerson et al. 1996; Heaton et al. 1994), there is a need to simplify treatment manuals and client materials. There is a vast range of ability and functioning in clients with SMI, and therefore the treatment must allow for considerable flexibility in order to meet the needs of individual clients. PTSD is one of a host of possible problems clients with SMI face, and it is critical that its treatment be carefully integrated into the overall treatment a client receives. Specifically, in order for PTSD to be effectively treated, there must be ongoing communication between the therapist and other members of the clients' treatment team, especially the case manager, whose role is to coordinate the various aspects of the client's treatment. This permits the therapist to be aware of critical issues the client is experiencing, and for the case manager, or other members of the treatment team, to support and reinforce the teaching that takes place in the CBT.

Based on the preceding considerations, we have developed a CBT intervention to address the problem of PTSD in clients with SMI (Mueser et al. 2004a). The programme involves 12–16 weeks of CBT that incorporates the following treatment elements: (1) orientation to the programme; (2) developing a crisis plan; (3) breathing retraining; (4) education about PTSD and associated symptoms; (5) cognitive restructuring; and (6) generalization training to ensure transfer of cognitive restructuring skills to clients' day-to-day lives. The treatment programme is delivered in the context of comprehensive mental health treatment, including elements such as pharmacological treatment, case management, and psychosocial rehabilitation. The programme has been standardized in a manual, pilot tested with promising results (Hamblen et al. 2004; Rosenberg et al. 2004), and is currently being evaluated in a randomized controlled trial.

Other considerations

Psychosis and PTSD

Prior to the inclusion of PTSD in the DSM-III in 1980 (American Psychiatric Association 1980), it was not uncommon for combat veterans exhibiting symptoms of PTSD, in addition to delusions and/or hallucinations, to be misdiagnosed with, and treated for, schizophrenia. Some combat veterans and other trauma survivors show a course and severity of PTSD that resembles a primary psychotic disorder. However, early conceptualizations of PTSD assumed that when psychotic symptoms were present, they were due to another comorbid disorder, such as schizophrenia or psychotic depression. Since the mid 1980s a wealth of evidence has emerged that severe PTSD can result in psychotic symptoms that are not apparently due to another disorder (Butler et al. 1996; Hamner 1997; Hamner et al. 1999; Mueser and Butler 1987; Oruc and Bell 1995; Sautter et al. 1999; Seedat et al. 2003), and some have proposed a psychotic subtype for PTSD that is distinct from a primary diagnosis of psychosis (Sautter et al. 2002).

The apparent overlap between psychotic experiences and PTSD has the potential to cause misdiagnosis and diagnostic conundrums. For example, Waldfogel and Mueser (1988) described a case of a male client with prominent psychotic difficulties (mainly paranoid delusions) that appeared related to PTSD following sexual assault in the military who had been diagnosed and treated for schizophrenia for many years at an inpatient Veterans Administration hospital. When the client was taken off antipsychotic medication and provided with cognitive-behavioral treatment for his PTSD, his problems rapidly abated and he was successfully discharged from the institution.

There is much that remains unknown regarding psychosis secondary to PTSD. For example, it is unclear whether the nature of these psychotic experiences are trauma related; some studies have found that they are, while others have not (Seedat et al. 2003). Similarly the present studies are inconclusive regarding whether severity of PTSD is related to the presence of psychosis. Nearly all studies examining psychosis associated with a primary diagnosis of PTSD have been conducted on veteran populations with combat-related PTSD, therefore significantly limiting its generalizability to other populations. It is therefore undetermined at this point how commonly psychotic problems are associated with PTSD in non-veteran populations.

Psychosis as a triggering traumatic event

There is a small but growing literature raising the question of whether PTSD can result from the experience of a psychotic episode (McGorry et al. 1991; Morrison et al. 2001; Mueser and Rosenberg 2003; Shaner and Eth 1989; Shaw et al. 1997; Shaw et al. 2002; Williams-Keeler et al. 1994). The basic thesis is that the psychosis itself, characterized by perceptual disturbances, frightening delusions, feelings of persecution, and other threats to the self, may be sufficiently terrifying to qualify as a 'traumatic event' according to criterion A of DSM-IV. This concept represents a modification of the traditional PTSD paradigm, which implies that the traumatic stressor is an external event.

Perhaps less controversial is the observation that the events related to the treatment of a major psychiatric illness may be traumatic and meet the criterion A definition in DSM-IV (Priebe et al. 1998). Psychiatric admissions often include law enforcement personnel, involuntary hospitalization, and may entail the use of restraints and seclusion, coerced medication, and exposure to other people in the throes of acute psychosis (Frueh et al. 2000; Meyer et al. 1999). For many clients, fear of or actual assault by other clients is the major trauma associated with commitment to inpatient care. Interpersonal violence or threat, psychosis itself, and treatment experiences in the early stages of illness, can evoke an extreme sense of threat to one's physical integrity, and be accompanied by feelings of fear, helplessness and horror. These evaluations may be heightened because clients are already in a state of crisis, coping resources have already been overwhelmed, and standard social supports are likely to be absent or reduced. More research is clearly needed to better understand in what ways the onset of psychosis is experienced by clients as traumatic, the similarities and differences between these events and more traditional criterion A events, and whether the psychological problems that result are PTSD in nature. Further research is also needed to develop interventions to treat early episode psychosis in order to better equip first episode clients with the knowledge and tools needed to manage their difficulties and make progress towards their own personal recovery.

Conclusion

In this chapter, we have attempted to present the many different potential relationships between trauma, PTSD and psychosis, with particular focus on PTSD as a comorbid condition with another major mental illness, such as a schizophrenia-spectrum disorder, bipolar disorder or refractory major depression. Trauma is extremely common in the lives of people with SMI, and people with SMI are much more likely to develop PTSD following trauma, as compared to the general population. The reasons for this heightened vulnerability are not entirely clear, but likely due to a combination of factors related to psychopathology itself and external circumstances common in the lives of people with SMI including poverty, housing instability, homelessness, and problems with substance use.

Trauma exposure and PTSD have also been associated with greater severity of psychiatric problems and increased use of acute care services. In this chapter, we proposed a model that identifies potential mechanisms to explain how trauma and comorbid PTSD might worsen the course of severe mental illness. We then discussed the implications of the proposed model on treatment and presented some possible adaptations for treating PTSD in people with SMI. Finally, we considered two additional relationships between PTSD and psychosis: psychotic experiences secondary to PTSD and a PTSD-like syndrome following an early psychotic episode. Clearly the relationships between trauma, PTSD and psychosis are complex, variable and multidetermined. Additional research is necessary to better understand these relationships and to guide treatment planning.

References

Allen, J. G. (1995) *Coping with trauma*. Washington, DC: American Psychiatric Association Press.

American Psychiatric Association (1980) *Diagnostic and statistical manual of mental disorders* (3rd edn). Washington, DC: APA.

American Psychiatric Association (1994) *Diagnostic and statistical manual of mental disorders (DSM-IV)* (4th edn – revised edn). Washington, DC: APA.

Aro, S., Aro, H., and Keskimäki, I. (1995) Socio-economic mobility among patients with schizophrenia or major affective disorder: A 17-year retrospective follow-up. *British Journal of Psychiatry, 166*, 759–767.

Astin, M. C., Ogland-Hand, S. M., Coleman, E. M., and Foy, D. W. (1995) Post-traumatic stress disorder and childhood abuse in battered women: Comparisons with maritally distressed women. *Journal of Consulting and Clinical Psychology, 63*, 308–312.

Avison, W. R., and Speechley, K. N. (1987) The discharged psychiatric patient: A review of social, social-psychological, and psychiatric correlates of outcome. *American Journal of Psychiatry, 144*, 10–18.

Bartels, S. J., Teague, G. B., Drake, R. E., Clark, R. E., Bush, P. W., and Noordsy, D. L. (1993) Substance abuse in schizophrenia: Service utilization and costs. *Journal of Nervous and Mental Disease, 181*, 227–232.

Bebbington, P., and Kuipers, L. (1992) Life events and social factors. In D. J. Kavanagh (ed.) *Schizophrenia: An overview and practical handbook* (pp. 126–144). London: Chapman and Hall.

Bebbington, P., and Kuipers, L. (1994) The predictive utility of expressed emotion in schizophrenia: An aggregate analysis. *Psychological Medicine, 24*, 707–718.

Beitchman, J. H., Zucker, K. J., Hood, J. E., de Costa, G. A., Akman, D., and Cassavia, E. (1992) A review of the long term effects of child sexual abuse. *Child Abuse and Neglect, 16*, 101–118.

Bell, M. D., Lysaker, P. H., and Milstein, R. M. (1996) Clinical benefits of paid work activity in schizophrenia. *Schizophrenia Bulletin, 22*, 51–67.

Bellack, A. S., Morrison, R. L., Wixted, J. T., and Mueser, K. T. (1990) An analysis of social competence in schizophrenia. *British Journal of Psychiatry, 156*, 809–818.

Bellack, A. S., Mueser, K. T., Wade, J. H., Sayers, S. L., and Morrison, R. L. (1992) The ability of schizophrenics to perceive and cope with negative affect. *British Journal of Psychiatry, 160*, 473–480.

Bellack, A. S., Sayers, M., Mueser, K. T., and Bennett, M. (1994) An evaluation of social problem solving in schizophrenia. *Journal of Abnormal Psychology, 103*, 371–378.

Berkson, J. (1949) Limitations of the application of four-fold tables to hospital data. *Biological Bulletin, 2*, 47–53.

Blake, D. D., Weathers, F. W., Nagy, L. M., Kaloupek, D. G., Charney, D. S., and Keane, T. M. (1995) *Clinician Administered PTSD Scale for DSM-IV*. Boston, MA: National Center for Posttraumatic Stress Disorder.

Blanchard, E. B., Jones-Alexander, J., Buckley, T. C., and Forneris, C. A. (1996) Psychometric properties of the PTSD Checklist (PCL). *Behaviour Research and Therapy, 34*, 669–673.

Bordin, E. S. (1976) The generalizability of the psychoanalytic concept of the working alliance. *Psychotherapy: Theory, Research and Practice, 16*, 252–260.

Brandon, S., Boakes, J., Glaser, D., and Green, R. (1998) Recovered memories of childhood sexual abuse: Implications for clinical practice. *British Journal of Psychiatry, 172*, 296–307.

Breslau, N., Davis, G. C., Andreski, P., and Peterson, E. (1991) Traumatic events and posttraumatic stress disorder in an urban population of young adults. *Archives of General Psychiatry, 48*, 216–222.

Breslau, N., Davis, G. C., Andreski, P., Peterson, E. L., and Schultz, L. R. (1997) Sex differences in posttraumatic stress disorder. *Archives of General Psychiatry, 54*, 1044–1048.

Breslau, N., Davis, G. C., and Schultz, L. R. (2003) Posttraumatic stress disorder and the incidence of nicotine, alcohol, and other drug disorders in persons who have experienced trauma. *Archives of General Psychiatry, 60*, 289–294.

Briere, J., Woo, R., McRae, B., Foltz, J., and Sitzman, R. (1997) Lifetime victimization history, demographics, and clinical status in female psychiatric emergency room patients. *Journal of Nervous and Mental Disease, 185*, 95–101.

Brown, P. J., Strout, R. L., and Gannon-Rowley, J. (1998) Substance use disorder PTSD comorbidity: Patient's perceptions of symptom interplay and treatment issues. *Journal of Substance Abuse Treatment, 15*, 445–448.

Browne, A., and Finkelhor, D. (1986) Impact of child sexual abuse: A review of the research. *Psychological Bulletin, 99*, 66–77.

Burnam, M. A., Stein, J. A., Golding, J. M., Siegel, J. M., Sorenson, S. B., Forsythe, A. B., and Telles, C. A. (1988) Sexual assault and mental disorders in a community population. *Journal of Consulting and Clinical Psychology, 56*, 843–850.

Butler, R. W., Mueser, K. T., Sprock, J., and Braff, D. L. (1996) Positive symptoms of psychosis in posttraumatic stress disorder. *Biological Psychiatry, 39*, 839–844.

Butzlaff, R. L., and Hooley, J. M. (1998) Expressed emotion and psychiatric relapse. *Archives of General Psychiatry, 55*, 547–552.

Carmen, E., Rieker, P. P., and Mills, T. (1984) Victims of violence and psychiatric illness. *American Journal of Psychiatry, 141*, 378–383.

Cascardi, M., Mueser, K. T., DeGiralomo, J., and Murrin, M. (1996) Physical aggression against psychiatric inpatients by family members and partners: A descriptive study. *Psychiatric Services, 47*, 531–533.

Chilcoat, H. D., and Breslau, N. (1998a) Investigations of causal pathways between PTSD and drug use disorders. *Addictive Behaviors, 6*, 827–840.

Chilcoat, H. D., and Breslau, N. (1998b) Posttraumatic stress disorder and drug disorders: Testing causal pathways. *Archives of General Psychiatry, 55*, 913–917.

Coverdale, J. H., and Grunebaum, H. (1998) Sexuality and family planning. In K. T. Mueser and N. Tarrier (eds) *Handbook of Social Functioning in Schizophrenia*. Needham Heights, MA: Allyn and Bacon.

Craine, L. S., Henson, C. E., Colliver, J. A., and MacLean, D. G. (1988) Prevalence of a history of sexual abuse among female psychiatric patients in a state hospital system. *Hospital and Community Psychiatry, 39*, 300–304.

Cresswell, C. M., Kuipers, L., and Power, M. J. (1992) Social networks and support in long-term psychiatric patients. *Psychological Medicine, 22*, 1019–1026.

Darves-Bornoz, J.-M., Lempérière, T., Degiovanni, A., and Gaillard, P. (1995) Sexual victimization in women with schizophrenia and bipolar disorder. *Social Psychiatry and Psychiatric Epidemiology, 30*, 78–84.

Davies-Netzley, S., Hurlburt, M. S., and Hough, R. (1996) Childhood abuse as a precursor to homelessness for homeless women in severe mental illness. *Violence and Victims, 11*, 129–142.

Dawson, M. E., and Nuechterlein, K. H. (1984) Psychophysiological dysfunctions in the developmental course of schizophrenic disorders. *Schizophrenia Bulletin, 10*, 204–232.

Dickerson, F., Boronow, J. J., Ringel, N., and Parente, F. (1996) Neurocognitive deficits and social functioning in outpatients with schizophrenia. *Schizophrenia Research, 21*, 75–83.

Dickey, B., and Azeni, H. (1996) Persons with dual diagnoses of substance abuse and major mental illness: Their excess costs of psychiatric care. *American Journal of Public Health, 86*, 973–977.

Drake, R. E., Osher, F. C., and Wallach, M. A. (1989a) Alcohol use and abuse in schizophrenia: A prospective community study. *Journal of Nervous and Mental Disease, 177*, 408–414.

Drake, R. E., Wallach, M. A., and Hoffman, J. S. (1989b) Housing instability and homelessness among aftercare patients of an urban state hospital. *Hospital and Community Psychiatry, 40*, 46–51.

Drake, R. E., Mueser, K. T., Clark, R. E., and Wallach, M. A. (1996) The natural history of substance disorder in persons with severe mental illness. *American Journal of Orthopsychiatry, 66*, 42–51.

Drossman, D. A., Leserman, J., Nachman, G., Li, Z., Gluck, H., Toomey, T. C., and Mitchell, C. M. (1990) Sexual and physical abuse in women with functional or organic gastrointestinal disorders. *Annals of Internal Medicine, 113*, 828–833.

Drury, V., Birchwood, M., Cochrane, R., and MacMillan, F. (1996) Cognitive therapy and recovery from acute psychosis: A controlled trial: I. Impact on psychotic symptoms. *British Journal of Psychiatry, 169*, 593–601.

Duncan, R. D., Saunders, B. E., Kilpatrick, D. G., Hanson, R. F., and Resnick, H. S. (1996) Childhood physical assault as a risk factor for PTSD, depression, and substance abuse: Findings for a national survey. *American Journal of Orthopsychiatry, 66*, 437–448.

Durham, R. C., Guthrie, M., Morton, R. V., Reid, D. A., Treliving, L. R., Fowler, D., and Macdonald, R. R. (2003) Tayside-Fife clinical trial of cognitive-behavioural therapy for medication-resistant psychotic symptoms: Results to 3-month follow-up. *British Journal of Psychiatry, 182*, 303–311.

Farina, A. (1998) Stigma. In K. T. Mueser and N. Tarrier (eds) *Handbook of social functioning in schizophrenia* (pp. 247–279). Boston, MA: Allyn and Bacon.

Figley, C. R. (ed.) (1985) *Trauma and its wake: The study and treatment of post-traumatic stress disorder*. New York: Brunner/Mazel.

Figueroa, E. F., Silk, K. R., Huth, A., and Lohr, N. E. (1997) History of childhood sexual abuse and general psychopathology. *Comprehensive Psychiatry, 38*, 23–30.

Foa, E. B., and Rothbaum, B. O. (1998) *Treating the trauma of rape: Cognitive-behavioral therapy for PTSD*. New York: Guilford Press.

Foa, E. B., Keane, T. M., and Friedman, M. J. (2000a) Guidelines for the treatment of PTSD. *Journal of Traumatic Stress, 13*, 539–555.

Foa, E. B., Keane, T. M., and Friedman, M. J. (eds) (2000b) *Effective treatments for PTSD*. New York: Guilford Press.

Franklin, C. L., and Zimmerman, M. (2001) Posttraumatic stress disorder and major depressive disorder: Investigating the role of overlapping symptoms in diagnostic comorbidity. *Journal of Nervous and Mental Disease, 189*, 548–551.

Freedy, J. R., Resnick, H. S., Kilpatrick, D. G., Dansky, B. S., and Tidwell, R. P. (1994) The psychological adjustment of recent crime victims in the criminal justice system. *Journal of Interpersonal Violence, 9*, 450–468.

Frueh, B. C., Dalton, M. E., Johnson, M. R., Hiers, T. G., Gold, P. B., Magruder, K. M., and Santos, A. B. (2000) Trauma within the psychiatric setting: Conceptual framework, research directions, and policy implications. *Administration and Policy in Mental Health, 28*, 147–154.

Gehrs, M., and Goering, P. (1994) The relationship between the working alliance and rehabilitation outcomes of schizophrenia. *Psychosocial Rehabilitation Journal, 18*, 43–54.

Golding, J. M., Stein, J. A., Siegel, J. M., Burnam, M. A., and Sorenson, S. B. (1988) Sexual assault history and use of health and mental health services. *American Journal of Community Psychology, 16*, 625–643.

Goodman, L. A., Dutton, M. A., and Harris, M. (1995) Physical and sexual assault prevalence among episodically homeless women with serious mental illness. *American Journal of Orthopsychiatry, 65*, 468–478.

Goodman, L. A., Dutton, M. A., and Harris, M. (1997a) The relationship between violence dimensions and symptom severity among homeless, mentally ill women. *Journal of Traumatic Stress, 10*, 51–70.

Goodman, L. A., Rosenberg, S. D., Mueser, K. T., and Drake, R. E. (1997b) Physical and sexual assault history in women with serious mental illness: Prevalence, correlates, treatment, and future research directions. *Schizophrenia Bulletin, 23*, 685–696.

Goodman, L. A., Thompson, K. M., Weinfurt, K., Corl, S., Acker, P., Mueser, K. T., and Rosenberg, S. D. (1999) Reliability of reports of violent victimization and PTSD among men and women with SMI. *Journal of Traumatic Stress, 12*, 587–599.

Goodman, L. A., Salyers, M. P., Mueser, K. T., Rosenberg, S. D., Swartz, M., Essock, S. M., et al. (2001) Recent victimization in women and men with severe mental illness: Prevalence and correlates. *Journal of Traumatic Stress, 14*, 615–632.

Goodwin, F. K., and Jamison, K. R. (1990) *Manic depressive illness*. New York: Oxford University Press.

Green, B. L. (1996) Trauma history questionnaire. In B. H. Stamm (ed.) *Measurement of stress, self-report trauma, and adaptation* (pp. 366–368). Lutherville, MD: Sidran Press.

Greenfield, S. F., Strakowski, S. M., Tohen, M., Batson, S. C., and Kolbrener, M. L. (1994) Childhood abuse in first-episode psychosis. *British Journal of Psychiatry, 164*, 831–834.

Hamblen, J., Jankowski, M. K., Rosenberg, S. D., and Mueser, K. T. (2004) Cognitive-behavioral treatment for PTSD in people with severe mental illness: Three case studies. *American Journal of Psychiatric Rehabilitation, 7*, 147–170.

Hamner, M. B. (1997) Psychotic features and combat-associated PTSD. *Depression and Anxiety, 5*, 34–38.

Hamner, M. B., Frueh, B. C., Ulmer, H. G., and Arana, G. W. (1999) Psychotic features and illness severity in combat veterans with chronic posttraumatic stress disorder. *Biological Psychiatry, 45*, 846–852.

Hamner, M. B., Frueh, B. C., Ulmer, H. G., Huber, M. G., Twomey, T. J., Tyson, C., and Arana, G. W. (2000) Psychotic features in chronic posttraumatic stress disorder and schizophrenia. *Journal of Nervous and Mental Disease, 188*, 217–221.

Harrison, G., Croudace, T., Mason, P., Glazebrook, C., and Medley, I. (1996) Predicting the long-term outcome of schizophrenia. *Psychological Medicine, 26*, 697–705.

Haywood, T. W., Kravitz, H. M., Grossman, L. S., Cavanaugh, J. L., Jr., Davis, J. M., and Lewis, D. A. (1995) Predicting the 'revolving door' phenomenon among patients with schizophrenic, schizoaffective, and affective disorders. *American Journal of Psychiatry, 152*, 856–861.

Heaton, R., Paulsen, J. S., McAdams, L. A., Kuck, J., Zisook, S., Braff, D., et al. (1994) Neuropsychological deficits in schizophrenics: Relationship to age, chronicity, and dementia. *Archives of General Psychiatry, 51*, 469–476.

Herman, J. L. (1992) *Trauma and recovery.* New York: Basic Books.

Hiday, V. A., Swartz, M. S., Swanson, J. W., Borum, R., and Wagner, H. R. (1999) Criminal victimization of persons with severe mental illness. *Psychiatric Services, 50*, 62–68.

Hutchings, P. S., and Dutton, M. A. (1993) Sexual assault history in a community mental health center clinical population. *Community Mental Health Journal, 29*, 59–63.

Jacobson, A. (1989) Physical and sexual assault histories among psychiatric outpatients. *American Journal of Psychiatry, 146*, 755–758.

Jacobson, A., and Herald, C. (1990) The relevance of childhood sexual abuse to adult psychiatric inpatient care. *Hospital and Community Psychiatry, 41*, 154–158.

Jacobson, A., and Richardson, B. (1987) Assault experiences of 100 psychiatric inpatients: Evidence of the need for routine inquiry. *American Journal of Psychiatry, 144*, 508–513.

Jacobson, L. K., Southwick, S. M., and Kosten, T. R. (2001) Substance use disorders in patients with posttraumatic stress disorder: A review of the literature. *American Journal of Psychiatry, 158*, 1184–1190.

Jordan, B. K., Marmar, C. R., Fairbank, J. A., Schlenger, W. E., Kulka, R. A., Hough, R. L., and Weiss, D. S. (1992) Problems in families of male Vietnam veterans with posttraumatic stress disorder. *Journal of Consulting and Clinical Psychology, 20*, 1776–1788.

Keane, T. M., and Wolfe, J. (1990) Comorbidity in post-traumatic stress disorder: An analysis of community and clinical studies. *Journal of Applied Social Psychology, 20*, 1776–1788.

Kelly, A. E., and McKillop, K. J. (1996) Consequences of revealing personal secrets. *Psychological Bulletin, 120*, 450–465.

Kessler, R. C., Sonnega, A., Bromet, E., Hughes, M., and Nelson, C. B. (1995) Posttraumatic stress disorder in the National Comorbidity Survey. *Archives of General Psychiatry, 52*, 1048–1060.

King, D. W., King, L. A., Foy, D. W., and Gudanowski, D. M. (1996) Prewar factors in combat-related posttraumatic stress disorder: Structural equation modeling with a national sample of female and male Vietnam veterans. *Journal of Consulting and Clinical Psychology, 64*, 520–531.

Kozaric-Kovacic, D., Folnegovic-Smalc, V., Folnegovic, Z., and Marusic, A. (1995) Influence of alcoholism on the prognosis of schizophrenic patients. *Journal of Studies on Alcohol, 56*, 622–627.

Lam, J. A., and Rosenheck, R. (1998) The effect of victimization on clinical outcomes of homeless persons with serious mental illness. *Psychiatric Services, 49*, 678–683.

Lauterbach, D., and Vrana, S. (1996) Three studies on the reliability and validity of a self-report measure of posttraumatic stress disorder. *Assessment, 3*, 17–26.

Linszen, D., Dingemans, P., and Lenior, M. (1994) Cannabis abuse and the course of recent onset schizophrenic disorders. *Archives of General Psychiatry, 51*, 273–279.

Lipschitz, D. S., Kaplan, M. L., Sorkenn, J. B., Faedda, G. L., Chorney, P., and Asnis, G. M. (1996) Prevalence and characteristics of physical and sexual abuse among psychiatric outpatients. *Psychiatric Services, 47*, 189–191.

Loftus, E., and Ketcham, K. (1994) *The myth of repressed memory*. New York: St Martin's Press.

Lysaker, P. H., Meyer, P. S., Evans, J. D., Clements, C. A., and Marks, K. A. (2001) Childhood sexual trauma and psychosocial functioning in adults with schizophrenia. *Psychiatric Services, 52*, 1485–1488.

McDonagh-Coyle, A., Friedman, M. J., McHugo, G. J., Ford, J. D., Sengupta, A., Mueser, K. T., et al. (2005) Randomized trial of cognitive behavioral therapy for chronic PTSD in adult female childhood sexual abuse survivors. *Journal of Consulting and Clinical Psychology, 73*, 515–524.

McFarlane, A. C. (1998) Epidemiologic evidence about the relationship between PTSD and alcohol abuse: The nature of the association. *Addictive Behaviors, 6*, 813–825.

McFarlane, A. C., Bookless, C., and Air, T. (2001) Posttraumatic stress disorder in a general psychiatric inpatient population. *Journal of Traumatic Stress, 14*, 633–645.

McGorry, P. D., Chanen, A., McCarthy, E., Van Riel, R., McKenzie, D., and Singh, B. S. (1991) Posttraumatic stress disorder following recent-onset psychosis: An unrecognized postpsychotic syndrome. *Journal of Nervous and Mental Disease, 179*, 253–258.

Marks, I., Lovell, K., Noshirvani, H., Livanou, M., and Thrasher, S. (1998) Treatment of posttraumatic stress disorder by exposure and/or cognitive restructuring. *Archives of General Psychiatry, 55*, 317–325.

Meadows, E., Jaycox, L., Stafford, J., Hambree, E., and Foa, E. (1995) Recognition of risk in revictimized women. Paper presented at the Poster session presented at the 29th Annual Meeting of the Association for the Advancement of Behavior Therapy, Washington, DC, November.

Meadows, E., Jaycox, L., Orsillo, S., and Foa, E. (1997) The impact of assault on risk recognition in ambiguous situations. Paper presented at the Poster session presented at the 31st Annual Meeting of the Association for the Advancement of Behavior Therapy, Miami Beach, FL, November.

Meyer, H., Taimenen, T., Vuori, T., Aijala, A., and Helenius, H. (1999) Posttraumatic stress disorder symptoms related to psychosis and acute involuntary hospitalization in schizophrenic and delusional patients. *Journal of Nervous and Mental Disease, 187*, 343–352.

Moeller, T. P., Bachman, G. A., and Moeller, J. R. (1993) The combined effects of physical, sexual, and emotional abuse during childhood: Long-term health consequences for women. *Child Abuse and Neglect, 17*, 623–640.

Morrison, A. P., Bowe, S., Larkin, W., and Nothard, S. (2001) The psychological impact of psychiatric admission: Some preliminary findings. *Journal of Nervous and Mental Disease, 189*, 250–253.

Morrison, A. P., Frame, L., and Larkin, W. (2003) Relationships between trauma and psychosis: A review and integration. *British Journal of Clinical Psychology, 42*, 331–353.

Muenzenmaier, K., Meyer, I., Struening, E., and Ferber, J. (1993) Childhood abuse and neglect among women outpatients with chronic mental illness. *Hospital and Community Psychiatry, 44*, 666–670.

Mueser, K. T., and Butler, R. W. (1987) Auditory hallucinations in combat-related chronic posttraumatic stress disorder. *American Journal of Psychiatry, 144*, 299–302.

Mueser, K. T., and Rosenberg, S. R. (2003) Treating the trauma of first episode psychosis: A PTSD perspective. *Journal of Mental Health, 12*, 103–108.

Mueser, K. T., Goodman, L. A., Trumbetta, S. L., Rosenberg, S. D., Osher, F. C., Vidaver, R., et al. (1998) Trauma and posttraumatic stress disorder in severe mental illness. *Journal of Consulting and Clinical Psychology, 66*, 493–499.

Mueser, K. T., Salyers, M. P., Rosenberg, S. D., Ford, J. D., Fox, L., and Cardy, P. (2001) A psychometric evaluation of trauma and PTSD assessments in persons with severe mental illness. *Psychological Assessment, 13*, 110–117.

Mueser, K. T., Rosenberg, S. D., Goodman, L. A., and Trumbetta, S. L. (2002) Trauma, PTSD, and the course of schizophrenia: An interactive model. *Schizophrenia Research, 53*, 123–143.

Mueser, K. T., Noordsy, D. L., Drake, R. E., and Fox, L. (2003) *Integrated treatment for dual disorders: A guide to effective practice.* New York: Guilford Press.

Mueser, K. T., Rosenberg, S. D., Jankowski, M. K., Hamblen, J., and Descamps, M. (2004a) A cognitive-behavioral treatment program for posttraumatic stress disorder in severe mental illness. *American Journal of Psychiatric Rehabilitation, 7*, 107–146.

Mueser, K. T., Salyers, M. P., Rosenberg, S. D., Goodman, L. A., Essock, S. M., Osher, F. C., et al. (2004b) Interpersonal trauma and posttraumatic stress disorder in patients with severe mental illness: Demographic, clinical, and health correlates. *Schizophrenia Bulletin, 30*, 45–57.

Neale, M. S., and Rosenheck, R. A. (1995) Therapeutic alliance and outcome in a VA intensive case management program. *Psychiatric Services, 46*, 719–721.

Neria, Y., Bromet, E. J., Sievers, S., Lavelle, J., and Fochtmann, L. J. (2002) Trauma exposure and posttraumatic stress disorder in psychosis: Findings from a first-admission cohort. *Journal of Consulting and Clinical Psychology, 70*, 246–251.

Nishith, P., Mechanic, M. B., and Resick, P. A. (2000) Prior interpersonal trauma: The contribution to current PTSD symptoms in female rape victims. *Journal of Abnormal Psychology, 109*, 20–25.

Norris, F. H., and Kaniasty, K. Z. (1996) Received and perceived social support in times of stress: A test of the social support deterioration deterrence model. *Journal of Personality and Social Psychology, 71*, 498–511.

North, C. S., Smith, E. M., and Spitznagel, E. L. (1997) One-year follow-up of survivors of a mass shooting. *American Journal of Psychiatry, 154*, 1696–1702.

Orr, S. P., and Kaloupek, D. G. (1997) Psychophysiological assessment of post-traumatic stress disorder. In J. P. Wilson and T. M. Keane (eds) *Assessing psychological trauma and PTSD* (pp. 69–97). New York: Guilford Press.

Oruc, L., and Bell, P. (1995) Multiple rape trauma followed by delusional parasitosis: A case report from the Bosnian war. *Schizophrenia Research, 16*, 173–174.

Penn, D. L., Corrigan, P. W., Bentall, R. P., Racenstein, J. M., and Newman, L. (1997) Social cognition in schizophrenia. *Psychological Bulletin, 121*, 114–132.

Polusny, M. A., and Follette, V. M. (1995) Long-term correlates of child sexual abuse: Theory and review of the empirical literature. *Applied and Preventive Psychology, 4*, 143–166.

Pope, H. G., Jr., and Hudson, J. I. (1995) Can memories of childhood sexual abuse be repressed? *Psychological Medicine, 25*, 121–126.

Priebe, S., and Gruyters, T. (1993) The role of the helping alliance in psychiatric community care: A prospective study. *Journal of Nervous and Mental Disease, 181*, 552–557.

Priebe, S., Broker, M., and Gunkel, S. (1998) Involuntary admission and post-traumatic stress disorder symptoms in schizophrenia patients. *Comprehensive Psychiatry, 39*, 220–224.

Rajkumar, S., and Thara, R. (1989) Factors affecting relapse in schizophrenia. *Schizophrenia Research, 2*, 403–409.

Rapkin, A. J., Kames, L. D., Darke, L. L., Stampler, F. M., and Naliboff, B. D. (1990) History of physical and sexual abuse in women with chronic pelvic pain. *Obstetrics and Gynecology, 76*, 92.

Read, J., Perry, B. D., Moskowitz, A., and Connolly, J. (2001) The contribution of early traumatic events to schizophrenia in some patients: A traumagenic neurodevelopmental model. *Psychiatry, 64*, 319–345.

Rector, N. A., Seeman, M. V., and Segal, Z. V. (2000) Cognitive therapy for schizophrenia: Treatment outcomes and follow-up effects from the Toronto Trial Study. Paper presented at the 160th Annual Meeting of the American Psychiatric Association, Chicago, May.

Regier, D. A., Farmer, M. E., Rae, D. S., Locke, B. Z., Keith, S. J., Judd, L. L., and Goodwin, F. K. (1990) Comorbidity of mental disorders with alcohol and other drug abuse: Results from the Epidemiologic Catchment Area (ECA) study. *Journal of the American Medical Association, 264*, 2511–2518.

Resick, P. A., Nishith, P., Weaver, T. L., Astin, M. C., and Feuer, C. A. (2002) A comparison of cognitive processing therapy with prolonged exposure and a waiting condition for the treatment of posttraumatic stress disorder in female rape victims. *Journal of Consulting and Clinical Psychology, 70*, 867–879.

Resnick, H. S., and Kilpatrick, D. G. (1994) Crime-related PTSD: Emphasis on adult general population samples. *PTSD Research Quarterly, 5*, 1–3.

Resnick, H. S., Kilpatrick, D. G., Dansky, B. S., Saunders, B. E., and Best, C. E. (1993) Prevalence of civilian trauma and post-traumatic stress disorder in a representative national sample of women. *Journal of Consulting and Clinical Psychology, 61*, 984–991.

Resnick, S. G., Bond, G. R., and Mueser, K. T. (2003) Trauma and posttraumatic stress disorder in people with schizophrenia. *Journal of Abnormal Psychology, 112*, 415–423.

Roesler, T. A., and McKenzie, N. (1994) Effects of childhood trauma on psychological functioning in adults sexually abused as children. *Journal of Nervous and Mental Disease, 182*, 145–150.

Rose, S. M., Peabody, C. G., and Stratigeas, B. (1991) Undetected abuse among intensive case management clients. *Hospital and Community Psychiatry, 42*, 499–503.

Rosenberg, H. J., Rosenberg, S. D., Williamson, P. J., and Wolford, G. L. (2000a) A comparative study of trauma and PTSD prevalence in epileptic and psychogenic non-epileptic seizure patients. *Epilepsia, 41*, 447–452.

Rosenberg, H. J., Rosenberg, S. D., Wolford, G. L., Manganiello, P. D., Brunette, M. F., and Boynton, R. A. (2000b) The relationship between trauma, PTSD and medical utilization in three high risk medical populations. *Psychiatry in Medicine, 30*, 247–259.

Rosenberg, S. D., Wolford, G. I., Jankowski, M. K., Rosenberg, H. J., Mueser, K. T., and Vidaver, R. (2002) Reliability, validity and diagnostic accuracy of the PCL for clients with severe mental illness. Manuscript.

Rosenberg, S. D., Mueser, K. T., Jankowski, M. K., Salyers, M. P., and Acker, K. (2004) Cognitive-behavioral treatment of posttraumatic stress disorder in severe mental illness: Results of a pilot study. *American Journal of Psychiatric Rehabilitation, 7*, 170–186.

Ross, C. A., Anderson, G., and Clark, P. (1994) Childhood abuse and the positive symptoms of schizophrenia. *Hospital and Community Psychiatry, 45*, 489–491.

Saunders, B. E., Villeponteaux, L. A., Lipovsky, J. A., Kilpatrick, D. G., and Veronen, L. J. (1992) Child sexual assault as a risk factor for mental disorders among women: A community survey. *Journal of Interpersonal Violence, 7*, 189–204.

Sautter, F. J., Brailey, K., Uddo, M. M., Hamilton, M. F., Beard, M. G., and Borges, A. H. (1999) PTSD and comorbid psychotic disorder: Comparison of veterans diagnosed with PTSD or psychotic disorder. *Journal of Traumatic Stress, 12*, 73–88.

Sautter, F. J., Cornwell, J., Johnson, J. J., Wiley, J., and Faraone, S. V. (2002) Family history study of posttraumatic stress disorder with secondary psychotic symptoms. *American Journal of Psychiatry, 159*, 1775–1777.

Seedat, S., Stein, M. B., Oosthuizen, P. P., Emsley, R. A., and Stein, D. J. (2003) Linking posttraumatic stress disorder and psychosis: A look at epidemiology, phenomenology, and treatment. *Journal of Nervous and Mental Disease, 191*, 675–681.

Sensky, T., Turkington, D., Kingdon, D., Scott, J. L., Scott, J., Siddle, R., et al. (2000) A randomized controlled trial of cognitive-behavioral therapy for persistent symptoms in schizophrenia resistant to medication. *Archives of General Psychiatry, 57*, 165–172.

Shaner, A., and Eth, S. (1989) Can schizophrenia cause posttraumatic stress disorder? *American Journal of Psychotherapy, 43*, 588–597.

Shaw, K., McFarlane, A., and Bookless, C. (1997) The phenomenology of traumatic reactions to psychotic illness. *Journal of Nervous and Mental Disease, 186*, 434–441.

Shaw, K., McFarlane, A. C., Bookless, C., and Air, T. (2002) The aetiology of postpsychotic posttraumatic stress disorder following a psychotic episode. *Journal of Traumatic Stress, 15*, 39–47.

Solomon, P., Draine, J., and Delaney, M. A. (1995) The working alliance and consumer case management. *Journal of Mental Health Administration, 22*, 126–134.

Southwick, S. M., Yehuda, R. T., and Charney, D. S. (1997) Neurobiological alterations in PTSD: Review of the clinical literature. In C. S. Fullerton and R. J. Ursano (eds) *Posttraumatic stress disorder: Acute and long-term responses to trauma* (pp. 241–266). Washington, DC: American Psychiatric Press.

Stein, M. B., Walker, J. R., Hazen, A. L., and Forde, D. R. (1997) Full and partial posttraumatic stress disorder: Findings from a community survey. *American Journal of Psychiatry, 154*, 1114–1119.

Stewart, S. H., Pihl, R. O., Conrod, P. J., and Dongier, M. (1998) Functional associations among trauma, PTSD, and substance-related disorders. *Addictive Behaviors, 6*, 797–812.

Straube, E. R., and Öhman, A. (1990) Functional role of the different autonomic nervous system activity patterns found in schizophrenia: A new model. In E. R. Straube and K. Hahlweg (eds) *Schizophrenia: Concepts, vulnerability, and intervention* (pp. 135–157). Berlin: Springer-Verlag.

Strauss, J. S., and Carpenter, W. T. J. (1972) The prediction of outcome in schizophrenia I. Characteristics of outcome. *Archives of General Psychiatry, 27*, 739–746.

Swartz, M. S., Swanson, J. W., Hiday, V. A., Borum, R., Wagner, H. R., and Burns, B. J. (1998) Violence and mental illness: The effects of substance abuse and nonadherence to medication. *American Journal of Psychiatry, 155*, 226–231.

Switzer, G. E., Dew, M. A., Thompson, K., Goycoolea, J. M., Derricott, T., and Mullins, S. D. (1999) Posttraumatic stress disorder and service utilization among urban mental health center clients. *Journal of Traumatic Stress, 12*, 25–39.

Tarrier, N., Pilgrim, H., Sommerfield, C., Faragher, B., Reynolds, M., Graham, E., and Barrowclough, C. (1999) Cognitive and exposure therapy in the treatment of PTSD. *Journal of Consulting and Clinical Psychology, 67*, 13–18.

Tarrier, N., Kinney, C., McCarthy, E., Humphreys, L., Wittkowski, A., and Morris, J. (2000) Two-year follow-up of cognitive-behavioral therapy and supportive counseling in the treatment of persistent symptoms in chronic schizophrenia. *Journal of Consulting and Clinical Psychology, 68*, 917–922.

Waldfogel, S., and Mueser, K. T. (1988) Another case of chronic PTSD with auditory hallucinations. *American Journal of Psychiatry, 145*, 1314.

Widom, C. S. (1999) Posttraumatic stress disorder in abused and neglected children grown up. *American Journal of Psychiatry, 156*, 1223–1229.

Williams-Keeler, L., Milliken, H., and Jones, B. (1994) Psychosis as precipitating trauma for PTSD: A treatment strategy. *American Journal of Orthopsychiatry, 64*, 493–498.

Wilson, A. E., Calhoun, K. S., and Bernat, J. A. (1999) Risk recognition and trauma-related symptoms among sexually revictimized women. *Journal of Consulting and Clinical Psychology, 67*, 705–710.

Wing, J. K., and Brown, G. W. (1970) *Institutionalism and schizophrenia*. Cambridge: Cambridge University Press.

Wolford, G. I. (1999) *Formats for assessing HIV risk in severely mentally ill people*. National Institute of Mental Health grant RO-1 MH60073.

Zahn, T. P. (1986) Psychophysiological approaches to psychopathology. In M. G. H. Coles, E. Donchin and S. W. Porges (eds) *Psychophysiology: Systems, processes and applications* (pp. 508–610). New York: Guilford Press.

Zayfert, C., and Becker, C. B. (2000) Implementing of empirically supported treatment for PTSD: Obstacles and innovations. *The Behavior Therapist, 23*, 161–168.

Zayfert, C., Dums, A. R., Ferguson, R. J., and Hegel, M. T. (2002) Health functioning impairments associated with posttraumatic stress disorder, anxiety disorders, and depression. *Journal of Nervous and Mental Disease, 190*, 233–240.

Chapter 5

The catastrophic interaction hypothesis

How do stress, trauma, emotion and information processing abnormalities lead to psychosis?

David Fowler, Daniel Freeman, Craig Steel, Amy Hardy, Ben Smith, Corrina Hackman, Elizabeth Kuipers, Philippa Garety and Paul Bebbington

Introduction

Severe interpersonal victimisation and its consequences can clearly contribute to the emotional distress of people with psychosis, as it does in other disorders. However, the degree to which trauma occurs, and can contribute to symptoms of psychosis is more controversial. In this chapter we attempt to clarify how psychological processes associated with reactions to trauma and threat memories may sometimes play a part in the maintenance of psychotic symptoms. In speculating about the pathway from stress and trauma to psychosis we consider four routes:

- Direct associations between intrusive memories of traumatic or stressful experiences and delusions and hallucinations.
- Indirect associations between trauma and persecutory delusions and hallucinations mediated by negative evaluations of self and others (the schema route).
- Indirect associations between trauma and hallucinations mediated by negative and self-critical rumination concerning relationship between the voice hearer and the voice identity.
- Speculations about potential catastrophic interactions between trauma processes and information processing abnormalities which characterise psychosis which may magnify vulnerability to psychosis.

We review existing evidence for each type of process, particularly highlighting our own recent studies and implications for future studies. We also draw out clinical implications.

Alice was a 35-year-old woman with a diagnosis of schizophrenia. She was severely thought disordered and initially the therapist had some problems making sense of her difficulties. Eventually it was possible to identify that among the problems that were most distressing to her was an experience she had every day when going off to sleep. Alice complained of hearing threatening voices coming from the loft. When she was going to sleep, she also had feelings of being sexually interfered with which were accompanied by visions of the rapist. She believed strongly that her father lived in the loft and was coming down to abuse her at night. Alice believed these to be real and current experiences and was scared to go to bed at night. The night-time events appeared to be linked to past experiences of being sexually abused both as an adult by past partners and as a child by her father.

Eric was a 40-year-old man with a diagnosis of paranoid schizophrenia. Seven years previous to his first contact with the therapist he had been functioning as a senior manager. He had now given up work and was living on benefit. He had spent much of his money moving house, four times in the past seven years. Each time he had reinforced the house with extensive security measures. He said that there was a conspiracy against him and that he was in danger of being killed. This conspiracy involved the government and the police. The origin of Eric's problems appeared to be an episode in which he had been severely beaten up by a gang who had been robbing a shop close to his place of work. This event had apparently shattered his previous view of the world as stable and safe. His conspiracy beliefs and sense of current threat appeared to evolve out of a sense that the world had become dangerous and an unpredictable place, a view reinforced by what Eric regarded as the inadequate reaction of the police.

Joe complained of hearing voices. He was scared in sessions as the voices told him not to talk about what had happened to him. The voices also shouted at him and told him he was disgusting. He was scared of the voices and believed them to be real. He became totally submissive when the voices occurred. Joe believed strongly in the truth of what they said and hence followed all their commands. Joe also complained of flashbacks, which he described as unbearable. At such times he became overwhelmed with fear and had visual and tactile images related to his experience of being sexually abused when a teenager. Joe said that on a day-to-day basis the voice threatened to rape him, and that the visual and tactile images were experiences of rape caused by the voices. They appeared to the therapist to reflect traumatic memories of the teenage abuse.

What is the nature of associations between trauma, stress and psychosis?

The study of the relationship between social crises, traumas and psychotic experiences has a long history. Since the early 1960s, various researchers have studied the impact of life events in the period before onset or relapse of psychosis. In general, these have supported the conclusion that stressful or personally significant events tended to cluster significantly in the few weeks or months before onset of psychosis (Bebbington et al. 1996). Some studies also clearly show that a history of trauma and victimisation is very common among people with psychosis and may both precede and accompany the course of psychotic disorder (Mueser et al. 1998). A substantive minority of people with psychosis report current problems associated with memories of such traumatic experience. Several large-scale studies carried out in the United States suggest that around 30–40 per cent of people with chronic psychosis report symptoms severe enough to qualify for a diagnosis of PTSD (see Mueser et al. 2002 for review), although notably the rates in non-affective psychosis (schizophrenia, delusional disorder) are considerably smaller than those in affective psychosis (depression, bipolar disorder).

In the United Kingdom we assessed trauma history in a sample of 228 people with non-affective psychosis who were recruited for a trial of cognitive behavioural therapy for psychotic relapse in London, Essex and Norfolk. The study used a detailed structured interview to assess trauma (the trauma history questionnaire), the same tool as used in the Mueser et al. (1998) study. PTSD symptoms were assessed by self-report questionnaire (Carlier et al. 1998). Trauma history and PTSD were assessed three months following an acute relapse. We found that 76 per cent of cases reported experiencing an event accompanied by extreme fear, 54 per cent reported that they currently avoided or had intrusive memories of the event and 13 per cent met diagnostic criteria for PTSD (Fowler et al. 2006). Fourteen cases (6 per cent) had experienced severe child sex abuse and thirty-eight cases (17 per cent) had experienced severe physical or emotional abuse in childhood. Twenty-four cases (10 per cent) had experienced severe sex abuse as an adult and seventy-two cases (30 per cent) had experienced severe physical abuse as an adult. Overall, the level of severe interpersonal victimisation in the sample was strikingly present in almost half the cases (47 per cent). A history of interpersonal victimisation was strongly associated with the presence of emotional distress, and sexual abuse was associated with more severe hallucinations. Psychological reactions associated with PTSD leading to intrusive memories and avoidance have also been found to follow adverse experiences associated with hospitalisation and the experience of psychotic symptoms (McGorry et al. 1991).

The degree of traumatic experience and stress which accompanies psychosis is high and represents a dimension of need which deserves to be recognised and addressed in clinical services. As with other disorders severe interpersonal victimisation is likely to contribute strongly to the presence of severe emotional distress in psychosis. However, speculations concerning links between interpersonal trauma and psychosis are still controversial and contested. The traditional tendency as represented by vulnerability stress models of psychotic disorder has been to interpret associations between trauma and psychosis as at best indicating only a triggering effect of life events on symptoms of psychosis, perhaps acting by increasing arousal, with this in turn being linked in a non-specific way with the emergence of positive symptoms. Mueser et al. (2002) have similarly suggested that hyperarousal associated with PTSD symptoms may affect psychosis, but expand to also provide a sophisticated analysis of how intrusive memories may act as an additional internal source of stress, with additional roles for avoidance and associated problems of drug abuse and social disability. Psychiatric opinion is however still dominated by the traditional view that the vulnerability to psychosis may be characterised by altered brain processes which have little to do with the sufferer's social environment following Kraeplin's view of schizophrenia. Indeed, often, psychotic experience has been regarded as not understandable as a consequence of psychological processes. The influential views of Jaspers (1913), that psychotic experiences were ultimately un-understandable, implied no possibility of a meaningful link between experience and the contents of psychotic thinking. To what degree should these traditional assumptions now be questioned?

The observations of those using cognitive behaviour therapy have provided a new perspective. Therapists from a number of groups have reported that many symptoms of psychosis have a content that can be meaningfully related to past personally significant experience (Fowler et al. 1998). Indeed helping people to make sense of their psychotic experience, at least partially, in the context of past events, stresses and psychological processes forms an important aspect of cognitive behaviour therapy for psychosis (Fowler et al. 1995). Furthermore users often seek explanations for their experience which suggests that psychosis arises partially from stress (Watson et al. 2006) and particularly highlight the need to recognise the impact that past psychological trauma and stress has had on their problems (Reeves 2000). Cases where there appears to be an obvious and understandable link between a social crisis and the onset of psychotic symptoms, such as those described in the introduction, suggest that there may sometimes be causal connections between trauma and psychotic symptoms. Potential causal links between stress, trauma and psychosis are also suggested by various studies which show links between severe trauma and the emergence of psychotic symptoms in a context where post-traumatic stress disorder of more ordinary form would be expected (Bebbington et al. 2004; Hamner et al. 1999). Trauma and the presence of PTSD symptoms also appear to be associated with the presence of more severe and chronic psychotic symptoms (specifically hallucinations) and potentially worse outcomes in a variety of domains including depression, negative symptoms, social outcomes, and comorbid drug abuse (see Mueser et al. 2002 for review).

These associations suggest that trauma and PTSD may potentially have a greater contributory role in the development and maintenance of psychosis than has usually been assumed. However, in making sense of such associations it is important to distinguish between traumatic experience and stress and to appreciate the complex nature of causal processes in psychosis. While cases where there are obvious direct links between PTSD and psychotic symptoms clearly occur, they may be relatively uncommon (we describe our studies on this phenomenon later in the chapter). Also while one can quite often observe meaningful links between the content of psychotic experiences and past stressful and personally significant events this does not necessarily imply simple causation. In fact the nature of the stresses which trigger most psychoses are often common life events (e.g. relationship breakdowns, interpersonal conflicts, problems at work) which alone do not make sense of the occurrence of severe symptoms of psychosis (it could be that people vulnerable to psychosis are sensitive to stress). In making sense of how psychosis occurs in reaction to stress it may be important to consider both psychological processes which are common to most mental health problems including neurotic disorders and distinct psychological processes which are specifically associated with psychosis such as information processing abnormalities and reasoning biases (Freeman and Garety 2003). In this chapter we consider ways in which interactions between these two types of processes may result in the catastrophic changes which lead to acute psychotic states. We consider the possibility that a characteristic of vulnerability to psychosis may be that it leads to problems in processing normal emotions and reactions to stress (such as the occurrence of intrusive memories and rumination). The consequence of psychosis may be that normal emotions (and reactions to trauma or day-to-day stress) may become distorted, exaggerated and difficult to inhibit. This type of understanding provides both new clinical insights and novel hypotheses for further research, which we try to highlight.

We have previously described a cognitive model of psychosis which makes sense of the experiences, beliefs and behaviours of people with psychosis; in terms of emotions, appraisals, related schematic structures and information processing abnormalities characteristic of psychosis (Fowler 2000; Fowler et al. 1995; Freeman et al. 2002; Garety et al. 2001). Our view is that psychosis is a complex experience that cannot be explained by one single factor. Instead, the complexity of the phenomena can only be fully appreciated by considering interactions between a number of psychological, social and biological factors.

Process 1: direct and indirect links between intrusive trauma memories and psychotic symptoms

The idea that forms of psychosis may arise as a direct consequence of PTSD has a long history. Cases where psychotic symptoms seem very obviously to be linked to past traumatic events, such as those described above, have often been regarded as arising from different causal processes than other psychoses and have been separated off as 'psychogenic' or 'reactive' psychoses, a diagnosis particularly favoured by Scandinavian psychiatrists (Lindvall et al. 1993). Traditionally, cases of this type have been regarded as relatively rare. However, there is still debate about prevalence. Some studies suggest that this type of syndrome, particularly occurring as a consequence of sexual abuse, may be quite common (Ellason et al. 1997; Read et al. 2003; see also Read, Chapter 9 in this volume). There is more consistent evidence from epidemiological studies that trauma history can increase risk of psychosis (Bebbington et al. 2004) and we found an association between severity of hallucinations and sexual abuse, even though the rate of child sex abuse was relatively low (6 per cent) (Fowler et al. 2006). In explaining such a link Morrison (2001) developed a cognitive model of hallucinations which places particular emphasis on intrusions. This model suggests that normal intrusive memories and images, such as occur in anxiety and other neurotic disorders, form the basis for most psychotic experience. This model suggests that it is the appraisal of intrusive memories and images as representing an external threat, which forms the basis for psychosis and particularly for hallucinations.

Clinical observations by cognitive therapists from several different groups have highlighted many cases in which people have reported voices or delusions which appear to reflect in some manner past traumatic experiences (e.g. Chadwick et al. 1996; Fowler et al. 1998; Kingdon and Turkington 1994). In a preliminary study, Fowler (1997) reported that fourteen of twenty-four people with distressing delusions and hallucinations who were receiving cognitive behaviour therapy as part of the London and East Anglia randomised controlled trial had problems associated with memories of past traumatic events. In four of these cases there was a direct connection between the traumatic event (two were rapes in adulthood, one child sexual abuse and one bullying) and the experience of hallucination. In all of these four cases the report was of hearing a voice appraised to be that of the abuser. Sometimes the content of the voices was suggestive that these were memories as the comments were similar to those made at the time of the abuse. However, it was also noted that most of the time the voices made general critical comments or comments about the person's day-to-day experiences. A particular aspect of such voices was that although the voices were appraised to be of the identity of an abuser from the past, the current experience of the voices was appraised as reflecting real experiences and current threat. In most of the other treatment trial cases where there had been a history of trauma, the therapists also reported what appeared to be meaningful connections between past trauma and current symptoms: but in these instances the connection was indirect, i.e. the voices and delusions might have a common theme or meaning (e.g. humiliation/threat) but there was no direct connection in terms of identity or content. We used the term 'syntonic' in an attempt to describe what appeared to be a similarity in themes between past trauma and the content of current delusions and hallucinations in some cases. This may be a specific instance of the broader idea that previous experiences and emotions shape much psychotic symptom content as suggested originally by Bleuler. We also noted that a consistency between the themes of past events and current psychotic symptoms could also be clinically observed in cases who had not experienced events which could be regarded as traumatic (e.g. not life threatening or associated with extreme fear or helplessness) but which were personally significant. For example, the threatening themes of hallucinations and delusions might sometimes reflect upbringing in difficult but not abusive family circumstances or emotional bullying which was perhaps personally significant but could not be regarded as either unusual or meeting the criterion of traumatic.

Morrison et al. (2002) described the images reported by people with psychosis in a small CBT case series. Various types of images were reported: some were associated with fears concerning hospitalisation; some were images concerning current fears associated with delusional beliefs; and some reflected past traumas. The cases described in this study also varied in the degree to which the images had a direct and indirect link with past events. Not all of the images associated with psychosis reflected trauma. Many of the images reflected idiosyncratic personally significant events or current goals, hopes or expectations. Images of this type have also been observed to occur in disorders such as depression, anxiety and social phobia (Hackman et al. 2000). The occurrence of such images and intrusive memories of stress in psychosis are consistent with contemporary views that the borderline between psychosis and neurosis may not be as distinct as has normally been assumed (Freeman and Garety 2003) and support the idea that intrusive memories and images might be of importance in understanding the content of psychosis (Morrison 2001).

Studies undertaken with small convenience samples by therapists do not provide a reliable indication of how common direct or indirect connections between the content and themes of psychotic symptoms and past traumatic events actually are in the wider population of people with psychosis. Furthermore, the suggestions of links in such studies are also compromised by the process of narrative creation, which is an intrinsic aspect of the work of cognitive therapy. The extent of links between trauma and psychosis may be exaggerated by therapist report. Hardy et al. (2005) have recently undertaken a systematic study of the relationship between traumatic experiences and hallucinations, which attempted to overcome some of these methodological flaws. The participants were seventy-five patients with non-affective psychosis who were recruited for a treatment trial of cognitive behaviour therapy (the Psychological Prevention of Relapse in Psychosis Trial). All patients with relapses of psychosis in identified clinical teams in London, Essex and East Anglia were approached to take part in the study. Systematic and reliable measures of trauma experience and of psychotic symptoms were used. Careful examination was made of the content of the patients' hallucinations in relation to the content of past traumas by raters who were independent of the patients' therapy context. Approximately half (55 per cent) of cases reported that they had current problems associated with past stressful experiences, although many of these stressful experiences did not meet criteria for trauma and only 26 per cent met criteria for PTSD. Strikingly, however, only a very small proportion (13 per cent of those who reported current problems associated with past stress and 7 per cent of the total) were rated as having direct relationships between current psychotic symptoms and trauma (i.e. rated has having both themes and content similar to that of past trauma). Around a third of cases (30 per cent of the total and 45 per cent of the stress subgroup) were rated as having some similar themes but not content related to their past trauma. The traumas most likely to have thematic relationships were sexual abuse and bullying. It is noteworthy that in 42 per cent of cases who reported having current problems associated with past trauma, there was *no* association of any kind between their hallucination content and past trauma.

At present what may be conservatively concluded from the clinical studies, is that while direct links between hallucinations and trauma can occur and are of interest they may actually be quite rare. A further study of direct links between the content of persecutory delusions and traumatic events is under-way. Indirect thematic links between hallucinations and traumatic experience appear to be more common but again are far from universal. Even among people who have hallucinations and report experiencing a trauma which is currently troubling them, many hallucinations occur which have little con-nection with past adverse experience. These observations are an important starting point for theorising. Trauma and PTSD process may in some cases contribute to hallucinations but they are neither necessary nor sufficient for either the formation or maintenance of hallucinations.

The idea that memories of stressful and traumatic past experiences *can* influence psychosis is important. It is also important to recognise that the intrusive memories, thoughts and images associated with trauma, threat and adversity occur in many psychiatric disorders including depression (Kuyken and Brewin 1994), social phobia (Hackmann et al. 2000) and PTSD (Brewin and Holmes 2003; Ehlers and Clark 2000) can also occur in psy-chosis. Furthermore, studies of non-clinical samples which have been used to examine the relationship between a tendency to experience hallucinations, intrusive memories and trauma, or between past trauma and risk of psychosis are indicative that intrusive memories of traumatic experience might be a contributory factor to a tendency to hallucinate. Morrison and Peterson (2003) found that a tendency to experience hallucinations was associated with a history of bereavement, physical assault and emotional abuse. More recently Gracie et al. (submitted) examined the association of traumatic experience PTSD symptoms and hallucinations in 246 students contacted via the internet. In this study only bereavement (and not sexual abuse, or physical assault or other traumas) was associated with an increase in hallucinatory experience. However, in a subsequent multiple regression, intrusive memories of traumatic experience were found to have a significant although small association with the presence of hallucinatory experience. Further studies using both clinical and non-clinical samples are required. It is important that attempts are made to recruit representative samples of patients and methodologies employed that are rigorous. This is basic groundwork needed for theoretical development. Direct links between intrusions associated with traumatic events and psychosis are only one route from trauma to psychosis, and the current evidence suggests that indirect factors may be more important in most cases. In the remainder of this chapter we theorise in detail about other potential psychological pathways that can link trauma and psychosis.

Process 2: the schema route to delusions and paranoia

Delusions can be conceptualised as explanations of experiences arising out of a search for meaning in the context of anomalous perceptions or threatening social events for which an explanation is not evident (Maher 1988). The acceptance of relatively implausible delusional explanations for these anomalous events or threatening experiences occurs in the context of a person's culturally conditioned own idiosyncratic beliefs and may be facilitated by biased reasoning processes (Garety et al. 2001). Recent advances in understanding delusions indicate that different types of processes may be associated with different dimensions of delusional thinking (e.g. content, conviction, preoccupation, distress, persistence). Although emotion may provide content to delusional ideation (Freeman et al. 2002), we have recently found evidence that reasoning biases associated with jumping to conclusions and extreme responding is most associated with belief flexibility (ability to recognise the possibility of being mistaken) and thereby to delusional conviction (Garety et al. 2005). Conversely, distress and preoccupation (although not conviction) of persecutory ideas is associated with emotional distress and negative beliefs about self and others (Smith et al. submitted).

Like other psychological theorists we suggest that distress and preoccupation with persecutory beliefs may be closely associated with beliefs about self and others. We have argued specifically that it is synthesising extreme beliefs about one's own personal characteristics that is important (beliefs that one is bad, weak, vulnerable, inadequate etc.). This idea came from clinical observations (Fowler et al. 1995). Studies using both detailed interview assessments of negative personal evaluation and a new self-report measure of evaluations of self and others show a specific association between negative self-evaluation and paranoia (Barrowclough et al. 2003; Smith et al. submitted). It is noteworthy that it is specifically, extreme negative personal evaluations rather than other aspects of self-esteem (e.g. autonomy concerns, need for control), conditional or predicative beliefs, dysfunctional assumptions or personality style, which may reliably show specific and strong associations with positive symptoms, paranoia and self-evaluation. The findings on the association between psychotic symptoms and other aspects of self and other appraisal and self-esteem are conflicting (see Bentall et al. 2001; Freeman et al. 1998 for review) and often show only modest associations with paranoid thinking (e.g. Bentall and Swarbrick 2003). Essentially we suggest that the synthesising of persecutory ideas in the context of a negative view of self and related negative emotions may lead to a vicious cycle type of maintenance process or gridlock, akin to that suggested in depression (e.g. Teasdale and Barnard 1993). If one's sense of self is that of badness or weakness then one might feel vulnerable or alert to persecution from others and in turn the experience of persecution may maintain views of self as bad or weak and negative emotions. Therefore, a combination of anxiety and negative self-evaluation may contribute directly to the experience of positive psychotic experiences and particularly paranoia and may lead to the persistence of delusional ideas.

We have also suggested that there may be an association between negative beliefs about others and persecutory ideas, independently of beliefs about self. For example, one may have a positive or normal sense of self but may learn to regard others as untrustworthy or dishonest. Persecutory ideas may arise in the context of an extreme form of negative beliefs about others and may be maintained because they are consistent with this core belief and related negative emotions such as anger. It is of interest here that anger often concerns judgments of the negative intentions of others, which is an important element of persecutory thinking. Our recent studies provide support for this idea that negative beliefs about others (in non-clinical and psychotic groups) are associated with paranoia (Fowler et al. 2006; Smith et al. submitted).

In general our approach is to emphasise a role for negative self and other evaluation as consistent with ongoing emotions such as anxiety and anger and thus may drive persecutory thinking. This model is then slightly different from those which suggest paranoia are defensive and associated with attempts to maintain self-esteem (Bentall et al. 2001; Trower and Chadwick; 1995). We believe our model is more parsimonious. A combination of extreme negative self and extreme negative other may represent a particularly catastrophic appraisal of social position. A social position in which the individual both appraises self negatively (as weak, vulnerable, inadequate) and others as threatening (devious, bad) is both vulnerable and dangerous (Gilbert 1992). We have recently found that this catastrophic combination of very extreme negative self and extreme negative other evaluation appears to be characteristic of people with psychosis compared to non-clinical controls in a study which compared the self and other evaluations of 100 people with relapsing psychosis recruited for a trial of cognitive therapy with 750 students (Fowler et al. 2006). Our recent studies also found that this combined pattern of negative self and other evaluation in association with anxiety is specifically and uniquely associated with paranoia, in both the clinical sample (Smith et al. submitted) and two separate large-scale studies of non-clinical students (Fowler et al. 2006; Gracie et al. submitted). The combined pattern of extreme self and other evaluation was associated with a history of humiliating trauma (bullying, assault, sexual abuse) and multiple regressions suggested that extreme self and other evaluations were the strongest mediator of the relationship between traumatic events and paranoia.

Akin with other theorists (e.g. Birchwood 2003; Brown and Harris 1989) our view is that a tendency to synthesise extreme negative beliefs about self and others probably derives from adaptation to humiliating social experience via social learning and the representation of such learning in schematic knowledge about self and others. We have found clear evidence to suggest that extreme negative evaluations of self and others are more likely to be present among people with psychosis who have been exposed to either ongoing social adversity or specific social humiliations such as rape or bullying. The way in which past traumatic and stressful experience may be linked to paranoia may then be via the mediation of negative self and others' evaluations. This can occur as a result of adaptation and social learning in a similar manner to that suggested by psychological theorists of PTSD (Dalgleish 2004; Foa and Rothbaum 1998). People who have been traumatised are more likely, from time to time, to synthesise extreme negative beliefs about self and others in association with related negative emotions (anger, depression, feelings of threat). When this occurs it may often be associated with persecutory ideas and may comprise an important process leading to the maintenance of the delusional ideas and the associated distress and preoccupation.

Process 3: critical and threatening voices: relationship to self-critical thinking and rumination concerning interpersonal relationships with abusive figures

There are important similarities between negative content of hallucinations and self-critical thinking in depression as described by Gilbert et al. (2001). Several studies have shown that distressing auditory hallucinations are often closely associated with depression and negative beliefs about self (Birchwood and Chadwick 1997; Birchwood et al. 2000, 2004; Close and Garety 1998). Hallucinations are regarded by many theorists as misattributions of our own thoughts or internal dialogue, possibly as a result of faulty source, or self-monitoring (Bentall 1990; Johns and McGuire 1999). In the context of faulty source or self-monitoring the emotional processes which can result in negative conscious thoughts or internal dialogue (e.g. I'm bad, useless, it's hopeless) may become experienced as hallucinations (you are bad, useless, it's hopeless). This switching of processes associated with language or thought production into voices is consistent with recent evidence from source monitoring experiments and fMRI studies (Johns and McGuire 1999; Johns et al. 2001; McGuire et al. 1993, 1996).

There is also evidence that beliefs about the voices, as well as voice content, underpin distress and preoccupation with voice hearing. Birchwood et al. (2000, 2004) in developing a model of auditory hallucinations have suggested that a childhood experience of social adversity leads to negative schemas involving social humiliation and subordination which fuel voices and paranoia. This is consistent with studies which show that distress is associated with beliefs about voices in particular appraisals of malevolence; and that voices can be regarded as internal signals appraised as powerful dominant shaming/insulting persecutors, and the self is seen as subordinated, shamed and inferior (Birchwood and Chadwick 1997; Birchwood et al. 2000, 2004). Vaughan and Fowler (2004) have similarly shown that distress is mediated by a person's appraisal of their relationship with voices; they identify two key appraisals associated with distressing voices: the appraisal that voices relate in an overly dominant and close manner and, further, the appraisal that the voice hearer is behaving in a submissive manner. In people who have had traumatic interpersonal experiences who hear voices it may be that rumination over the relationship with abuse figures drives expectations concerning hearing a voice. It may be evaluations of self in interaction with others (and related appraisals of subordination, humiliation, dominance etc.) which are important in understanding links between traumatic and stressful events and voice hearing rather than the occurrence of absolute negative evaluations of self and others.

Further investigation of the way in which past experience may shape voice hearing is needed. Patterns of interpersonal relating to voices may reflect general social and interpersonal learning about self in relation to others; and dysfunctional patterns are likely to be associated with difficult interpersonal circumstances. Ruminating about difficult interpersonal traumas and events is a common reaction to trauma and stress (Ehlers and Clark 2000). People who have been traumatised and are vulnerable to having hallucinations might sometimes experience the products of such rumination as voices, i.e. their thinking or rumination about their interactions with their abuser occurring as voices rather than as ruminative thoughts or the experience of internal dialogue. That the content of voice hearing might reflect altered experience of rumination about the trauma (thinking about oneself in relation to the abuser) rather than a direct intrusive image of the trauma event may also be consistent with the observation that even in cases where voices are identified as being past abuse figures, the content of the voice does not always directly reflect exactly what the voice said in the past. Often such voices criticise with respect to what the voice hearer is saying currently. In psychosis the abuser is often appraised as a figure who is current and real. Voice content may then sometimes reflect patterns of rumination or internal dialogue about self in relationship to what a shaming and insulting abuser might say about one's current actions. Such a view would be consistent with the observations of those who have studied voice hearing in both normal and clinical populations which suggest that often the content of voices reflects what would normally be internal dialogue regarding ongoing events (Leudar et al. 1997; Nayani and David 1996).

Process 4: the catastrophic interaction hypothesis: how might psychosis exaggerate and distort the experience of emotion and current personally significant experience and memories of past events?

Kapur (2003) has usefully emphasised that the underlying information processing abnormalities associated with psychosis occur in the very processes that underpin our experiences of motivation, novelty, and salience, and modulate our experience of affect. The consequences of such information processing abnormalities may be in distortions in our experience of self and the world, non-significant external events may feel personally significant (e.g. déjà vu), the products of cognitive processing of internal origin such as thoughts or images may feel as if they are of external origin thus providing the basis for altered experiences of thought and hallucinations (Hemsley 1994). The degree to which such experience is appraised as threatening or exciting or neutral may depend on the association of psychosis with emotion and the way such experience is appraised by the individual. As discussed above distressing psychotic experience sometimes occurs in the context of a background of traumatic events (Mueser et al. 1998), and typically occurs in the context of recent personally significant events (Bebbington et al. 1996). The emotional reaction and appraisal associated with psychosis may then depend in turn on the nature of such recent and past stressful or traumatic events. In the following we develop a hypothesis that it is the interaction between information processing abnormalities and normal processes associated with the emotional reaction to stress and trauma, which may form the catastrophic change observed as acute psychotic states. Such a catastrophic change may be understood in terms of both the way information processing abnormalities may distort and exaggerate the experience of the products of emotional processing, and how extreme emotion may exaggerate information processing abnormalities. The idea that psychosis exaggerates emotional responses deserves further investigation but is consistent with longitudinal observations of the build up of emotion in combination with unusual symptoms in psychotic relapse (e.g. Birchwood et al. 1989) and with observations that the occurrence of rare and unusual symptoms of psychosis are associated with the occurrence of common symptoms of emotional disturbance (Freeman et al. 2005).

The experience of emotion in the context of acute psychotic experience may be altered. Emotional experience in psychosis may be both affectively valent (e.g. threatening) but also have a peculiar quality of being personally significant, current and real. These characteristics may be explained by the nature of the information processing abnormalities that occur (Hemsley 1994). We noted above that the feeling of the reality of current threat associated with psychosis occurs even when such experience can be meaningfully related to past events. For example when people hear voices which are appraised as being of the abuser, these are often not recognised or appraised as a memory or emotion relating to past events, and instead they are regarded as being current events in the real world. This is also true of threatening delusional experience. For example, a young man who had been assaulted and threatened by a gang with a knife some months previously developed a severe paranoia in the context of acute psychosis which was associated with the terror of being stabbed. His extreme fear at the time of being psychotic was of an immediate current threat rather than a rumination about the past event. These qualities of psychotic experience may then have some phenomenological commonalities with re-experiencing or reliving symptoms in PTSD. As noted by Ehlers and Clark (2000) a characteristic of PTSD is that the anxiety associated with a past event becomes appraised as a current real threat. Contemporary theories of PTSD suggest that this type of clinical phenomena may be best understood with reference to disorders of memory processing. Theories of PTSD suggest that problems in placing trauma memories in the context of autobiographical knowledge (Ehlers and Clark 2000) and a tendency to process information in a data-driven rather than a contextual manner may explain the clinical phenomena.

Steel et al. (2005) have put forward an information processing account of trauma-related intrusions which are argued to occur within psychosis. They draw on existing information processing models of both PTSD (Brewin 2001; Ehlers and Clark 2000) and psychosis (Hemsley 1994) and highlight the similarities within the processes argued to underlie the development of intrusions within both disorders.

With reference to psychosis, Hemsley (1994) suggests that individuals who experience problems in placing moment to moment experiences within an appropriate context may be vulnerable to experiencing the positive symptoms of psychosis. Thus, it is argued that a failure to integrate incoming information with either co-occurring external events, or with memories of past experience, results in memories being stored within a context that leaves them vulnerable to being triggered involuntarily at a later date. This process of 'temporal contextual integration' is a basic cognitive process, and occurs outside of conscious awareness. Efficient 'temporal contextual integration' contributes to our development of an awareness of meaningful relationships between events occurring over time, and consequently how our attentional resources are allocated towards events which reach our conscious awareness. Being aware of the origin of the contents of our consciousness would seem crucial in distinguishing between events which arise from the external world and those that arise from internal cognitive processes (e.g. images, memories, thoughts).

Steel et al. (2005) note the similarities between Hemsley's information processing account and an information processing account of PTSD (Brewin 2001; Ehlers and Clark 2000). Thus, contemporary PTSD theory suggests that the flashbacks associated with a diagnosis of PTSD are the product of a failure to integrate traumatic information (e.g. the moment an individual thought he was going to die during a car crash) within a temporal context of the previous and subsequent events. This results in a traumatic memory which cannot be accessed voluntarily, but is vulnerable to being triggered involuntarily by stimuli which are associated with that of the traumatic event (e.g. seeing a car similar to the one that was crashed into). Thus, within the development of PTSD it is argued that there is a failure to efficiently contextually integrate information, for short periods of time, during the worst moments of the traumatic events (Holmes et al. 2005).

At a neurological level, it has been suggested that the hippocampus serves to bind the individual features of incoming information within a spatial and temporal context, thus forming a coherent whole (Eichenbaum 1997; Squire 1992). Information is thought to be integrated within the hippocampus before being processed by the amygdala, which governs emotional regulation and biological reactions to stress (LeDoux et al. 1988). On this basis, PTSD theory (Brewin 2001) suggests that information is processed directly within the amygdala during intensely traumatic events (an information processing 'shortcut' which facilitates a faster emotional response) resulting in poor contextual integration of specific traumatic information. Interestingly, Hemsley (1994) suggests that individuals diagnosed with psychosis suffer from continuous problems with hippocampal functioning, and consequently poor contextual integration, during a psychotic episode. There is strong evidence for structural changes in the hippocampi preceding and accompanying the early psychotic episodes as well as in chronic schizophrenia (e.g. Phillips et al. 2002).

Steel et al. (2005) conclude by suggesting that the same processes seem to underlie the development of intrusive experiences within both PTSD and psychosis. It is also argued that there would seem to be a continuum within which people are vulnerable to developing intrusions, which is based upon an individual's ability to contextually integrate information. On the basis of PTSD theory it would seem that individuals may shift along this continuum (termed 'temporal context integration continuum') during traumatic or stressful events. Therefore, one individual with strong temporal context integration may suffer intrusions only if they have been exposed to severely traumatic events. Other individuals such as those suffering from, or vulnerable to suffering from, psychosis may experience frequent intrusions of relatively mild stressful events, such as an argument. Factors which affect neurobiology may also influence where a person is on such a continuum. High vulnerability may be conferred from genetic or constitutional factors, there may also be neurodevelopmental factors. Finally, street drugs which influence dopaminergic pathways may also affect ability to place ongoing experience in context, and potentially neuroleptic medication may moderate feelings of salience and threat (Kapur 2003).

This approach to understanding is important as it provides a link between the body of evidence relating to information processing abnormalities in psychosis and how people process personally significant threat and emotion. As described above, problems in contextual processing associated with vulnerability to psychosis may then have the capacity to distort or exaggerate personally significant threat, related anxiety and a range of emotions. An understanding of the emotional reactions of people with psychosis, in response to day-to-day stresses, might then be facilitated with reference to models of how extreme trauma memories are processed in PTSD. In acute psychosis the experience of emotions and related memories may occur without being placed in an appropriate autobiographical context, and without effective processing past stress may continue to be appraised as real and current threats. The need to create a personal narrative and autobiographical context for distorted emotional experience associated with personally significant events may be associated with delusion formation. This has clinical implications as it provides a justification for the actions of cognitive behaviour therapists carefully placing psychotic experience in context by cognitive behavioural assessment and formulation which is at the basis of our approach to cognitive behaviour therapy for psychosis (Fowler et al. 1995).

This understanding also provides an explanation for why, in the subgroup of people with psychosis who have had traumatic events, the experience of the combination of psychosis with trauma might be particularly catastrophic. The catastrophic interaction hypothesis can provide an explanation for why people with psychosis appear to have higher rates of PTSD after being exposed to a trauma than people without psychiatric problems, and that cases who have a combination of PTSD and psychosis have a particularly poor outcome (see Mueser et al. 2002). Psychological reactions to trauma associated with PTSD such as dissociation, absorption, preferential data-driven processing, and avoidance might in turn exacerbate pre-existing contextual processing problems (i.e. trauma can itself exaggerate information processing abnormalities thus magnifying psychotic symptoms). Such a hypothesis is consistent with current findings which suggest associations between dissociation, schizotypy and psychotic symptoms (Ellason et al. 1997; Morrison and Peterson 2003). A further hypothesis worth investigation is that cases that present with both PTSD and psychosis might have more severe information processing abnormalities.

The catastrophic interaction hypothesis suggests other hypotheses for further research and insights which have clinical implications. It suggests that the effective processing of day-to-day stress may be inhibited in the presence of psychosis by contextual processing problems. The hypothesis that people vulnerable to psychosis may be more likely to experience intrusions following exposure to a stressful event is open to empirical test, and a study by Holmes and Steel (2004) provides evidence in support of this idea. They found that people rated with high positive symptom schizotypy reported more intrusions after being exposed to a stressful film during the following week than people with low schizotypy scores. The film paradigm is only one of many which may be used to assess how people with psychosis respond to stressful events. We are also examining how people who are vulnerable to psychosis react to virtual reality environments, and are looking in detail at their experience of memories of stress events. The hypothesis suggests not only that people who have higher levels of contextual processing type problems will have more intrusions in response to stress but also that it is possible that people with psychosis will have more vivid intrusions which are more likely to be appraised as real than those of other disorders when exposed to similar stressors. Severe contextual processing problems may also lead to alterations in the experience of intrusions. In particular, the latter may not be experienced as the products of one's own consciousness, but rather as voices or persecutory ideas originating in the external world. We are investigating this in detailed phenomenological studies. An inability to effectively place stress event in context of autobiographical memory would suggest people are unable to inhibit stress response. This is consistent with clinical observations of extreme emotional sensitivity and hyperarousal among people with psychosis. It remains to be demonstrated that emotional sensitivity is specifically associated with context processing problems.

The catastrophic interaction hypothesis suggests that the experience of being less able to process or moderate emotional reactions effectively as a result of contextual processing problems may result in any emotional experience being aversive. This in turn may lead to extreme patterns of avoiding emotion and possibly certain aspects of negative symptoms such as flat affect may be interpreted in this light. In relation to clinical practice, we have previously described common problems associated with extreme sensitivity to emotion associated with psychosis which can occur in therapy sessions and have recommended care in discussing and managing emotions associated with traumatic events because of this (Fowler et al. 1995). Like others (Mueser et al. 2004) we do not recommend the use of techniques which result in extreme emotion in sessions because people may be less able to inhibit their emotional responses. In cognitive behaviour therapy, often gentle approaches to facilitating disclosure are required during the engagement process to help the person bring emotional experience to mind in a safe and non-threatening context. Possibly, clinical observations of people avoiding discussion of their difficulties which may be regarded as patterns of 'sealing over' may also be interpreted in the light of attempts to recover without the aversive experience associated with the triggering of emotion in psychosis. The catastrophic interaction hypothesis suggests that investigations of the association between information processing abnormalities and emotional processing with respect to clinical patterns of avoidance, negative symptoms and withdrawal may be promising.

Conclusion

In this chapter we have argued that people with psychosis can have intrusive thoughts, images and memories akin to those occurring in emotional disorders. Further, we have noted that traumatic events might affect beliefs about the self in relation to others in a manner akin to that suggested for other emotional disorders and this may be associated with paranoia and persecutory delusions. The way individuals appraise abuse figures and ruminate over their interactions with such figures may be associated with hallucinations. We have also argued that people with psychosis may have a vulnerability which may be characterised by information processing abnormalities associated with the ability to place moment-to-moment experience in context, and furthermore we proposed that it may be a catastrophic distortion of emotional processing of personally significant events in the presence of contextual processing problems associated with acute psychosis that gives rise to the altered experiences associated with psychosis. These different types of processes can sometimes occur independently but most often in severe cases they occur in combination and interact often catastrophically to give rise to acute psychotic states. The catastrophic interaction hypothesis provides a new basis for understanding novel clinical insights and suggests hypotheses for research. People with psychosis are sometimes attempting to adapt to traumatic past events but almost always are adapting to day-to-day personally significant stress. However, their problems may be fully understood only by examining how their attempt to adapt to trauma and stress might be affected by information processing abnormalities. Psychosis is a complex disorder frequently associated with processing and storing of traumatic and emotional information. However, in psychosis it may be that desynchrony in the processing of information at different levels, can lead to the processing of trauma and emotional information being experienced as voices, anomalies of subjective experiences, and delusions.

As clinicians, we need to recognise that people with psychosis can have both emotional problems (sometimes relating to past trauma), and problems with contextual processing and reasoning. We have argued that, as a consequence of contextual processing problems, people with psychosis can come to experience the products of their own emotional processing as external events rather than as images, memories or thoughts, and that this has important clinical implications. People with psychosis may have little awareness of the problem in contextual processing that underpins their altered experience. They are likely to react to changes in momentary conscious experiences as if their cognitive processes were working normally. Conscious experience originating as emotions, memories and thoughts can become experienced as current real experiences and this is likely to be regarded by others as loss of insight or awareness. Moreover, as people with psychosis are less able to place emotion in the context of autobiographical information, they are less likely to be able to resolve emotional problems. As illustrated in the cases at the beginning of this chapter, a key problem of people with psychosis is that they may appraise voices and delusions as real experiences even when they may have their origins either in past memories of threatening experience or in day-to-day stresses. It is confusion about the origin of emotional experience that may mark a key difference between people with anxiety and depression and those with psychosis, even when the processes underpinning emotional difficulties may be common. This insight has important implications for cognitive behaviour therapy. Assisting people with psychosis to become aware of their emotional experience and its connection with psychotic experiences, to place it in an appropriate context in relation to past experience, current goals, hopes and expectations, and to compensate for a tendency to regard such experience as an external threat may be an important target in cognitive therapy for psychosis. This is consistent with the specific approach to cognitive therapy for psychosis adopted by our group in which making sense of psychotic experience in terms of psychological processes and helping people to adopt a less distressing shared formulation or personal narrative for their difficulties is at centre stage (Fowler et al. 1995).

References

Barrowclough, C., Tarrier, N., Humphreys, L., Ward, J., Gregg, L., and Andrews, B. (2003) Self-esteem in schizophrenia: Relationships between self-evaluation, family attitudes and symptomology. *Journal of Abnormal Psychology, 112*, 92–99.

Bebbington, P., Wilkins, S., Sham, P., and Jones, P. (1996) Life events before psychotic episodes: Do clinical and social variables affect the relationship? *Social Psychiatry and Psychiatric Epidemiology, 31*, 122–128.

Bebbington, P. E., Bhugra, D., Brugha, T., Singleton, N., Farrell, M., Jenkins, R., et al. (2004) Psychosis, victimisation and childhood disadvantage: Evidence from the second British National Survey of Psychiatric Morbidity. *British Journal of Psychiatry, 185*, 220–226.

Bentall, R. P. (1990) The illusion of reality: A review and integration of psychological research on hallucinations. *Psychological Bulletin, 107*, 82–85.

Bentall, R. P., and Swarbrick, R. (2003) The best laid schemas of paranoid patients: Autonomy, sociotropy and need for closure. *Psychology and Psychotherapy: Theory, Research and Practice, 76*, 163–171.

Bentall, R. P., Corcoran, R., Howard, R., Blackwood, R., and Kinderman, P. (2001) Persecutory delusions: A review and theoretical integration. *Clinical Psychology Review, 21*, 1143–1192.

Birchwood, M. (2003) Pathways to emotional dysfunction in first-episode psychosis. *British Journal of Psychiatry, 182*, 373–375.

Birchwood, M., and Chadwick, P. D. J. (1997) The omnipotence of voices: Testing the validity of a cognitive model. *Psychological Medicine, 27*, 1345–1353.

Birchwood, M., Smith, J., Macmillan, F., Hogg, B., Prasad, R., Harvey, C., and Bering, S. (1989) Predicting relapse in schizophrenia: The development and implementation of an early signs monitoring system using patients and families as observers. *Psychological Medicine, 19*, 649–656.

Birchwood, M., Meaden, A., Trower, P., Gilbert, P., and Plaistow, J. (2000) The power and omnipotence of voices: Subordination and entrapment by voice and significant others. *Psychological Medicine, 30*, 337–344.

Birchwood, M., Gilbert, P., Gilbert, J., Trower, P., Meaden, A., Hay, J., et al. (2004) Interpersonal and role-related schema influence the relationship with the dominant voice in schizophrenia: A comparison of three models. *Psychological Medicine, 34*, 1–10.

Brewin, C. R. (2001) A cognitive neuroscience account of posttraumatic stress disorder and its treatment. *Behaviour Research and Therapy, 38*, 373–393.

Brewin, C. R., and Holmes, E. A. (2003) Psychological theories of posttraumatic stress disorder. *Clinical Psychology Review, 23*, 339–376.

Brown, G. W., and Harris, T. O. (1989) *Life events and illness*. New York: Guilford Press.

Carlier, I. V., Lamberts, R. D., Van Uchelen, A. J., and Gersons, B. P. (1998) Clinical utility of a brief diagnostic test for posttraumatic stress disorder. *Psychosomatic Medicine, 60*, 42–47.

Chadwick, P. D. J., Birchwood, M., and Trower, P. (1996) *Cognitive therapy for delusions, voices and paranoia*. Chichester: John Wiley.

Close, H., and Garety, P. (1998) Cognitive assessment of voices: Further developments in understanding the emotional impact of voices. *British Journal of Clinical Psychology, 37*, 173–188.

Dalgleish, T. (2004) Cognitive approaches to posttraumatic stress disorder: The evolution of multirepresentational thinking. *Psychological Bulletin, 130*, 228–260.

Ehlers, A., and Clark, D. M. (2000) A cognitive model of posttraumatic stress disorder. *Behaviour Research and Therapy, 38*, 319–345.

Eichenbaum, H. (1997) Declarative memory: Insights from cognitive neurobiology. *Annual Review of Psychology, 48*, 547–572.

Ellason, J., Ross, C., and Fuchs, D. (1997) Lifetime Axis 1 and Axis II comorbidity and childhood trauma history in dissociative identity disorder. *Psychiatry, 59,* 255–266.

Foa, E. B. and Rothbaum, B. O. (1998) Treating the trauma of rape: Cognitive behavioral therapy for PTSD. New York: Guilford Press.

Fowler, D. (1997) Direct and indirect links between the content of psychotic symptoms and past traumatic experience: Evidence from therapists reports from the London-East Anglia study of cognitive behaviour therapy for psychosis. Paper presented at the British Association of Behavioural and Cognitive Psychotherapy Annual Conference, Southport, July.

Fowler, D. (2000) Psychological formulation of early episodes of psychosis: A cognitive model. In M. Birchwood, D. Fowler, and C. Jackson (eds) *Early intervention in psychosis* (pp. 101–127). New York: John Wiley.

Fowler, D., Garety, P. A., and Kuipers, E. (1995) *Cognitive behaviour therapy for psychosis.* New York: John Wiley.

Fowler, D., Garety, P., and Kuipers, E. (1998) Understanding the inexplicable: A cognitive approach to delusions. In C. Perris and P. McGorry (eds) *A handbook of cognitive psychotherapy for psychosis.* Chichester: John Wiley.

Fowler, D., Freeman, D., Smith, B., Kuipers, E., Bebbington, P., Bashforth, H., et al. (2006) The Brief Core Schema Scales (BCSS): Psychometric properties and associations with paranoia and grandiosity in non-clinical and psychosis samples. *Psychological Medicine, 36,* 749–759.

Freeman, D., and Garety, P. A. (2003) Connecting neurosis and psychosis: The direct influence of emotion on delusions and hallucinations. *Behaviour Research and Therapy, 41,* 923–947.

Freeman, D., Garety, P. A., Fowler, D., Kuipers, E. K., Dunn, G., Bebbington, P., and Hadley, C. (1998) The London-East Anglia randomised controlled trial of cognitive-behaviour therapy for psychosis IV: Self-esteem and persecutory delusions. *British Journal of Clinical Psychology, 37,* 415–430.

Freeman, D., Garety, P. A., Kuipers, E., Fowler, D., and Bebbington, P. E. (2002) A cognitive model of persecutory delusions. *British Journal of Clinical Psychology, 41,* 331–347.

Freeman, D., Dunn, G., Garety, P. A., Bebbington, P., Slater, M., Kuipers, E., et al. (2005) The psychology of persecutory ideation 1: A questionnaire survey. *Journal of Nervous and Mental Disease, 193,* 302–308.

Garety, P., Kuipers, E., Fowler, D., Freeman, D., and Bebbington, P. (2001) A cognitive model of the positive symptoms of psychosis. *Psychological Medicine, 31,* 189–195.

Garety, P. A., Freeman, D., Jolley, S., Dunn, G., Bebbington, P. E., Fowler, D., et al. (2005) Reasoning, emotions and delusional conviction in psychosis. *Journal of Abnormal Psychology, 114,* 373–384.

Gilbert, P. (1992) *Depression: The evolution of powerlessness.* Hove: Erlbaum.

Gilbert, P., Birchwood, M., Gilbert, J., Trower, P., Hay, J., Murray, E., et al. (2001) An exploration of evolved mental mechanisms for dominant and subordinate behaviour in relation to auditory hallucinations in schizophrenia and critical thoughts in depression. *Psychological Medicine, 31,* 1117–1127.

Gracie, A., Fowler, D., Freeman, D., Garety, P. A., Kuipers, E., and Bebbington, P. E. (submitted) The pathway between traumatic experience, paranoia and hallucinations: A test of two routes in a non-clinical sample. Submitted to *Acta Psychiatrica Scandinavica.*

Hackmann, A., Clark, D. M., and McManus, F. (2000) Recurrent images and early memories in social phobia. *Behaviour Research and Therapy, 38*, 601–610.

Hamner, M. B., Frueh, B., Umer, H. G., and Arana, G. W. (1999) Psychotic features of illness severity in combat veterans with chronic post traumatic stress disorder. *Biological Psychiatry, 45*, 846–852.

Hardy, A., Fowler, D., Freeman, D., Smith, B., Steel, C., Evans, J., et al. (2005) Trauma and hallucinatory experience in psychosis. *Journal of Nervous and Mental Disease, 193*, 501–507.

Hemsley, D. R. (1994) A cognitive model for schizophrenia and its neural basis. *Acta Psychiatric Scandinavia, 90*, 80–86.

Holmes, E. A., and Steel, C. (2004) Schizotypy as a vulnerability factor for traumatic intrusions: An analogue investigation. *Journal of Nervous and Mental Disease, 192*, 28–34.

Holmes, E. A., Grey, N., and Young, K. A. D. (2005) Intrusive images and 'hotspots' of trauma memories in posttraumatic stress disorder: Emotions and cognitive themes. *Journal of Behavior Therapy and Experimental Psychiatry, 36*, 3–17.

Jaspers, K. (1913) Kausale und verstandliche zusammenhange zwischen schicksal and psychose bei der dementia praecox (schizophrenie). *Zeitschrift fur die Gesammelte Neurologie und Psychiatrie, 14*, 158–263.

Johns, L. C., and McGuire, P. K. (1999) Verbal self monitoring and auditory hallucinations in schizophrenia. *Lancet, 353*, 469–478.

Johns, L. C., Russel, J., Ahmed, F., Frith, C. D., Hemsley, D., Kuipers, E., and McGuire, P. K. (2001) Verbal self monitoring and auditory hallucinations in patients with schizophrenia. *Psychological Medicine, 31*, 705–715.

Kapur, S. (2003) Psychosis as a state of aberrant salience: A framework linking biology, phenomenology and pharmacology in schizophrenia. *American Journal of Psychiatry, 160*, 13–23.

Kingdon, D., and Turkington, D. (1994) *Cognitive behavioural therapy of schizophrenia*. New York: Guilford Press.

Kuyken, W., and Brewin, C. R. (1994) Intrusive memories of childhood abuse during depressive episodes. *BRAT, 32*, 525–528.

LeDoux, J. E., Iwata, J., Cicchetti, P., and Reis, D. J. (1988) Different projections of the central amygdaloid nucleus mediate autonomic and behavioural correlates of conditioned fear. *Journal of Neuroscience, 8*, 2517–2529.

Leudar, I., Thomas, P., McNally, D., and Glinski, A. (1997) What voices can do with words: Pragmatics of verbal hallucinations. *Psychological Medicine, 27*, 885–898.

Lindvall, M., Axelsson, R., and Oehman, R. (1993) Incidence of cycloid psychosis: A clinical study of first admission psychotic patients. *European Archives of Psychiatry and Clinical Neuroscience, 242*, 197–202.

McGorry, P. D., Chanen, A., McCarthy, E., van Riel, R., McKenzie, D., and Singh, B. (1991) Posttraumatic stress disorder following recent-onset psychosis: An unrecognized postpsychotic syndrome. *Journal of Nervous and Mental Disease, 179*, 253–258.

McGuire, P. K., Syed, G. M. S., and Murray, R. M. (1993) Increased blood flow in Brocas area during auditory hallucinations in schizophrenia. *Lancet, 342*, 703–706.

McGuire, P. K., Sibersweig, D. A., and Frith, C. D. (1996) Functional neuroanatomy of verbal self monitoring. *Brain, 119*, 907–917.

Maher, B. A. (1988) Anomalous experience and delusional thinking: The logic of explanations. In T. F. Oltmanns and B. A. Maher (eds) *Delusional beliefs* (pp. 15–33). New York: John Wiley.

Morrison, A. P. (2001) The interpretation of intrusions in psychosis: An integrative cognitive approach to psychotic symptoms. *Behaviour and Cognitive Psychotherapy, 29*, 257–276.

Morrison, A. P., and Peterson, T. (2003) Trauma, metacognition and predisposition to hallucinations in non-patients. *Behavioural and Cognitive Psychotherapy, 31*, 235–246.

Morrison, A. P., Beck, A. T., Glentworth, D., Dunn, H., Reid, G., Larkin, W., and Williams, S. (2002) Imagery and psychotic symptoms: A preliminary investigation. *Behaviour Research and Therapy, 40*, 1053–1062.

Mueser, K. T., Trumbetta, S. L., Rosenberg, S. D., Vivader, R., Goodman, L. B., Osher, F. C., et al. (1998) Trauma and post-traumatic stress disorder in severe mental illness. *Journal of Consulting and Clinical Psychology, 66*, 493–499.

Mueser, K. T., Rosenberg, S. D., Goodman, L. A., and Trumbetta, S. L. (2002) Trauma, PTSD, and the course of severe mental illness: An interactive model. *Schizophrenia Research, 53*, 123–143.

Mueser, K. T., Salyers, M. P., Rosenberg, S. D., Goodman, L. A., Essock, S. M., Osher, F. C., et al. (2004) Interpersonal trauma and posttraumatic stress in patients with severe mental illness: Demographic clinical and health correlates. *Schizophrenia Bulletin, 30*, 45–57.

Nayani, T. H. and David, A. S. (1996) The auditory hallucination: A phenomenological survey. *Psychological Medicine, 26*, 177–189.

Phillips, L., Velakoulis, D., Pantelis, C., Wood, S., Yuen, H. P., Yung, A., et al. (2002) Non-reduction in hippocampal volume is associated with higher risk of psychosis. *Schizophrenia Research, 58*, 145–158.

Read, J., Agar, K., Argyle, N., and Aderhold, V. (2003) Sexual and physical abuse during childhood and adulthood as predictors of hallucinations, delusions and thought disorder. *Psychology and Psychotherapy: Theory, Research and Practice, 76*, 1–22.

Reeves, A. (2000) Creative journeys of recovery: A survivor perspective. In M. Birchwood, D. Fowler, and C. Jackson (eds) *Early intervention in psychosis: A guide to concepts, evidence and interventions*. Chichester: John Wiley.

Smith, B., Fowler, D., Freeman, D., Bebbington, P. E., Bashforth, H., Garety, P. A., et al. (submitted) Emotion and psychosis: Direct links between schematic beliefs about self and others, emotion and delusions and hallucinations. *Schizophrenia Research* (under review).

Squire, L. (1992) Memory and the hippocampus: A synthesis from findings with rats, monkeys and humans. *Psychological Review, 99*, 195–231.

Steel, C., Fowler, D., and Holmes, E. (2005) Trauma related intrusions and psychosis: An information processing account. *Cognitive and Behavioural Psychotherapy, 33*, 139–152.

Teasdale, J., and Barnard, P. (1993) *Affect, cognition and change: Remodelling depressive thought*. Hillsdale, NJ: Erlbaum.

Trower, P., and Chadwick, P. D. J. (1995) Pathways to defense of the self: A theory of two types of paranoia. *Clinical Psychology: Science and Practice, 2*, 263–278.

Vaughan, S., and Fowler, D. G. (2004) The distress experienced by voice hearers is associated with the perceived relationship between voice hearer and the voice. *British Journal of Clinical Psychology, 43*, 143–153.

Watson, P. W., Garety, P. A., Weinman, J., Dunn, G., Bebbington, P. E., Fowler, D., et al. (2006) Emotional dysfunction in schizophrenia spectrum psychosis: The role of illness perceptions. *Psychological Medicine, 36*, 761–770.

Part II

Specific populations

Chapter 6

Trauma and first episode psychosis

Chris Jackson and Max Birchwood

Trauma and first episode psychosis: is there a link?

The onset of psychosis, for some, can be a devastating and harrowing event in the life of a young person and their family. For others it may emerge as a more positive experience, an opportunity to 'take stock', learn lessons and rebuild. In this chapter we will argue that there is no simple cause and effect relationship between psychosis and trauma. Instead we will put the case for a model, which puts at its heart the role of mediating variables: cognitive appraisals and coping style. We will also argue that the relationship between early trauma (sexual, physical, emotional abuse) and the first episode of psychosis is again not a simple one but one that is influenced by a complex array of interacting psychobiosocial factors including emotional dysfunction which arises as a result of disruption to a person's developmental trajectory (Birchwood 2003). Lastly we will argue that a new approach is needed to the assessment and treatment of trauma in people experiencing psychosis for the first time: one which questions current psychiatric conceptualisations of the link between psychosis, PTSD and co-morbidity and tests out newly developed and adapted psychological interventions for PTSD and trauma.

The trauma of first episode psychosis

Since 1994 and a revision of the DSM criteria for PTSD, an individual's subjective experience has become more important in how a traumatic event is defined than whether the event is unusual or unexpected, i.e. war or disaster (Joseph and Bailham 2003). As a consequence, since the early 1990s, there has been an upsurge in research into the traumatic nature of a number of relatively common but stressful life events including medical conditions and procedures such as childbirth (Bailham and Joseph 2003), cancer (Brewin et al. 1998) and head injury (Wright and Telford 1996). It is against this background of research into the traumatic nature of medical procedures, disorders and illnesses that, since the early 1990s, a number of studies have proposed that the diagnosis and experience of psychosis may also qualify as a traumatic event in its own right (McGorry et al. 1991; Morrison et al. 2003; Priebe et al. 1998; Seedat et al. 2004; Shaw et al. 1997; see also Chapter 3 in this book).

Yet despite an increased willingness for clinicians and researchers to recognise the subjective nature of traumatic events, and the availability of anecdotal (Lundy 1992) and empirical evidence (Shaw et al. 2002) which attests to the traumatic nature of psychosis, there still remains a number of unresolved issues with its diagnostic status as a PTSD triggering event (Jackson and Iqbal 2000; C. Jackson et al. 2004a).

In order to fulfil the DSM-IV criteria for a diagnosis of PTSD, an identifiable stressor which is potentially life threatening needs to be defined and the content of the symptoms should refer to the stressor (Breslau et al. 2002). PTSD type symptoms on their own (intrusive re-experiencing, avoidance, hyper-arousal etc.), without a connection to the stressor (criterion A in DSM-IV) would not qualify for a PTSD diagnosis (Green et al. 1985). (They may, however, be indicative of other comorbid emotional disorders such as depression or anxiety which can overlap with PTSD (Bleich et al. 1997).) According to DSM-IV (APA 1994), to qualify for a diagnosis of PTSD, the patient must have experienced an event defined by criterion A:

> The person has been exposed to a traumatic event in which both of the following are present: (1) the person experienced, witnessed, or was confronted with an event or events that involved actual or threatened death or serious injury, or a threat to the physical integrity of self or others; (2) the person's response involved intense fear, helplessness, or horror.
>
> (APA 1994: 427–428)

In criterion A, the emphasis is clearly placed upon threats to *physical* and not psychological integrity. Given that the candidate traumas associated with psychosis are related either to the content of the psychotic symptoms (Frame and Morrison 2001), the pathways to care (e.g. police involvement, use of Mental Health Act etc.; McGorry et al. 1991) or experience of treatment (Priebe et al. 1998), it is likely that the current operational definitions of PTSD will miss these potentially traumatic stressors entirely.

We still have relatively little information about whether non-life-threatening, 'objective' events such as police involvement or compulsory admission are actually related to the PTSD (traumatic) symptoms often observed in psychotic populations. There is some evidence that this link may be tenuous. Priebe et al. (1998) found no relationship between PTSD symptoms in 105 community-care patients suffering from multiple episode schizophrenia, and a history of involuntary admissions; nor did Frame and Morrison (2001). This would be important to establish, for, as pointed out above, it is difficult to make a case even for meeting the current criteria for PTSD diagnosis if there is no link between the PTSD type symptoms and the experience of 'objective' psychosis related events which are assumed to form part of the trauma.

Given the evidence reported by many studies of traumatic symptoms in psychosis, this calls into question whether the current operational definition of PTSD in DSM-IV and ICD-10 can be meaningfully applied to the experience of first episode psychosis. Adherence to the framework of DSM-IV and ICD-10 may mean we could be overlooking genuine traumatic symptoms and, accordingly, denying some patients with first episode psychosis therapies and interventions (usually psychological) which may be helpful and therapeutic. A large number of patients appraise their first episode of psychosis as extremely stressful (C. Jackson et al. 2004a). Chadwick and Birchwood (1994) and latterly Morrison (1998) have argued that many people with psychosis may initially make catastrophic misinterpretations of their psychotic symptoms. For instance, perceiving their voices as a threat to their life or physical and/or psychological well-being (see also Freeman and Garety 2003). It is imperative therefore, that in the future, research, assessment and treatment of PTSD in psychosis should move away from a simple 'traumatic event causes PTSD' model to one which takes account of cognitive mediation (C. Jackson et al. 2004a; Ehlers and Clark 2000).

McGorry et al. (1991) in the only published study to date of first episode psychosis noted that 35 per cent of a sample of young adults, eleven months after a first episode, were so traumatised by their experience of the symptoms of psychosis that they reported signs of trauma consistent with some of the diagnostic criteria for PTSD (see Chapter 3 in this book). The majority of the sample (65 per cent), however, were not sufficiently traumatised by their experiences. Such observations naturally lead to the question: why do some people become traumatised by their first episode of psychosis while others do not?

There is no doubt that patients' experience of the onset of psychosis varies greatly with regard to type of symptoms, management/treatment and pathways to care (Birchwood et al. 2000b; McGorry and Jackson 1999). Despite this, evidence to date suggests that variation in the objective experience of a first episode alone can not account for the aetiology of PTSD and trauma related symptoms. For example, we (C. Jackson et al. 2004a) found no relationship between involuntary admission and PTSD symptoms in a first episode cohort. Further variation is introduced since the same kind of symptom or diagnosis may be appraised differently by those experiencing them.

The role of cognitive appraisal and coping style in trauma and first episode psychosis

Psychotic symptoms (or the memory of the psychotic symptoms in the case of PTSD), as we have touched on already, may be appraised differently by different people. For instance, voice hearers may experience the same kind of voice in form and content but experience different emotions (fear, depression, anxiety, joy, anger) linked to how they perceive/appraise the hallucination (Chadwick and Birchwood 1994; Romme and Escher 1989). Birchwood et al. (2000c) have shown that those who view their voices as malevolent and omnipotent and feel subordinate in their relationship with their voices are more likely to become depressed and anxious and report that they feel 'down ranked' in other interpersonal relationships. In contrast people who appraise their voices as benevolent, less omnipotent and helpful reported no such interpersonal problems. Romme and Escher in a now well-documented body of work (Honig et al. 1998; Romme and Escher 1989) have expanded this theme to argue that people's decision to seek help from mental health services for their voices may be ultimately dictated by such an appraisal process.

Thus during a first episode of psychosis people will have experienced different symptoms for different amounts of time under different circumstances but most importantly they will have appraised those symptoms and their diagnostic interpretation in different ways. Indeed current models of PTSD place at their heart the role of psychological appraisals of traumatic events and coping mechanisms (Ehlers and Clark 2000; Joseph et al. 1997) as there are often large individual differences in response to the same traumas.

In relation to psychosis and the first episode of psychosis in particular, we have less knowledge about the mediating effects on traumatic symptoms of the appraisal of the diagnosis, individual symptoms and the nature of the treatment of psychosis and the events that surround it (e.g. the degree to which the patient appraised an admission to hospital as stressful and how s/he coped with it). In our study (C. Jackson et al. 2004a) we looked at this issue in a sample (N = 35) of early psychosis patients. People in the sample who had been admitted to a psychiatric hospital for the first time were asked about the degree to which they perceived the ward during their admission to be stressful as measured by the Experiences of Admission Questionnaire (McGorry et al. 1991). The usual objective traumas were documented including involuntary admission, police involvement etc.

Results from the study (see Table 6.1) showed that approximately one-third of patients experiencing a first episode of psychosis fulfilled DSM-IV criteria for a diagnosis of 'PTSD' where that diagnosis was made on the basis of DSM criteria B, C and D (intrusive re-experiencing, avoidance and increased arousal) but in the absence of criterion A (life-threatening trauma).

The study did not indicate, however, that these traumatic symptoms were linked to the presence of any pathway or treatment event including police involvement, involuntary detention and presence on a secure ward.

The levels of intrusive re-experiencing (12.7) and avoidance (15.0) on the IES were, however, comparable with non-psychotic traumatised clinical samples at a similar time point. For instance, Joseph et al. (1993) found intrusion and avoidance scores of 11.2 and 11.8 respectively for traumatised

Table 6.1 Impact of Events Scale (IES) and Hospital Anxiety and Depression Scale (HADS) for the PTSD groups

	Scale range	PTSD (N = 11) mean (SD)	Non-PTSD (N = 24) mean (SD)	P
IES				
Intrusion	0–35	21.4 (3.5)	8.7 (7.5)	<0.001
Avoidance	0–40	19.5 (8.8)	12.9 (9.9)	0.06
Total	0–75	40.9 (9.2)	21.6 (13.2)	<0.001
HADS				
Depression	0–21	7.4 (4.7)	6.8 (4.4)	NS
Anxiety	0–21	9.5 (5.4)	6.1 (3.4)	<0.05

Source: C. Jackson et al. 2004a

survivors of the *Jupiter* shipping disaster, nineteen months after the event. The degree of clinically significant anxiety (64 per cent) and depression (45 per cent) in the PTSD group also confirmed the extent of comorbid symptomatology often found in PTSD and first episode samples (Birchwood et al. 2000b; Bleich et al. 1997; Strawkoski et al. 1995).

This finding that there was no direct relationship between traumatic symptoms and candidate traumas, is consistent with other studies (McGorry et al. 1991; Priebe et al. 1998). Frame and Morrison (2001), for example, in their letter reported that 'experience in hospital' explained only 6 per cent of the variance in PTSD scores in their multiple episode sample.

These results, however, point to the role of psychological mediating factors as described by Ehlers and Clark's (2000) model of PTSD. Those who were admitted to hospital and retrospectively perceived their admission as particularly 'stressful', were significantly more likely to meet a diagnosis of 'PTSD' (without criterion A) and to report higher levels of intrusions. This is consistent with the idea that individual appraisals may be more important than more 'objective' events. Perceived stressfulness of their stay on the ward correlated specifically with intrusive memories about the first episode of psychosis (r = 0.61; p = 0.002) and although this finding should be treated with caution in view of the fact that appraisals were made approximately eighteen months after the first psychotic episode, this correlation remained significant even after controlling for time elapsed since first episode (r = 0.64; p = 0.001).

Further ongoing research, however, is needed to test the true relationship between appraisals of a first episode of psychosis and its traumatic impact through a study into peri-traumatic processing (i.e. appraisals during the first episode) and the longitudinal relationship between such appraisals and trauma symptoms (Holmes et al. 2004).

An individual's adaptation to 'traumatic events' will also bear upon the development of traumatic symptoms. A patient's recovery style (sealing over versus integration) may influence the traumatic impact of the first episode of psychosis (McGlashan 1987). People who 'seal over' adopt cognitive and behavioural strategies to help them avoid thinking about the diagnosis and experience of psychosis. 'Integrators', on the other hand, tend to acknowledge the significance of psychosis and remain curious about it. They make active attempts to cope by seeking out information, knowledge and support from others.

In our study, as can be seen from Table 6.2, the importance of psychological processes is further highlighted by the link identified between recovery style and severity of traumatic symptoms. The most marked difference between these two recovery styles was the avoidance of intrusions in 'sealers'. Sealers, by definition, avoid thinking about their first episode more than integrators, and appear therefore to use sealing strategies to 'ward off' painful memories and thoughts from that time. This lends support to McGlashan's original hypothesis that 'sealers' are often unable to access memories of their psychotic episode (McGlashan 1987). These findings are consistent with models of assimilation and trauma (Brewin et al. 1996; Horowitz 1986; Williams et al. 1999) which advocate that some people ward off unwanted thoughts and images because they anticipate the catastrophic consequences of recollection. Under some circumstances experiences may even become inaccessible to memory retrieval altogether (Stiles et al. 1990).

What is not so clear is what factors motivate such warding-off and inhibition of unwanted thoughts in the 'sealing over' group. We have argued elsewhere that sealers are a particularly vulnerable group psychologically (Drayton et al. 1998) and that the onset of psychosis and its implications for future aspirations and identity (Birchwood et al. 2000a), renders patients unable to deal with ('face up to') the diagnosis. In two studies (Hall et al. 2001; Tait et al. 2003) it has been found that 'sealers' have a low level of engagement with services suggesting, perhaps, that they may wish to avoid further trauma.

In the cognitive framework it is argued that the process of appraisal and

Table 6.2 Trauma and recovery style

	Sealing over N = 9 (26%)	Integrating N = 26 (74%)	t or χ^2
PTSD			
Diagnosis	22%	35%	$\chi^2 = 0.48$*
Total (IES)	29.0 (16.3)	27.2 (14.9)	t = 0.31
Intrusion (IES)	9.3 (8.3)	14.2 (8.6)	t = −1.76
Avoidance (IES)	20.7 (10.2)	13.1 (9.2)	t = 2.08
Anxiety (HADS)	6.2 (4)	7.5 (4.5)	t = −0.73
Depression (HADS)	6.7 (5)	7.1 (4.3)	t = −0.26

Source: C. Jackson et al. 2004b

the individual differences are influenced by the individual's attachment experience and developmental trajectory. Although further research into the reasons why people 'seal over' following an episode of psychosis is still needed, there is some evidence to support the hypothesis that sealers may be psychologically 'fragile' and feel overwhelmed when made to 'face up to' (integrate) the episode. Two studies seem to bear this out. Drayton et al. (1998) interviewed thirty-six people with a recent onset of psychosis. These authors argued that such fragility would be manifest in (a) negative self-evaluation and (b) ambivalent or negative early attachment experience leading to low self-confidence and self-definition. The sample according to McGlashan's (1987) original conceptualisation were then divided into a sealing over group, an integrating group and a mixed group (displaying evidence of both sealing over and integrating). The findings indicated that 'sealers' (compared to the other two groups) were more likely to view themselves in negative ways but not necessarily view others or think that others viewed them negatively. They also had a tendency to rate their parents as being less caring than the integration group.

Further evidence for the psychological fragility of 'sealers' is evident in another study by Tait et al. (2004). Dividing their sample of fifty young people with psychosis into 'sealing over', 'integration' and 'mixed' groups, Tait et al. (2004) found that compared with 'integrators', those who used a 'sealing-over' recovery style reported more negative early childhood experiences, more insecure adult attachment, more negative self-evaluative beliefs and an insecure identity (as measured by the Self and Other Scale: Dagnan et al. 2002).

Overall, therefore, it seems that 'sealers' are psychologically vulnerable individuals who might be motivated to 'seal over' following traumatic events. In line with this and findings from our study (C. Jackson et al. 2004a), it is feasible to suggest that 'sealers' may be consciously or unconsciously 'warding off' the perceived painful realities of having a psychotic episode (Williams et al. 1999).

To test this hypothesis Tait et al. (2003) using a longitudinal prospective design assessed their sample of fifty young multiple-episode patients (68 per cent of the sample had experienced psychosis for five years or less) on measures of recovery style, psychotic symptoms, insight and service engagement during an acute episode of psychosis and at three- and six-month follow-ups. Of the forty-two who completed the study 28 per cent were classified as 'sealing over' during their acute episode. By six months, however, this figure had more than doubled to 60 per cent suggesting that as people recovered after an acute episode of psychosis, and they became more aware of what has happened to them and what may be the long-term implications of their psychosis, they were more likely to develop a 'sealing-over' recovery style (see Figure 6.1).

In this study, recovery style proved to be a better predictor of engagement

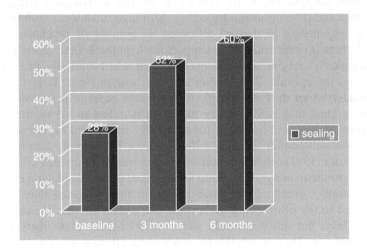

with services than either symptoms or insight. In fact Tait et al. (2003) argue, that when insight and symptoms improve, individuals may become overly aware of the impact and negative consequences of the psychosis which thus motivates sealing over.

They further postulate that patients who seal over may be those who have witnessed greater loss and shame in their psychosis and as a consequence are more motivated to enter into denial (Birchwood et al. 2000a).

This raises the possibility that the appraisal of psychosis and its secondary consequences (especially during the early phase or critical period: Birchwood et al. 1998) when coupled with pre-morbid psychological factors such as view of self and early care may give rise to a coping style which ultimately influences the course of the disorder (Harrison et al. 2001; Thompson et al. 2003). This points to the need to understand the traumatic nature of first episode psychosis and how people appraise and cope with it. Moreover, it also points to the need to develop interventions for the treatment and prevention of traumatic symptoms which take such factors into account (Jackson and Birchwood 1996). The therapeutic implications of this would be as follows:

- modification of the appraisals associated with a first episode
- focusing on the patient's developmental history and interpersonal functioning
- although sealing may be adaptive initially, it may not in the long term.

The following case study illustrates this potential therapeutic model.

Case study

J. was a 21-year-old African-Caribbean man who developed psychosis following a period of withdrawal, depression and anxiety. J. had had a difficult childhood. His father had died of a drugs overdose when he was 14, leaving J. and his younger brother to be brought up by their mother. J. found it difficult to talk about his father's death and generally coped with premorbid aversive life events and traumas by keeping quiet and avoiding any conversation about them. He was a naturally socially anxious and shy child and this eventually extended into early adulthood.

Following the emergence of his psychotic symptoms (including voices, thought broadcast and paranoia) and a period of non-adherence to medication, J. began to deteriorate and he was eventually admitted to a psychiatric hospital under the 1983 Mental Health Act. Here he was treated with anti-psychotic medication and after just less than four weeks was discharged. Overall, he found his first experience of psychosis and how it was managed to be very traumatic and stressful. However, he initially refused to discuss anything to do with his psychosis (including his admission) and after a few months, having made a good symptomatic recovery, he gradually became increasingly angry and upset about how he had been treated during his stay in hospital. He started to experience flashbacks and intrusive thoughts and images related to his admission. Although he initially refused to discuss these PTSD type symptoms with anybody in any detail, approximately a year later after building up rapport and trust with his CPN/case manager, he began to discuss his experiences. He questioned his perceived lack of control over the treatment process and his inability to assert himself within the mental health system.

Childhood trauma, the onset and course of psychosis: the role of emotional dysfunction

It is now well known that the reported prevalence of early trauma (childhood sexual abuse, emotional abuse, childhood neglect and physical abuse) in general adult psychiatric populations is high (Allen 2001; see also Chapter 2 this book). It is also evident that a large percentage of patients experiencing such childhood trauma will go on to develop psychosis (Jannsen et al. 2004; Read 1997) and co-occurring emotional dysfunction such as depression, anxiety and PTSD (Birchwood 2003; Roy 1982). That is, childhood trauma can be a risk factor for (a) psychosis (Janssen et al. 2004), (b) emotional dysfunction (Iqbal et al. 2004) and (c) PTSD in psychosis (Brewin et al. 2000).

Yet despite this, little is still known about the longitudinal relationship between childhood trauma, the onset of psychotic symptoms, its subsequent course and its relationship to other comorbid features of psychosis and schizophrenia such as post-psychotic depression, suicidality, PTSD, anxiety and problematic drug and alcohol use. Emotional dysfunction in psychosis has resurfaced as a problem in its own right. Early trauma and other psychosocial developmental anomalies in people who go on to develop psychosis may also act as a vulnerability factor for such difficulties as post psychotic depression and PTSD (Iqbal et al. 2004).

Most studies which explore the link between early trauma and psychosis tend to rely on correlational cross-sectional designs and sample inpatients with long histories of psychosis and schizophrenia (Read et al. 2003). This has a tendency to produce biased and distorted findings and may lead to an overestimate of the prevalence of childhood trauma among people with psychosis and an oversimplification of its aetiological role (Goodman et al. 1997). Older, more chronic samples by their nature tend to have a larger number of poor prognosis patients with greater levels of comorbidity including childhood abuse (Mueser et al. 1998). Very little research has studied the prevalence of early trauma in first episode samples. Neria et al. (2002), for example, found lower rates of childhood abuse than a similar study conducted by Friedman and Harrison (1984) in an older multiple episode sample. Similarly Varma et al. (1997) noted the prevalence of reported childhood trauma in a large-scale survey of patients experiencing their first admission for psychosis in the United States was lower than the prevalence for patients who had been ill for some time. However, both the Neria and Varma studies sampled people who had been admitted to hospital. This would exclude those with less severe first episodes which could be managed in the community, again overemphasising the relationship between childhood trauma and the onset of psychosis (Greenfield et al. 1994; Varma et al. 1997).

Yet despite these arguments that different sampling procedures and methodologies may have overestimated the link between childhood trauma and the development of psychosis in the current literature, the idea that early trauma may contribute to the onset of psychosis is hard to dismiss (Bentall 2003; Janssen et al. 2004). What is less clear is *how* it may influence the onset of psychosis and whether other factors (i.e. social deprivation, age at which it occurred, social and emotional support, type, frequency and duration, appraisal etc.) may mediate this relationship. Again it is quite clear from the literature that while not everyone who develops a psychotic illness will report a history of early trauma, not everyone who has been physically, sexually and/ or emotionally abused as children will go on to develop psychosis or a co-occuring emotional dysfunction. One way of explaining such an observation may be through a cognitive framework which posits that traumatic histories and developmental anomalies may influence the cognitive schemas that govern the processing of self and social information (Birchwood 2003). Developmental trauma may act as a risk factor for adult emotional disorder in general. For example, as has been documented in this book already, there is now a large body of evidence to suggest that childhood abuse and neglect may predispose people to low self-esteem, depression, PTSD, substance abuse and other psychological problems in adulthood (Allen 2001; Beitchman et al. 1992; Boney-McCoy and Finkelhor 1996). We know that first episode psychosis is often preceded by social difficulty and emotional disorder (as well as low level psychotic experience) which often begins in early adolescence (Poulton et al. 2000). People who have been traumatised in childhood may be more susceptible to the development of 'at risk mental states' (Yung et al. 1996) in the first place. Second, they may have a greater chance of making a transition to psychosis because they have not developed the appropriate coping strategies and/or elicited adequate emotional support to prevent them making such transition.

This raises the possibility that psychological intervention with people who are at risk of making a transition to psychosis which targets the appraisal of early trauma and the associated dysfunctional schema may help delay (or possibly prevent) the onset of psychosis (Morrison et al. 2004).

Once psychosis has developed, early traumatic experiences may make young first episode patients more resistant to treatment (Fowler 1999) and more vulnerable to relapse (Doering et al. 1998). They may also experience more comorbid problems such as drug and alcohol abuse (Patterson n.d.), PTSD (Neria et al. 2002), depression and suicidal thinking (Birchwood and Iqbal 1998) which in turn may also increase the risk of early relapse and suicide (Birchwood 2003).

Many of these issues are illustrated in the following case study.

Case study

L. was a 26-year-old Caucasian man who first experienced symptoms of psychosis just after his twenty-third birthday. Auditory hallucinations, paranoia and referential thinking began following a period of problematic drug and alcohol use, arguments with his family and homelessness. Bouts of depression, social anxiety, self-harm and suicide attempts were evident both *before* and *after* his first episode of psychosis but became a significant issue for him only after the psychotic symptoms had emerged. As a result L. initially experienced numerous admissions to hospital and home treatment following suicide attempts and relapse of his psychotic symptoms.

Following a psychological assessment it soon became apparent that L. had experienced a number of traumatic experiences both as a child and young adult. During his early teens, on a number of occasions, he witnessed his mother being severely hit and kicked by her boyfriend. On one occasion when L. was 11 years old he attempted to protect his mother by retaliating against the boyfriend, who was much taller and heavier than L. Unfortunately he too received a severe physical beating followed by a further two years of psychological and physical bullying. He decided to leave home when he was 16. Three years later after L. had been made homeless, he was raped by a man who had befriended him and offered him a place to stay.

As a result L. experienced a number of related intrusive thoughts and images. These often led to feelings of shame and guilt (Lee et al. 2001) as they were appraised as memories and images of events that he should have been able to control (i.e. he believed that he could have prevented the physical assaults on his mother and sexual assault on himself despite the fact they were carried out by men who were significantly stronger than he was). Such painful re-experiencing was often antecedent to his suicide attempts and psychotic symptoms. Although he used 'crack' cocaine and other illicit substances to control the intrusions, low mood and psychotic symptomatology his main coping strategy was to drink large amounts of alcohol (12–15 pints a night, five or six nights a week). To fund his drink and drug habit he often resorted to petty crime, including theft and burglary, for which he was usually caught and prosecuted. L. also became violent and aggressive after drinking, leading to fights between him and his brothers and as a result his relationship with his mother and family significantly worsened. He was often evicted from the family home and asked not to return (although he often did) leading to a significant number of changes of accommodation (usually emergency hostels which had to be arranged by his case manager over a short space of time).

Only through addressing these earlier traumatic events through psychological therapy, as part of an integrated early intervention approach, did L. start to break these unhelpful patterns of behaviour and symptoms. Upon discharge from the service his rate of admission and relapse had significantly reduced as had his problematic drink and drug use, criminal behaviour and need for emergency accommodation. He eventually moved in with his new girlfriend and started a training course at his local further education college.

This case study serves to illustrate how, for some people, early (and later) trauma can have an influence on the trajectory of psychotic and comorbid symptomatology. It also suggests that other variables and factors (cognitive appraisal, emotional support, familial relationships) may mediate the relationship between trauma, psychosis and emotional dysfunction, and that ultimately this will have implications for the nature of psychological interventions for trauma that will be part of an integrated treatment approach to early intervention.

The treatment of traumatic symptoms in first episode populations

As yet there are very few empirically evaluated interventions to help people overcome PTSD and trauma following an episode of psychosis (Morrison et al. 2003). This is especially true for those experiencing their first episode of psychosis although some interventions are currently being developed and evaluated.

Henry Jackson et al. (1998, 2000) evaluated a trial of cognitively orientated psychotherapy specifically designed for people recovering from early psychosis (COPE). This approach has four phases of which the final phase is aimed at the treatment of secondary morbidity (co-morbidity/emotional dysfunction). This includes psychological interventions to alleviate PTSD and trauma symptoms whether they have occurred prior to, during or after the initial episode of psychosis (H. Jackson et al. 2000). For example, H. Jackson et al. (2000) illustrate this aspect of their intervention with a case study of a 28-year-old man who developed psychotic symptoms following a PTSD reaction to two armed robberies on the bank where he was working. Both robberies, which had occurred six years prior to his first episode of psychosis, within a two-week period of each other, included a direct threat of violence towards the subject (a gun was held to his head on both occasions). In this instance cognitive therapy was aimed at the subject's experiences *prior* to the first episode, during and after the bank robberies. It was hypothesised that the psychotic episode had 'compounded and masked the PTSD symptoms'. Imaginal and in vivo exposure was successfully utilised in order to expose the patient to the physical, emotional and cognitive triggers which he had been avoiding for so long and which had ultimately inhibited his emotional processing of the event. Similar approaches were used with patients who had developed their trauma symptoms as a result of their psychosis.

Early outcome results from the COPE trial indicated that overall, when compared with two control conditions (a group offered but who refused COPE and a group never offered COPE), there was little advantage to those receiving the intervention in terms of depression, anxiety, relapse, psychotic symptoms or quality of life at post treatment (H. Jackson et al. 1998) or after one year follow-up (H. Jackson et al. 2001). There was, however, no direct measure of PTSD or trauma and so it is difficult to evaluate what specific impact the intervention had on traumatised individuals. On the sealing over/ integration measure there was some evidence to suggest that those receiving COPE did better (i.e. they integrated their experiences more) than those not receiving the intervention. This would suggest that the intervention may have encouraged emotional processing and discouraged avoidance (one of the symptoms of PTSD) although other explanations are also feasible (i.e. people have become more willing to discuss their psychotic symptoms during therapy). Direct measures of intrusive re-experiencing of the trauma, avoidance of the behavioural and emotional cues associated with the trauma and hyper-arousal would have provided more concrete proof of the efficacy of COPE to reduce PTSD and trauma-like symptoms.

Moreover, the efficacy of the COPE intervention was investigated using an open uncontrolled trial design. That is, not under randomised control trial

(RCT) conditions. Conducting an RCT would be important because every patient would have an equal chance of receiving the intervention or the control condition thus reducing bias (patients being unwittingly selected or selecting themselves for one group or the other) and threats to validity.

Taking a slightly different approach to the problems of PTSD and emotional dysfunction in first episode psychosis, we and our colleagues have proposed a treatment model based on our previous research (Birchwood et al. 2000a; Jackson and Iqbal 2000) and that of others (Ehlers and Clark 2000; Gilbert and Allan 1998). In this model (C. Jackson et al. 2004b) we have argued that emotional dysfunction and problems of psychological adaptation following a first episode of psychosis occur as a direct result of key appraisals people make about themselves, their psychosis and their world. For instance, those who believe that they have experienced loss, humiliation and entrapment as a result of their psychosis (symptoms, diagnosis, management) are more likely to feel 'down ranked' and left struggling to reaffirm an identity (Rooke and Birchwood 1998). This will lead to not only a lowering of self-esteem and higher rates of depression but also vulnerability to other types of emotional dysfunction involving threats to self (i.e. anxiety and PTSD). Such appraisals, of course, do not occur in isolation and here it is argued that they will be influenced by both pre and post first episode factors such as early trauma, culture, residual psychotic symptoms and the opportunity within the person's social environment to fulfil roles and goals. In view of this and in contrast to the COPE intervention, the psychological intervention will focus upon such key appraisals and their maintaining influences.

In a randomised control trial conducted by us and our colleagues (C. Jackson et al. 2004b), sixty-seven patients experiencing a first episode of psychosis in the previous eighteen months were randomly assigned to one of two conditions: (a) treatment as usual or (b) our cognitive therapy-based recovery intervention (CARF-Cognitive therapy to promote Adjustment and Recovery following a First episode of psychosis). The recovery intervention, which adopted a formulation-based modular approach to cognitive therapy, was designed to reduce the degree of co-morbidity and emotional dysfunction (post-psychotic depression, low self-esteem, trauma) by challenging people's appraisals of their first episode of psychosis (loss, humiliation, entrapment, the self as vulnerable, the world as unsafe etc.). Each module was designed to address different aspects of emotional dysfunction including trauma and PTSD.

Results revealed (C. Jackson et al. 2004b) that nearly 90 per cent of those who received the CARF intervention and who completed the follow-up assessments had significantly lower PTSD symptoms (intrusions and avoidance as measured by the Impact of Events Scale: IES) twelve months later compared to only 55 per cent of those in the treatment as usual condition (TAU). Moreover, only two people (11 per cent) became either worse (i.e. PTSD symptoms increased) or remained the same compared to those in the control condition (TAU) where 45 per cent of the sample experienced worsening trauma symptoms (or no change) over the course of the year (see Figure 6.2).

Although there was no evidence for concomitant changes in depression or self-esteem for those receiving the cognitive therapy intervention (CARF), the experimental group did report a significantly greater reduction in positive (p<0.01) and negative (p<0.01) psychotic symptoms (as rated on the PANSS) at six months although not at twelve months.

Other interventions for trauma, already developed and evaluated on non-psychotic populations, may also be efficacious for those who have experienced a first episode of psychosis. For example, writing about the episode and its related aspects in an emotional way may be a simple and cost-effective method of helping people to 'come to terms' or emotionally process what they have been through. Evidence already exists to suggest that expressive writing can have beneficial physical and psychological effects for a wide range of non-psychotic populations (Smyth 1998).

The brief written emotional expression task used in these studies is usually based on the original exercise developed by Pennebaker which asks experimental subjects to write an essay that expresses their feelings about a traumatic experience in their life (e.g. 'Write about your deepest thoughts and feelings about a trauma'). Control subjects, in contrast, are asked to write about an innocuous topic such as their plans for the day (Pennebaker and Beall 1986).

We have recently conducted a small (N = 22) randomised control trial to test whether such an intervention, with some modifications, can be applied to patients who have experienced a first episode of psychosis (Bernard and Jackson, in preparation). Expressive writing may be useful for some people who find talking about their psychosis and the consequences of it relatively daunting. Shame, fear and a sealing-over recovery style may ultimately inhibit emotional expression through more traditional verbal

	CARF N=19	TAU N=22
PTSD symptoms worse or same	11%	45%
PTSD symptoms better	89%	55%

Figure 6.2 Improvements in 'PTSD' symptoms for TAU and CARF at 12 months' follow-up (chi square = 6.01; p = 0.01; phi = 0.38; Jackson et al. 2004b)

channels (i.e. talking about their experiences to a mental health professional) and may eventually lead to poor engagement with services (Hall et al., submitted; Tait et al. 2003). Writing on their own over a short period of time may aid the process whereby emotional expression facilitates cognitive processing of the traumatic memory and leads to affective and physiological change (Pennebaker 1993).

Results from our study (Bernard and Jackson, in preparation) indicated that those randomised to the written emotional expression group were significantly (p<0.05) more likely to benefit in terms of reduced PTSD symptoms (as measured by the Revised Impact of Events Scale Total) two months later than those assigned to the control writing condition. Most of this change appears to have been attributable to the reduction in the avoidance of thoughts, images and reminders of their initial episode of psychosis (p<0.01) that the written emotional expression task brought about.

In addition, when giving feedback about the study some people with psychosis reported that they found such an approach preferable to talking-based interventions. Despite this, research into psychological interventions for trauma with first episode patients still remains in its infancy.

Conclusion

In this chapter we have argued that people experiencing a first episode of psychosis may be at particular risk of developing trauma symptoms and other emotional difficulties. However, this is not inevitable and is dictated to a large extent by how people appraise the events surrounding the first episode as traumatic. Second, we believe that the current conceptualisation of trauma (and its diagnosis) that follows a first episode of psychosis is too narrow and prohibitive and that it should be expanded to take into account more subjective experiences such as the appraisal of the threat of persecutors (e.g. voices and delusions) and other aspects of the experience which challenge the psychological integrity of the event (Allen 2001). Third, we have made the case for those experiencing a first episode (or those at risk of developing a first episode of psychosis) as having higher reported levels of childhood trauma than you would find or expect in the general population (Greenfield et al. 1994). The link between childhood trauma and the onset of psychosis, however, is complex and still poorly understood. For instance, the term childhood trauma is an 'umbrella' term given to a wide range of incident-specific events or chronic harmful interpersonal interactions which may have differential effects on the susceptibility to and/or the eventual development of psychotic symptomatology. Childhood neglect (lack of parental care and nurturance), for example, which surprisingly still remains a poorly researched topic (Rutter and Stroufe 2000) may have long-term risk consequences for the development of serious mental health problems over and above those caused by childhood physical and/or sexual abuse (Hildyard and Wolfe 2002). Discovering what impact which types of childhood trauma have, and in which contexts, may unveil important clues as to the psycho-bio-social vulnerabilities and risk factors involved in the development and onset of psychosis.

References

Allen, J. G. (2001) *Traumatic relationships and serious mental disorders*. Chichester: John Wiley.

American Psychiatric Association (1994) *Diagnostic and statistical manual of mental disorders* (4th edn). Washington, DC: APA.

Bailham, D., and Joseph, S. (2003) Post-traumatic stress following childbirth: A review of the emerging literature and directions for research and practice. *Psychology, Health and Medicine, 8*, 159–168.

Beitchman, J. H., Zucker, K. J., Hood, J. E., daCosta, G. A., Akman, D., and Cassavia, E. (1992) A review of the long term effects of child sexual abuse. *Child Abuse and Neglect, 16*, 101–118.

Bentall, R. (2003) *Madness explained*. London: Penguin.

Bernard, M. and Jackson, C. (in preparation) Written disclosure following first episode psychosis: Effects on symptoms of PTSD.

Birchwood, M. J. (2003) Pathways to emotional dysfunctioning in first-episode psychosis. *British Journal of Psychiatry, 182*, 373–375.

Birchwood, M., and Iqbal, Z. (1998) Depression and suicidal thinking in psychosis: A cognitive approach. In T. Wykes, N. Tarrier and S. Lewis (eds) *Outcome and innovation in psychological treatment of schizophrenia*. Chichester: John Wiley.

Birchwood, M., Todd, P., and Jackson, C. (1998) Early intervention in psychosis: The critical period hypthesis. *British Journal of Psychiatry, 172* (suppl. 33), 53–59.

Birchwood, M. J., Iqbal, Z., Chadwick, P., and Trower, P. (2000a) A cognitive approach to depression and suicidal thinking in psychosis. I: The ontogeny of post-psychotic depression. *British Journal of Psychiatry, 177*, 516–521.

Birchwood, M. J., Fowler, D., and Jackson, C. (2000b) *Early intervention in psychosis*. Chichester: John Wiley.

Birchwood, M. J., Meaden, A., Trower, P., Gilbert, P., Meaden, A., and Plaistow, J. (2000c) The power and omnipotence of voices: Subordination and entrapment by voices and significant others. *Psychological Medicine, 30*, 337–344.

Bleich, A., Koslowsky, M., Dolev, A., and Lerer, B. (1997) Post-traumatic stress disorder and depression: An analysis of co-morbidity. *British Journal of Psychiatry, 170*, 479–482.

Boney-McCoy, S., and Finkelhor, D. (1996) Is youth victimization related to trauma symptoms and depression after controlling for prior symptoms and family relationships? A longitudinal prospective study. *Journal of Consulting and Clinical Psychology, 64*, 1406–1416.

Breslau, N., Chase, G. A., and Anthony, J. C. (2002) The uniqueness of the DSM definition of post-traumatic stress disorder: Implications for research. *Psychological Medicine, 32*, 573–576.

Brewin, C. R., Dalgleish, T., and Joseph, S. (1996) A dual representation theory of post-traumatic stress disorder. *Psychological Review, 103*, 670–686.

Brewin, C., Watson, M., McCarthy, S., Hyman, P., and Dayson, D. (1998) Memory processes and the course of anxiety and depression in cancer patients. *Psychological Medicine, 28*, 219–224.

Brewin, C. R., Andrews, B., and Valentine, J. D. (2000) Meta-analysis of risk factors for post-traumatic stress disorder in trauma-exposed adults. *Journal of Consulting and Clinical Psychology, 68*, 748–766.

Chadwick, P., and Birchwood, M. J. (1994) The omnipotence of voices: A cognitive approach to auditory hallucinations. *British Journal of Psychiatry, 164*, 190–201.

Dagnan, D., Trower, P., and Gilbert, P. (2002) Measuring vulnerability to threats to self-construction: The self and other scale. *Psychology and Psychotherapy: Theory, Research and Practice, 75*, 279–293.

Doering, S., Muller, E., Kopcke, W., Pietzcker, A., Gaebel, W., Linden, M., et al. (1998) Predictors of relapse and rehospitalization in schizophrenia and schizoaffective disorder. *Schizophrenia Bulletin, 24*, 87–98.

Drayton, M., Birchwood, M., and Trower, P. (1998) Early attachment experience and recovery from psychosis. *British Journal of Clinical Psychology, 37*, 269–284.

Ehlers, A., and Clark, D. M. (2000) A cognitive model of post-traumatic stress disorder. *Behaviour Research Therapy, 38*, 319–345.

Fowler, D. (1999) The relationship between trauma and psychosis. Paper presented at the Merseyside Psychotherapy Institute, Liverpool, May.

Frame, L., and Morrison, A. P. (2001) Causes of PTSD in psychosis. *Archives of General Psychiatry, 58*, 305–306.

Freeman, D., and Garety, P. A. (2003) Connecting neurosis and psychosis: The direct influence of emotion on delusions and hallucinations. *Behaviour Research and Therapy, 41*, 923–947.

Friedman, S., and Harrison, G. (1984) Sexual histories, attitudes and behaviour of schizophrenic and 'normal' women. *Archives of Sexual Behaviour, 13*, 555–567.

Gilbert, P., and Allan, S. (1998) The role of defeat and entrapment (arrested flight) in depression: An exploration of an evolutionary view. *Psychological Medicine, 28*, 585–598.

Goodman, L. A., Rosenberg, S. D., Mueser, K. T., and Drake, R. E. (1997) Physical and sexual assault history in women with serious mental illness: Prevalence, correlates, treatment, and future research directions. *Schizophrenia Bulletin, 23*, 685–696.

Green, B. L., Lindy, J. D., and Grace, M. C. (1985) Posttraumatic stress disorder: Toward DSM-IV. *Journal of Nervous and Mental Disorders, 173*, 406–411.

Greenfield, S. F., Strawkowski, S. M., Tohen, M., Batson, F. C., and Kolbrener, M. L. (1994) Childhood abuse in first episode psychosis. *British Journal of Psychiatry, 164*, 831–834.

Hall, M., Smith, J., Meaden, A., and Jones, C. Engagement with assertive outreach services: The importance of early parental experiences, the therapeutic relationship and recovery style. Submitted for publication.

Harrison, G., Hopper, K., Craig, T., Laska, E., Siegel, C., Wanderling, J., et al. (2001) Recovery from psychotic illness: A 15 and 25 year international follow-up study. *British Journal of Psychiatry, 178*, 506–517.

Hildyard, K. L., and Wolfe, D. A. (2002) Child neglect: Developmental issues and outcomes. *Child Abuse and Neglect, 26*, 679–695.

Holmes, E. A., Brewin, C. R., and Hennessy, R. G. (2004) Trauma films, information processing and intrusive memory development. *Journal of Experimental Psychology Gen., 133*, 3–22.

Honig, A., Romme, M. A., Ensink, B. J., Escher, S. D., Pennings, M. H., and deVries, M. W. (1998) Auditory hallucinations: A comparison between patients and non-patients. *Journal of Nervous and Mental Disease, 186*, 646–651.

Horowitz, M. J. (1986) *Stress response syndromes* (2nd edn). Northvale, NJ: Jason Aronson.

Iqbal, Z., Birchwood, M., Hemsley, D., Jackson, C., and Morris, E. (2004) Auto-biographical memory and postpsychotic depression in first episode psychosis. *British Journal of Clinical Psychology, 43*, 97–104.

Jackson, C., and Birchwood, M. J. (1996) Early intervention in psychosis: Opportunities for secondary prevention. *British Journal of Clinical Psychology, 35*, 487–502.

Jackson, C., and Iqbal, Z. (2000) Psychological adjustment to early psychosis. In M. Birchwood, D. Fowler and C. Jackson (eds) *Early intervention in psychosis*. Chichester: John Wiley.

Jackson, C., Knott, C., Skeate, A., and Birchwood, M. J. (2004a) The trauma of first episode psychosis: The role of cognitive mediation. *Australian and New Zealand Journal of Psychiatry, 38*, 327–333.

Jackson, C., Smith, J., Birchwood, M., Trower, P., Reid, I., Townend, M., et al. (2004b) Preventing the traumatic sequelae of first episode psychosis: A randomised controlled trial. Paper presented to the Fourth International Conference on Early Psychosis, Vancouver, Canada, September.

Jackson, H., McGorry, P., Edwards, J., Hulbert, C., Henry, C., Francey, S., et al. (1998) Cognitively-oriented psychotherapy for early psychosis (COPE). *British Journal of Psychiatry, 172*, (suppl. 33), 93–100.

Jackson, H., Hulbert, C. A., and Henry, L. (2000) The treatment of secondary morbidity in first episode psychosis. In M. Birchwood, D. Fowler and C. Jackson (eds) *Early intervention in psychosis: A guide to concepts, evidence and interventions*. Chichester: John Wiley.

Jackson, H., McGorry, P., Henry, L., Edwards, J., Hulbert, C., Harrigan, S., et al. (2001) Cognitively oriented psychotherapy for early psychosis (COPE): A 1 year follow-up. *British Journal of Clinical Psychology, 40*, 57–70.

Jannsen, I., Krabbendam, L., Bak, M., Hanssen, M., Vollebergh, W., De Graaf, R., and Van Os, J. (2004) Childhood abuse as a risk factor for psychotic experiences. *Acta Psychiatrica Scandinavia, 109*, 38–45.

Joseph, S., and Bailham, D. (2003) Post-traumatic stress following childbirth: A review of the emerging literature and directions for research and practice. *Psychology, Health and Medicine, 8*, 159–168.

Joseph, S., Yule, W., and Williams, R. (1993) Crisis support in the aftermath of disaster: A longitudinal perspective. *British Journal of Clinical Psychology, 32*, 177–185.

Joseph, S., Williams, R., and Yule, W. (1997) *Understanding post-traumatic stress*. Chichester: John Wiley.

Lee, D. A., Scragg, P., and Turner, S. (2001) The role of shame and guilt in traumatic events: A clinical model of shame-based and guilt-based PTSD. *British Journal of Medical Psychology, 74*, 451–466.

Lundy, M. S. (1992) Psychosis-induced post traumatic stress disorder. *American Journal of Psychotherapy, 46*, 435–491.

McGlashan, T. H. (1987) Recovery style from mental illness and long-term outcome. *Journal of Nervous and Mental Disease, 175*, 681–685.

McGorry, P. D., and Jackson, H. J. (eds) (1999) *The recognition and management of early psychosis: A preventive approach.* New York: Cambridge University Press.

McGorry, P., Chanen, A., McCarthy, E., Van Riel, R., McKenzie, D., and Singh, B. (1991) Post-traumatic stress disorder following recent onset psychosis: An unrecognised post psychotic syndrome. *Journal of Nervous and Mental Disease, 179*, 253–258.

Morrison, A. P. (1998) A cognitive analysis of auditory hallucinations: Are voices to schizophrenia what bodily sensations are to panic? *Behavioural and Cognitive Psychotherapy, 26*, 289–302.

Morrison, A. P., Frame, L., and Larkin, W. (2003) Relationships between trauma and psychosis: A review and integration. *British Journal of Clinical Psychology, 42*, 331–352.

Morrison, A. P., French, P., Walford, L., Lewis, S. W., Kilcommons, A., Green, J., et al. (2004) Cognitive therapy for the prevention of psychosis in people at ultra-high risk: Randomised controlled trial. *British Journal of Psychiatry, 185*, 291–297.

Mueser, K. T., Goodman, L. B., Trumbetta, S. L., Rosenberg, S. D., Osher, C., Vidaver, R., et al. (1998) Trauma and posttraumatic stress disorder in severe mental illness. *Journal of Consulting and Clinical Psychology, 66*, 493–499.

Neria, Y., Bromet, E. J., Sievers, S., Lavelle, J., and Fochtmann, L. J. (2002) Trauma exposure and posttraumatic stress disorder in psychosis: Findings from a first-admission cohort. *Journal of Consulting and Clinical Psychology, 70*, 246–251.

Patterson, P. J. (n.d.) Sexual trauma and psychosis in the development of comorbid symptoms. Unpublished manuscript.

Pennebaker, J. W. (1993) Putting stress into words: Health, linguistic and therapeutic implications. *Behaviour Research and Therapy, 31*, 539–548.

Pennebaker, J. W., and Beall, S. K. (1986) Confronting a traumatic event: Toward an understanding of inhibition and disease. *Journal of Abnormal Psychology, 95*, 274–281.

Poulton, R., Caspi, A., Moffitt, T. E., Cannon, M., Murray, R., and Harrington, H. (2000) Children's self reported psychotic symptoms and adult schizophreniform disorder: A 15 year longitudinal study. *Archives of General Psychiatry, 57*, 1053–1058.

Priebe, S., Broker, M., and Gunkel, S. (1998) Involuntary admission and post-traumatic stress disorder symptoms in schizophrenia patients. *Comprehensive Psychiatry, 39*, 220–224.

Read, J. (1997) Child abuse and psychosis: A literature review and implications for professional practice. *Professional Psychology Research and Practice, 28*, 448–456.

Read, J., Agar, K., Argyle, N., and Aderhold, V. (2003) Sexual and physical abuse during childhood and adulthood as predictors of hallucinations, delusions and thought disorder. *Psychology and Psychotherapy: Theory, Research and Practice, 76*, 1–22.

Romme, M. A., and Escher, A. D. (1989) Hearing voices. *Schizophrenia Bulletin, 15*, 209–216.

Rooke, O., and Birchwood, M. (1998) Loss, humiliation and entrapment as appraisals of schizophrenic illness: A prospective study of depressed and non-depressed patients. *British Journal of Clinical Psychology, 37*, 259–268.

Roy, A. (1982) Risk factors for suicide in psychiatric patients. *Archives of General Psychiatry, 39*, 1089–1095.

Rutter, M., and Stroufe, L. A. (2002) Developmental psychopathology: Concepts and challenges. *Development and Psychopathology, 12*, 265–296.

Seedat, S., Stein, M. B., Oosthuizen, P. P., Emsley, R. A., and Stein, D. J. (2004) Linking posttraumatic stress disorder and psychosis: A look at epidemiology, phenomenology, and treatment. *Journal of Nervous and Mental Disease, 191*, 675–681.

Shaw, K., McFarlane, A., and Bookless, C. (1997) The phenomenology of traumatic reactions to psychotic illness. *Journal of Mental Disease, 185*, 434–441.

Shaw, K., McFarlane, A. C., Bookless, C., and Air, T. (2002) The aetiology of postpsychotic posttraumatic stress disorder following a psychotic episode. *Journal of Traumatic Stress, 15*, 39–47.

Smyth, J. M. (1998) Written emotional expression: Effect sizes, outcome types and moderating variables. *Journal of Consulting and Clinical Psychology, 66*, 174–184.

Stiles, W. B., Elliott, R., Llewelyn, S. P., Firth-Cozens, J. A., Margison, F. R., Shapiro, D. A., and Hardy, G. (1990) Assimilation of problematic experiences by clients in psychotherapy. *Psychotherapy, 27*, 411–420.

Strakowski, S. M., Keck, P. E., and McElroy, S. L. (1995) Chronology of comorbid and principle syndromes in first-episode psychosis. *Comprehensive Psychiatry, 36*, 106–112.

Tait, L., Birchwood, M., and Trower, P. (2003) Predicting engagement with services for psychosis: Insight, symptoms and recovery style. *British Journal of Psychiatry, 182*, 123–128.

Tait, L., Birchwood, M., and Trower, P. (2004) Adapting to the challenge of psychosis: Personal resilience and the use of sealing over (avoidant) coping strategies. *British Journal of Psychiatry, 185*, 410–415.

Thompson, K. N., McGorry, P. D., and Harrigan, S. M. (2003) Recovery style and outcome in first episode psychosis. *Schizophrenia Research, 62*, 31–36.

Varma, V. K., Wig, N. N., Phookun, H. R., Misra, A. K., Khare, C. B., Tripathi, B. M., et al. (1997) First-onset schizophrenia in the community: Relationship of urbanization with onset, early manifestations and typology. *Acta Psychiatrica Scandinavia, 96*, 431–438.

Weiss, D. S., and Marmar, C. R. (1997) The impact of events scale-revised. In J. P. Wilson and T. M. Keane (eds) *Assessing psychological trauma and PTSD* (pp. 399–411). New York: Guilford Press.

Williams, J. M. G., Stiles, W. B., and Shapiro, D. A. (1999) Cognitive mechanisms in the avoidance of painful and dangerous thoughts: Elaborating the assimilation model. *Cognitive Therapy and Research, 23*, 285–306.

Wright, J. C., and Telford, R. (1996) Psychological problems following minor head injury: A prospective study. *British Journal of Clinical Psychology, 35*, 399–412.

Yung, A. R., McGorry, P. D., McFarlane, C. A., Jackson, H. J., Patton, G. C., and Rakkar, A. (1996) Monitoring and care of young people at incipient risk of psychosis. *Schizophrenia Bulletin, 22*, 283–303.

Chapter 7

Childhood trauma and psychosis in the major depressive disorders

Paul Hammersley and Ruth Fox

Introduction

The bulk of the content of this book is taken up with analysis of the importance of trauma in the context of a diagnosis of 'schizophrenia'. This chapter is slightly different in that we turn our attention to the relationship between childhood trauma and psychotic symptom profile in the affective disorders, namely psychotic depression and bipolar disorder type-1.

The fact that childhood trauma, particularly sexual abuse, is a significant risk factor in the subsequent development of adult depression is viewed by many as no longer a subject of debate. There is not yet enough evidence to suggest that the relationship is causal; however, it is certainly robust (Beitchman et al. 1992; Mullen et al. 1993). One of the strongest findings was reported by Kendler et al. (2002), who found that in a group of 1942 female twins interviewed four times over a nine-year period, childhood sexual abuse was associated with depression even after controlling for parental loss and adverse family environment. In addition, Hill et al. (2000), in a questionnaire-based population study of 862 women, found childhood sexual abuse by a non-relative to be strongly associated with depression.

Despite these findings little is known of the relationship (if any) between childhood trauma and depressive disorders in which psychotic symptoms (hallucinations and delusions) are present. There are a number of reasons why such an analysis may be important. Of these the most important is suicide. The best efforts of health care providers on both sides of the Atlantic since the mid 1980s have done little to slow the incidence of suicide, particularly in young men. Increasing suicide rates are becoming something of an emergency. Childhood trauma is known to be associated with attempted suicide (Read et al. 2001), and there is also strong evidence that the presence of psychotic symptoms in depression significantly increases risk of suicide (Black et al. 1988; Vythilingam et al. 2003). As such an examination of the possible relationship between childhood traumas, psychotic symptoms in depression and the consequences of any such relationship in terms of suicidality may offer important insights in this crucial area.

The presence of psychotic symptoms in unipolar depression may negatively affect course of illness in other areas such as severity of symptoms, poorer prognosis, poor treatment response (Schatzburg 2003), or less time between episodes, and fewer weeks with minimal symptoms (Coryell et al. 1996). The presence of psychotic symptoms in bipolar disorder can have similar negative consequences and have been associated with earlier onset of illness (Rosen et al. 1983a), greater global severity (Rosen et al. 1983b) and both more admissions to hospital and less time between episodes. Keck et al. (2002) have questioned these findings: in their study of hallucinations in 353 patients with bipolar disorder, psychotic symptoms had no effect on prognosis or illness course. However, they state that this may be due to the high morbidity and poor functional outcome of a large percentage of their cohort.

A final reason for investigating childhood traumas and psychosis in depression is that increasing evidence links childhood trauma with psychotic symptoms. If similar patterns can be shown to exist in psychotic depression, it suggests the possibility of a cross-diagnostic phenomenon in which environmental influence (abuse) is a central feature.

Psychotic symptoms in bipolar affective disorder

Bipolar disorder is a major mental health problem that occurs in approximately 1–1.5 per cent of the population (Lam et al. 1999). It is characterised by extreme episodic swings of mood and once diagnosed is commonly viewed as a lifelong condition. There are a number of forms of bipolar disorder and any patient who experiences psychotic symptoms during episodes must be categorised as suffering from bipolar disorder type-1 according to DSM-IV.

Psychotic symptoms occur relatively frequently during the lifetime of patients suffering from bipolar disorder type-1. Goodwin and Jamison (1990) estimated that over 50 per cent of bipolar disorder patients reported experiencing at least one psychotic symptom during their illness. Keck et al. (2002) found the percentage to be even higher at 68 per cent with mood congruent delusions being reported most commonly followed by mood incongruent or bizarre delusions, hallucinations and symptoms of catatonia, disorganised behaviour or negative symptoms respectively. Hammersley et al. (2003) also found delusions to be the most commonly reported psychotic symptom in bipolar disorder patients but reported a higher lifetime prevalence of hallucinations: forty-five individuals reported experiencing hallucinations out of a sample of ninety-six representing almost half the participants.

Visual hallucinations are more common in bipolar disorder than in schizophrenia and are significantly associated with manic episodes. Other psychotic experiences may occur in bipolar disorder including Schneiderian first rank symptoms such as thought broadcast and ideas of reference that were thought in the past to be exclusive to schizophrenia. Delusions in bipolar disorder are usually mood congruent (Bentall 2003), themes of guilt or impending doom often occur in the depressed state while mania is more normally accompanied by grandiosity. The picture with hallucinations is less clear: some researchers have suggested that bipolar hallucinations more closely resemble hallucinations of organic origin rather than schizophrenic hallucinations in that they have heightened psychosensory experience at their core. Silberman et al. (1985) took this line of reasoning further and compared visual hallucinations in affective disorder patients with visual hallucinations in epileptic patients who experienced complex-partial seizures and found them to be 'remarkably similar'.

Lowe (1973) compared hallucinations in patients with schizophrenia, paranoid disorder, bipolar disorder and organic psychosis and reported bipolar hallucinations to be brief, less real, less frequent and less controllable than schizophrenic hallucinations, and also more common in women. In a little reported study from 1973, Lowe reported that bipolar hallucinations differed from hallucinations in schizophrenia in that 50 per cent of bipolar disorder patients hallucinated only when alone compared to only 6 per cent of schizophrenia patients. The evidence we do have to date about hallucinations in bipolar disorder is scant and contradictory. If it is possible to distinguish bipolar disorder hallucinations from hallucinations in other disorders then no one has yet come up with a reliable method of doing so.

Childhood trauma and symptom profile in bipolar disorder

Analysis of childhood trauma and psychosis in bipolar disorder is very new and there are few studies. Some studies in the past have looked at childhood adversity in groups of psychotic patients in general including bipolar disorder patients (e.g. Goodman et al. 1997), but very few have looked at bipolar disorder patients specifically.

Levitan et al. (1998) examined the relationship between childhood trauma and symptom profile in 653 individuals with major depression including bipolar disorder and found physical and sexual abuse in childhood to be associated with reversed neurovegetative symptoms (i.e., increased appetite, weight gain and hypersomnia). This association remained even when manic subjects were included in the analysis. Patients with a lifetime history of depression and mania had a significantly greater rate of childhood abuse than other depressed patients. The study also reported a strong association between physical abuse and mania, and noted that women were particularly affected by sexual abuse.

Hyun et al. (2000) investigated whether sexual abuse was more common in the histories of bipolar disorder patients compared with unipolar depressed patients in a sample of 333 cases. Results showed significantly higher rates of sexual abuse in the bipolar patients, with bipolar patients also showing a trend for higher rates of combined physical and sexual abuse. Male bipolar disorder patients were shown to be 29 times more likely to have experienced both sexual and physical abuse compared to the other groups.

Leverich et al. (2002) examined the association between childhood physical and sexual abuse in a group of 661 bipolar disorder patients and found the abused group to have an earlier illness onset, and higher levels of comorbid anxiety, eating disorders, substance and alcohol misuse, personality disorder (particularly cluster B) and PTSD. In addition the abused group displayed, faster cycling of episodes and once again a significantly higher risk of suicide, with the physically abused group being more at risk of suicide in mania and the sexually abused group being more at risk when depressed.

Holmes (1997) had previously reported a robust effect of childhood abuse along with parental psychopathology on frequency of occurrence of bipolar episodes positively associated with a more severe illness course and functional deterioration.

Childhood trauma and psychotic symptoms in bipolar disorder

Until recently only one study to date has looked directly at childhood traumas and specific psychotic symptoms in bipolar disorder. That study was our own and was completed as an adjunct to the Medical Research Council multi-site randomised control trial into cognitive-behavioural therapy for bipolar disorder (Hammersley et al. 2003). Ninety-six patients from the treatment arm of the trial, from four geographically distinct areas (Manchester, Liverpool, Cambridge and Glasgow) participated in the study. Any spontaneous self-reports of childhood traumas made by the participants during six months of therapy were carefully noted by the trial therapists and subsequently categorised using the Trauma History Questionnaire (Green 1996). Inter-rater reliability for this categorisation was almost perfect. Symptom data relating to hallucinations and delusions were collected by research assistants attached to the trial using the Structured Clinical Interview for DSM-IV (First et al. 1996). The research assistants were blind to the hypothesised association between trauma and psychotic symptoms. Associations between childhood traumas and adult psychotic symptoms were analysed. Our results showed no association between childhood trauma and delusions in bipolar disorder patients. However, there was a significant association between reports of childhood traumas and hallucinations. Further analysis showed that this association was almost entirely explained by one factor, a highly significant association between auditory hallucinations often of a critical nature and sexual abuse in childhood. Severity of sexual abuse was also an important factor (severity defined as occurring if the abuser was a blood relative, if there were multiple abusers, if the sexual abuse involved violence, if the abuse occurred before the victim's sixth birthday or if there were multiple incidents of abuse), only one of the severely abused participators did not report auditory hallucinations.

These observations are consistent with the observations made in research into childhood trauma and psychotic symptoms in schizophrenia. The link between childhood sexual abuse and auditory hallucinations is consistently the most reliable finding.

A single study of this nature can be interesting, but can often be dismissed as something of a curiosity without replication. However, a study by Fox and Reid (in preparation) reported similar findings. This study assessed childhood trauma histories in bipolar disorder and examined the relationship between different forms of abuse, including emotional abuse and neglect, and particular symptom profiles. The study had a sample size of seventy-one participants, forty-one of which were outpatients with a diagnosis of bipolar disorder recruited through Bolton, Salford and Trafford Mental Health Trust and through the Manic Depression Fellowship in the north-west of England. The remaining thirty participants were from a non-clinical population, recruited through local contacts. Individuals with substance misuse as a primary diagnosis or evidence of an organic illness were excluded from the study, as were individuals in an acute affective episode. To obtain information about current symptomatology and history (including psychotic symptoms), participants in the clinical sample were interviewed using the Comprehensive Assessment of Symptoms and History (CASH: Andreasen et al. 1992), which is a structured clinical interview designed for use in research studies of psychoses and affective disorders. Almost half of participants in the clinical sample had experienced lifetime symptoms of psychosis, while 30 per cent reported lifetime history of hallucinations. All participants completed the Childhood Trauma Questionnaire (CTQ), developed by Bernstein and Fink (1998), and the Parental Bonding Instrument (Parker et al. 1979). The CTQ is a retrospective self-report questionnaire that measures five types of childhood maltreatment – emotional, physical and sexual abuse and emotional and physical neglect. It has been validated with a number of clinical samples including adult psychiatric outpatients (Bernstein and Fink 1998) and it has also previously been used with bipolar clinical samples (Garno et al. 2005; Holowka et al. 2003). Although there has been some concern about the use of self-report measures in psychotic samples, studies have shown that reports of trauma history in patients with severe mental illness are generally reliable (Goodman et al. 1997). Furthermore, research has also shown that when reports are unreliable, they are mostly the result of underreporting of maltreatment rather than false positives (Fergusson et al. 2000). Participants' scores on the CTQ subscales were categorised according to severity, ranging from none, through to mild, moderate and severe. In order to reduce false-positive reports of abuse, the cut scores of 'moderate' and 'severe' (as opposed to 'mild') were used to detect cases of abuse. The study found that over 70 per cent of participants in the clinical sample reported a history of childhood trauma of some form, compared to 20 per cent of participants in the control group. Within (non-mutually exclusive) subcategories of moderate or severe abuse, 44 per cent of the clinical sample reported a history of emotional abuse, 32 per cent physical abuse, 22 per cent sexual abuse, 39 per cent emotional neglect and 37 per cent physical neglect. Of participants in the control group, 7 per cent reported a history of moderate or severe emotional abuse, 13 per cent physical abuse, 4 per cent sexual abuse, 13 per cent emotional neglect and 7 per cent physical neglect. Multiple forms of abuse occurred in approximately half the clinical sample compared to 13 per cent of participants in the control group. Participants in the clinical sample also described significantly more adverse parent–child interactions, characterised by low maternal and paternal care and high maternal and paternal protection/control than those in the control group. With regards to symptom profiles of bipolar disorder, the study found that a history of childhood sexual abuse, above any other form of abuse, was the only significant predictor of lifetime history of hallucinations and this remained significant even after controlling for potential effects of early parent–child interactions. However, sexual abuse was not predictive of lifetime history of delusions. This finding is consistent with that from the psychosis literature. For example, Read et al. (2003) found, in a sample of 200 community patients, that hallucinations but not delusions were significantly related to a history of childhood sexual abuse. Furthermore, the findings also support those from Hammersley et al.'s (2003) study and, taken together, suggest that childhood sexual abuse may impact upon the symptom profile of patients with bipolar disorder, increasing their vulnerability to experiencing hallucinations.

A further study currently in preparation warrants attention. Reid et al. (in preparation) conducted an analogue study which tested for a possible association between early trauma and vulnerability to affective symptoms of bipolar disorder in 108 non-clinical participants. The study examined possible relationships using the Childhood Trauma Questionnaire, the Hypomanic Personality Questionnaire (HPQ: Eckbald and Chapman 1986) and the Beck Depression Inventory (Beck et al. 1961). The study found significant associations between emotional abuse, physical abuse and neglect, and elevated HPQ scores. There was no association between childhood sexual abuse and hypomanic traits. This is consistent with previous findings showing sexual abuse to be associated with psychological distress in the depressed phase of bipolar disorder, leading the authors to conclude:

> When considered alongside the findings of Hammersley et al. (2003), and Fox et al. (2005 in prep), these results are consistent with the notion that there may be a specific relationship between CSA and the development of auditory hallucinatory experiences, and possibly a relationship between emotional abuse and affective symptoms rather than a global relationship between early trauma and psychological symptoms per se.
>
> (Reid et al., in preparation)

Childhood trauma and unipolar psychotic depression

The presence of psychotic symptoms in unipolar depression (major depression without episodes of mania) was once thought to be very rare. Some research has shown this not to be the case. Ohayon and Schatzberg (2002), following a five-year multinational study into mental illness and sleep disorders in 19,000 individuals, reported that after excluding subjects with substance abuse, bipolar disorder or non-affective psychosis, 19 per cent of patients with major depression had experienced psychotic symptoms at some point in their illness. Interestingly the study found that the presence of psychotic symptoms was not determined by the severity of the depression.

There is plentiful evidence that the presence of psychotic symptoms in depression worsens the course of the depression (Coryell 1996). Delusions are again the most prominent psychotic symptom reported with persecutory delusions being most common. Grandiosity unsurprisingly almost never occurs in psychotic depression. There appears to be little difference in the presentation of psychotic depression and the presentation of psychosis in the depressed phase of bipolar disorder. Benazzi (1999) compared patients from each of the two groups and found them to be essentially the same, prompting him along with other researchers to speculate that psychotic depression may in fact constitute a distinct clinical entity.

As in bipolar disorder hallucinations in unipolar psychotic depression are less common than delusions. An Australian study by Parker et al. (1991) found the prevalence to be 97 per cent and 20 per cent for delusions and hallucinations respectively. It is possible that this trend is subject to cultural variation. In a study of psychotic depression conducted in Thailand by Saipanish and Lotrakul (1999) hallucinations were far more common, occurring in 77 per cent of the sample compared with delusions in 49 per cent. This study also showed low levels of mood incongruent delusions and the almost complete absence of delusions of guilt in comparison with western subjects.

Analysis of the relationship between childhood trauma and psychotic symptoms in subsequent adult depression is sparse. However, the literature examining hallucinations or delusions in depressed adolescents with a history of childhood trauma is both illuminating and consistent.

Glenn et al. (1988) examined data from fifty-four consecutive admissions to the adolescent inpatient unit at Vancouver General Hospital. Of these individuals 33 per cent experienced major depressive disorder, 45 per cent of whom displayed psychotic symptoms. The authors reported a highly significant association between childhood sexual abuse and psychosis, adding 'a predominance of hallucinations over delusions'.

Mundy et al. (1990) interviewed ninety-six homeless adolescents in Los Angeles, again finding a history of childhood abuse to be significantly associated with psychotic symptoms. Specifically, they found that adolescents who had experienced extra-familial sexual abuse frequently reported auditory hallucinations. Interestingly this research group did not assess for paranoia as they realistically recognised that paranoid symptoms would be generally elevated in their subjects as a result of the stress of street life as opposed to biological vulnerability.

Quinlan et al. (1997) interviewed 150 adolescents with major depression from a total of 265 consecutive admissions to the adolescent psychiatry inpatient programme at a large American university medical centre. Major (psychotic) depression was found in 10 per cent of the participants. The researchers found psychotic features in depressed adolescents to be significantly associated with an increase in comorbid PTSD, noting that traumatic events may result in perceptual distortions in adolescents that may be expressed as psychosis, PTSD or both conditions.

The one study that has examined childhood trauma in psychotic depression in adults has revealed similar findings. Zimmerman and Mattia (1999) interviewed 500 psychiatric outpatients using the Structured Clinical Interview for DSM-IV. Almost half of the sample had non-bipolar major depressive disorder, 19 per cent of whom also had comorbid posttraumatic stress disorder. When the patients with psychotic depression were compared with the patients with non-psychotic depression, it was found that the psychotic group were four times more likely to be suffering from PTSD. When the events that caused the PTSD were examined, it transpired that the two most commonly reported events were sexual assault by a family member or someone known to the patient or sexual assault by someone unknown to the patient. These two groups totalled 62 per cent or almost two-thirds of the traumatised group. Finally, Zimmerman and Mattia (1999) conducted an explanatory analysis to determine differences between those with psychotic depression with PTSD and those with psychotic depression without PTSD. The differentiating factor was that individuals with psychotic depression and PTSD were significantly more likely to have experienced auditory hallucinations. Therefore once again a potential association between sexual abuse and auditory hallucinations is suggested this time in a clinical group entirely separate from schizophrenia or bipolar disorder patients.

A further point that can be made in connection with the observations of Zimmerman and Mattia (1999) is that patients with psychotic depression are consistently found to have much higher blood cortisol levels than controls (Belanoff et al. 2001). Such an observation has also been commonly reported in sexual abuse survivors; in fact Heim et al. (2001) reported that women with a history of childhood abuse had a tendency to hypersecrete corticotrophin-releasing factor (CRF) on re-exposure to stress under experimental conditions.

Obviously some caution must be exercised when making claims about a potential association between childhood trauma and psychotic symptoms in the major depressive disorders on the basis of such a small number of studies that have all been criticised for methodological shortcomings. Future researchers might be best advised to concentrate on the area where the evidence seems strongest. This is quite clearly the relationship between severe sexual abuse in childhood and auditory hallucinations of a critical nature in adulthood. As yet we have no complete theory to explain why this association appears with such frequency. Possible suggestions (mentioned elsewhere in this book) include the mediating effects of dissociation, posttraumatic stress disorder and comorbid substance misuse. With this in mind, we are currently conducting research with a larger number of hallucinating and non-hallucinating bipolar disorder patients along with non-psychiatric controls and will be measuring levels of dissociation and PTSD. Should our original observations be confirmed the next step will be to develop acceptable psychological treatments for the substantial subgroup of patients with major depressive disorders for whom sexual abuse was a past reality and auditory hallucinations a significant source of current distress.

Towards the future

Until very recently the possibility of a relationship between childhood trauma and symptom profile in psychotic mood disorders has been largely ignored. There is some evidence that this is changing. The highly influential Stanley Foundation Bipolar network in the United States reported in a study into outcome correlates for bipolar disorder patients in August 2004 that childhood abuse should be considered among other factors in determining prognosis and future treatment goals (Nolen et al. 2004).

More significantly Nemeroff and colleagues (2003: 14, 293) examined outcomes in 681 patients with major depression offered antidepressant medication (nefedazone), cognitive-behavioural analysis system of psychotherapy or a combination of the two and reported that in patients with a history of childhood trauma, psychotherapy was superior to medication. Furthermore combination of psychotherapy and medication was only marginally superior to psychotherapy alone, leading the authors to conclude 'Psychotherapy may be an essential element in the treatment of patients with chronic forms of major depression and a history of childhood trauma'.

Evidence is now suggesting that the case for offering individual psychotherapy to patients with a psychotic mood disorder and an abuse history may form an important part of any agreed treatment plan. This is a treatment option that has been denied to many for years.

An important concern in the future is to establish which psychotherapeutic approaches offer most promise in terms of the reduction of distress. Ross and O'Carroll (2004) reviewed outcome studies into cognitive-behavioural interventions for both short- and long-term effects of childhood sexual abuse based on reliving and confronting the experiences and reported significant benefits to both the abused and the non-abusing carers.

Cognitive-behavioural therapy is far from being the only option available.

In a comprehensive review of individual psychotherapy outcomes for adult survivors of childhood sexual abuse, Price et al. (2001) identified significant improvements derived from CBT, experiential therapy, psychodynamic/interpersonal therapy, psychoeducation and supportive therapy. The obvious conclusion to be drawn is that for those who wish to talk, 'talking helps', and that as professionals our previous reluctance to discuss trauma and abuse issues with patients experiencing a disorder of mood with psychotic symptoms has been

- discriminatory practice of the worst kind (denial of a treatment option open to others on the basis of an often questionable diagnosis)
- a complete disregard of current outcome research (Read et al. 2004)
- neglect of duty of care that can amount to professional cowardice.

The last point is stated strongly and deserves further explanation. Since the late 1990s, when lecturing or offering seminars or discussion groups to health professionals of all disciplines on the subject of childhood trauma and psychosis, the reason most commonly offered by professionals for reluctance or caution in discussing childhood trauma with psychotic patients is a lack of specialised training or experience. However, the same reluctant professionals seem quite happy to refer trauma survivors on to the dedicated band of volunteers (survivors' groups, ChildLine, Samaritans etc.) many of whom have far less training or experience. This makes no sense at all.

For a number of years we were also personally reluctant to discuss trauma issues with patients distressed by psychotic symptoms. During our training for example we were told that delusions are held with 100 per cent conviction, and then also told that discussing delusions with psychotic patients would reinforce or increase belief in the delusion.

How can you believe something 150 per cent? Even the maths doesn't add up.

Careful collaborative therapy aimed at addressing the consequences of childhood trauma with psychotic patients is often a liberating experience. Individuals with no understanding of their current overwhelming distress can start to make sense of it. PTSD models (Meuser et al. 2002), intrusive thought models (Morrison 2001) and discussion of dissociative responses (Allen 2001) can all be used to normalise and explain the critical auditory hallucinations that frequently follow severe childhood abuse. Delusional thinking can similarly be examined using the idea of delusion as a metaphor for real experience (Bannister 1985; Rhodes and Jakes 2004).

Conclusion

The significance of childhood traumas in psychotic mood disorder has only recently been recognised. As evidence grows, trauma can often be seen not just as significant, but central. This appears to apply most consistently to auditory hallucinations. We certainly need more research into psychosis in the major mood disorders, but first we need the courage to listen and respond fairly to this group of patients, who to date have been consistently marginalised, stigmatised and often retraumatised by a system that refuses to recognise the reality of their experience and prefers to medicalise it.

References

Allen, J. G. (2001) *Traumatic relationships and serious mental disorders*. Chichester: John Wiley.

Andreasen, N., Flaum, M., and Arndt, S. (1992) The comprehensive assessment of symptoms and history (CASH): An instrument for assessing diagnosis and psychopathology. *Archives of General Psychiatry, 49*, 615–623.

Bannister, D. (1985) The psychotic disguise. In W. Dryden (ed.) *Therapists' dilemmas*. London: Sage.

Beck, A. T., Ward, C. H., Mendleson, M., Mock, J., and Erbaugh, J. (1961) An inventory for measuring depression. *Archives of General Psychiatry, 41*, 53–63.

Beitchman, J. H., Zucker, K. J., Hood, J. E., Da Costa, G. A., Akman, D., and Cassavia, E. (1992) A review of the long term effects of child sexual abuse. *Child Abuse and Neglect, 16*, 101–118.

Belanoff, J. K., Kalehzan, M., Sund, B., Fleming Ficek, S. K., and Schatzberg, A. F. (2001) Cortisol activity and cognition changes in psychotic major depression. *American Journal of Psychiatry, 158*, 1612–1616.

Benazzi, F. (1999) Bipolar versus unipolar psychotic outpatient depression. *Journal of Affective Disorders, 55*, 63–66.

Bentall, R. P. (2003) *Madness explained*. London: Allen Lane, Penguin Press.

Bernstein, D., and Fink, L. (1998) *The Childhood Trauma Questionnaire: A retrospective self report*. San Antonio, TX: The Psychological Corporation and Harcourt Brace.

Black, D. W., Winokur, G., and Nasrallah, A. (1988) Effect of psychosis on suicide risk in 1,593 patients with unipolar and bipolar affective disorders. *American Journal of Psychiatry, 145*, 849–852.

Coryell, W., Leon., A., Winokur, G., Endicot, J., Keller, M., Akiskal, H., and Solomon, D. (1996) Importance of psychotic features to long term course in major depressive disorder. *American Journal of Psychiatry, 153*, 483–489.

Eckbald, M., and Chapman, L. (1986) Development and validation of a scale for hypomanic personality. *Journal of Abnormal Psychology, 95*, 214–222.

First, M. B., Spitzer, R. L., Gibbon, M., and Williams, J. B. W. (1996) *Structured Clinical Interview for DSM-IV (SCID)*. New York: Biometric T Research.

Fox, R. M., and Reid G. S. (in preparation) A study of the relationship between childhood trauma and symptom profiles in bipolar disorder.

Fergusson, D. M., Horowood, L. J., and Woodward, L. J. (2000) The stability of child abuse reports: A longitudinal study of the reporting behaviour of young adults. *Psychological Medicine, 30*, 379–385.

Garno, J. L., Goldberg, J. F., Ramirez, P. M., and Ritzler, B. A. (2005) Impact of childhood abuse on the clinical course of bipolar disorder. *British Journal of Psychiatry, 186*, 121–125.

Glenn, M. T., Haley, M. A., Fine, S., and Marriage, K. (1988) Psychotic features in adolescents with major depression. *Journal of the American Academy for Child and Adolescent Psychiatry, 27*, 489–493.

Goodman, L. A., Rossenberg, S. G., Meuser, K., and Drake, R. E. (1997) Physical and sexual assault history in women with serious mental illness: Prevalence, correlates, treatment and future research directions. *Schizophrenia Bulletin, 23*, 685–696.

Goodwin, D. W., Rosenberg, S. G., and Rosenthal, R. (1971) Clinical significance of hallucinations in psychiatric disorders: A study of 116 patients. *Archives of General Psychiatry, 24*, 76–80.

Goodwin, F. K., and Jamison, K. R. (1990) *Manic depressive illness*. New York: Oxford University Press.

Green, B. J. (1996) The Trauma History Questionnaire. In B. Hudnall Stamm (ed.) *Measurement of stress, trauma and adaptation*. Lutherville, MD: Sidran Press.

Hammersley, P. A., Dias, A., Todd, G., Bowen Jones, K., Reiley, B., and Bentall, R. P. (2003) Childhood trauma and hallucinations in bipolar affective disorder: A preliminary investigation. *British Journal of Psychiatry, 182*, 543–547.

Heim, C., Newport, J., Bonsall, R., Miller, A. H., and Nemeroff, C. B. (2001) Altered pituitary adrenal axis responses to provocative challenge tests in adult survivors of childhood abuse. *American Journal of Psychiatry, 158*, 575–581.

Hill, J., Davis, R., Byatt, M., Burnside, E., Rollinson, L., and Fear, S. (2000) Childhood sexual abuse and affective symptoms in women: A general population study. *Psychological Medicine, 30*, 1283–1291.

Holmes, C. A. (1997) The psychological correlates of the recurrence of bipolar disorder from the national co-morbidity survey. *Dissertations-Abstracts-International-Section-A-Humanities-and-Social-Sciences, 57* (11-A), 4496.

Holowka, D. W., King, S., Saheb, B., Pukall, M., and Brunet, A. (2003) Childhood abuse and dissociative symptoms in adult schizophrenia. *Schizophrenia Research, 60*, 87–90.

Hyun, M., Friedman, S. D., and Dunner, D. L. (2000) Relationship of childhood physical and sexual abuse to adult bipolar disorder. *Bipolar Disorders, 2*, 131–135.

Keck, P. E., McElroy, S. L., Rochussen Havens, J., Altshuler, L. L., Nolen, W. A., Frye, M. A., et al. (2002) Psychosis in bipolar disorder: Phenomenology and impact on morbidity and course of illness. *Comprehensive Psychiatry, 44*, 263–269.

Kendler, K. S., Gardner, G. O., and Prescot, C. (2002) Towards a comprehensive developmental model of major depression in women. *American Journal of Psychiatry, 159*, 133–145.

Lam, D. H., Jones, S. H., Haywood, P. and Bright, J. A. (1999) *Cognitive therapy for bipolar disorder: A therapist's guide to concepts, methods and practice*. Chichester: John Wiley.

Lam, D. H., Watkins, E. R., Edwards, R., Haywood, P., Bright, J., Wright, K., et al. (2003) A randomised control trial of cognitive therapy for relapse prevention in bipolar disorder: Outcome of the first year. *Archives of General Psychiatry, 60*, 145–152.

Leverich, G. S., McElroy, S. L., Suppes, T., Keck, P. E., Denicoff, K. D., Nolen, W., et al. (2002) Early physical and sexual abuse associated with an adverse course of bipolar disorder. *Biological Psychiatry, 51*, 288–297.

Levitan, R. D., Parikh, S. V., Lesage, A. D., Hegadoren, K. M., Adams, M., Kennedy, S. H., and Goering, P. N. (1998) Major depression in individuals with a history of childhood physical or sexual abuse: Relationship to neurovegetative features, mania and gender. *American Journal of Psychiatry, 155,* 1746–1752.

Lowe, G. (1973) The phenomenology of hallucinations as an aid to diagnosis. *British Journal of Psychiatry, 123,* 612–633.

Meuser, K. T., Rosenberg, S., Goodman, L. A., and Trumbetta, L. (2002) Trauma, PTSD and the course of serious mental illness: An interactive model. *Schizophrenia Research, 53,* 123–143.

Morrison, A. P. (2001) The interpretation of intrusions in psychosis: An integrative approach to hallucinations and delusions. *Behavioural and Cognitive Psychotherapy, 29,* 257–276.

Mullen, P. E., Martin, J. L., Anderson, J. C., Romans, S. E., and Herbison, G. P. (1993) Childhood sexual abuse and mental health in adult life. *British Journal of Psychiatry, 163,* 721–732.

Mundy, P., Robertson, M., Robertson, J., and Greenblatt, M. (1990) The prevalence of psychotic symptoms in homeless adolescents. *Journal of the American Academy of Child and Adolescent Psychiatry, 29,* 724–731.

Nemeroff, C. B., Heim, C. M., Thase, M. E., Klein, D. N., Rush, A. J., Schatzburg, A. F., et al. (2003) Differential responses to psychotherapy versus pharcomacotherapy in patients with chronic forms of major depression and childhood trauma. *Proceedings of the National Academy of Sciences of the United States of America, 100,* (suppl. 2), 14,293–14,296.

Nolen, W. A., Luckenbaugh, D. A., Altshuler, L. L., Suppes, T., McElroy, S. L., Frye, M. A., et al. (2004) Correlates of one-year prospective outcome in bipolar disorder: Results from the Stanley Foundation Bipolar Network. *American Journal of Psychiatry, 161,* 1447–1454.

Ohayon, M. M., and Schatzberg, A. F. (2002) Prevalence of depressive episodes with psychotic features in the general population. *American Journal of Psychiatry, 159,* 1855–1861.

Parker, G., Tupling, H., and Brown, L. B. (1979) A Parental Bonding Instrument. *British Journal of Medical Psychology, 52,* 1–10.

Parker, G., Hadzi-Pavlovic, D., Hickie, I., Boyce, P., Mitchell, P., Wilheim, K., and Brodarty, H. (1991) Distinguishing psychotic and non-psychotic melancholia. *Journal of Affective Disorders, 22,* 135–148.

Price, J. L., Hilsenroth, M. J., Petretic-Jackson, P. A., and Bonge, D. (2001) A review of psychotherapy outcomes for adult survivors of childhood sexual abuse. *Clinical Psychology Review, 21,* 1095–1121.

Quinlan, P. E., King, C. A., Hanna, G. L., and Ghaziuddin, N. (1997) Psychotic versus nonpsychotic depression in hospitalized adolescents. *Depression and Anxiety, 6,* 40–42.

Read, J., Agar, K., Berker-Collo, S., Davies, E., and Moskowitz, A. (2001) Assessing suicidality in adults: Integrating childhood trauma as a major risk factor. *Professional Psychology: Research and Practice, 32,* 367–372.

Read, J., Agar, K., Argyle, N., and Aderhold, V. (2003) Sexual and physical abuse during childhood as predictors of hallucinations and delusions. *Psychology and Psychotherapy: Theory, Research and Practice, 76,* 1–22.

Read, J., Mosher, L. R., and Bentall, R. P. (eds) (2004) *Models of madness*. Hove: Brunner Routledge.

Reid, G. S., Morrison, A. P., Greenhall, K., Hartwell, R., and Marshall, N. (in preparation) Relationships between early trauma, beliefs about depression and hypomanic personality in a non-clinical sample.

Rhodes, J. E., and Jakes, S. (2004) The contribution of metaphor and metonymy to delusions. *Psychology and Psychotherapy Research and Practice, 77*, 1–17.

Rosen, A. M., Rosenthal, N. E., Dunner, D. L., and Feve, R. R. (1983a) Social outcome compared in psychotic and non-psychotic bipolar 1 patients. *Journal of Nervous and Mental Disease, 171*, 272–275.

Rosen, A. M., Rosenthal, N. E., Dunner, D. L., and Feve, R. R. (1983b) Age at onset and number of psychotic symptoms in bipolar 1 and schizoaffective disorder. *American Journal of Psychiatry, 140*, 1523–1524.

Ross, G., and O'Carroll, P. (2004) Cognitive behavioural psychotherapy intervention in childhood sexual abuse: Identifying new directions from the literature. *Child Abuse Review, 13*, 51–64.

Saipanish, R., and Lotrakul, M. (1999) Cross-cultural aspects of psychotic symptoms in Thai major depression. *Journal of the Psychiatric Association of Thailand, 44*, 19–29.

Schatzburg, A. F. (2003) New approaches to managing psychotic depression. *Journal of Clinical Psychiatry, 64* (suppl 1), 19–23.

Silberman, E. K., Post, R. E., Nurnberger, J., Theodore, W., and Boulenger, J. P. (1985) Transient sensory, cognitive and affective phenomena in affective illness: A comparison with complex partial epilepsy. *British Journal of Psychiatry, 146*, 81–89.

Vythilingam, M., Chen, J., Douglas Bremner, J., Mazure, C. M., Maciejewski, P. K., and Nelson, J. C. (2003) Psychotic depression and mortality. *American Journal of Psychiatry, 160*, 574–576.

Zimmerman, M., and Mattia, J. (1999) Psychotic subtyping of major depressive disorder and post-traumatic stress disorder. *Journal of Clinical Psychiatry, 60*, 311–314.

Chapter 8

Trauma and hearing voices

Marius A. J. Romme and Sandra D. M. Escher

Since the mid 1980s, there has been a growing body of research showing that many people with psychosis have suffered from traumatic experiences. Mueser (1998) reported that in a population of psychotic patients, nearly everybody (98 per cent) had experienced trauma, while in the case history, only seldom (2 per cent) was this acknowledged and reported. It does seem that trauma does not get enough attention as an aetiological factor in the development of psychosis. This is also the case with people hearing voices. In psychiatry this experience is called 'auditory hallucinations' and is interpreted as a psychotic illness.

In this chapter we will show from our own research, and that of others, that hearing voices is not only apparent in psychotic patients, but also common in the general population, in people without formal psychiatric diagnosis. There are many people who can cope well with their voices and use them to their advantage. However, in both the patient and the non-patient group, voices are frequently related to traumatic experiences. It is not specifically the kind of trauma, but rather the consequences of the trauma that influence the outcome. We found that the non-patients could overcome them, while in the patient group, the trauma had detrimental consequences that were harder to manage. We found that this applied to children hearing voices as well as adults.

In this chapter we will describe:

1 The current tradition in the diagnosis and treatment of psychosis (highlighting some reasons why traumatic experiences are neglected)
2 Research exploring the relationship between trauma and hearing voices
3 The history of trauma
4 Pathways from trauma to psychosis
5 Psychological theories needed in understanding the process of people hearing voices and/or experiencing psychosis
6 Important elements in treatment.

The current tradition in the diagnosis and treatment of psychosis

There are a number of reasons why, in clinical psychiatry, traumatic experiences are not seen as influential in the development of psychosis. One of these reasons is the reductionist way trauma is defined within the diagnostic system. The *Diagnostic and Statistical Manual* (DSM-IV: APA 1994) defines trauma only in the context of posttraumatic stress disorder (PTSD). To qualify for this diagnosis one must have experienced an event defined by the following criteria:

> The person has been exposed to a traumatic event in which both of the following are present.
>
> 1 The person experienced, witnessed, or was confronted with an event or events that involved actual or threatened death, serious injury, or a threat to the physical integrity of self or others.
> 2 The person's response involved intense fear, helplessness or horror.
>
> (APA 1994: 427–428)

The greatest problem with this definition is that it requires a threat to the physical integrity of the individual. This exclusive focus on physical integrity is too narrow and might well have been the consequence of a political influence. If you look at this definition, it fits very well the experience of war, and that is also its origin. The PTSD concept in DSM-IV is strongly influenced by the Veterans' Administration, an association of war veterans in the United States. They wanted a clear diagnosis for their members and were not happy with the existing DSM psychosis categories. Contemporary research has indeed shown that so-called chronic PTSD has many diagnostic similarities to the diagnosis of schizophrenia. In chronic PTSD, negative symptoms are common, as are delusions and hallucinations (Hamner et al. 2000). The relationship between trauma arising from war and the existing psychosis categories in DSM-IV are politically very sensitive. It is very unpleasant, when as a result of traumatic war experiences, you come to suffer from something that is diagnosed as schizophrenia. Neither would it be politically attractive to identify schizophrenia as a traumatic reaction pattern. This would show the weaknesses in our society, but it could also harm the image of the profession as medical specialists, treating biological illnesses.

A second reason why the influence of trauma is neglected in the development of psychosis is the way the DSM system works. A diagnosis in the DSM is based on the observable behaviour and mental experience of the person, in which all elements are seen as a consequence, or symptoms of an illness. There is no differentiation into primary or secondary reactions. However, when one studies a person's reactions to traumatic experiences, there is indeed a differentiation. For example, if a person reacts to an overwhelming trauma by hearing voices, because of the inability to cope with this trauma, the voices might be seen as a primary reaction. When the signal function of the voices is not perceived, the voices might become the main problem. However, the inability to cope with the voices might result in a number of secondary reactions, for example concentration difficulties (because of the disturbing influence of the voices), delusions (as an attempt to explain this strange experience), inappropriate affect (laughing because the voices say something funny while they are involved in a serious discussion) and negative symptoms (they might isolate themselves or stay in bed to try to avoid performing the aggressive acts the voices command them to do). These secondary reactions can mimic a full picture of the schizophrenia spectrum (Bock 2000; Coleman 1999). As there is no differentiation in the DSM between primary and secondary reactions, all elements in behaviour and experience are seen as the direct consequence of the illness. In this way, the reaction pattern quality of such diagnosis is denied. As a consequence, the influence of trauma is often denied.

A third reason for neglecting the influence of trauma in the development of psychosis is that dissociative experiences are not measured by most diagnostic instruments. An example is the often-used Brief Psychiatric Rating Scale (BPRS: Lukoff et al. 1986; Overall and Gorham 1962) where these experiences are not taken into account. A second example is found in the DSM. Even though dissociative experiences are one of the most frequent reactions to trauma, they are not listed within the symptoms of psychotic diagnoses in the DSM. Research has shown that many schizophrenic patients also experience dissociative symptoms (Spitzer et al. 1997).

There is another problem. Although there are quite a number of people (42 per cent) with dissociative disorders who hear voices (Ensink 1992), this phenomenon is not listed within the DSM-IV category of dissociative disorders. Neither is dissociation listed within the symptoms of schizophrenia or other psychosis categories. These factors mystify the relationship between trauma, hearing voices and psychosis.

Researchers have been peculiarly faithful to the diagnostic categories within the DSM. This faithfulness we meet in research on trauma and psychosis, when they refer to the posttraumatic stress disorder category. They suggest that there could be a double disorder of schizophrenia and PTSD (Morrison et al. 2003a; Mueser et al. 1998), instead of suggesting the possibility that trauma may lead to a reaction pattern that is called schizophrenia in the DSM.

In studying the relationship between trauma and psychosis we should not become prisoners of the DSM diagnostic system, but openly evaluate the reaction pattern people show as a consequence of their experienced trauma. We should then also study all the experiences people report to us as consequences of their experienced trauma. Second, we should use a less narrow and more generally accepted definition of trauma, as we might find in encyclopaedia or dictionaries. For example, in the *Oxford English Dictionary*, trauma is defined as 'a psychic injury, caused by emotional shock, the memory of which may be either repressed and unresolved, or disturbingly persistent: a state or condition resulting from this'.

Research exploring the relationship between trauma and hearing voices

In psychiatry, a high percentage of voice hearers are placed within the diagnostic category of schizophrenia. It is, therefore, commonly identified with this diagnosis and not with trauma. Research that shows a relationship between trauma and schizophrenia could be seen as evidence of the relationship between trauma and psychosis. It is also a first indication of the possible relationship with hearing voices. We will present a selection of such studies also focusing on populations of patients diagnosed with schizophrenia. Table 8.1 gives such a selection.

In Table 8.1, there is a diminishing percentage of trauma in the listed order. This is the result of the kind of trauma included in the research. The first four studies used the DSM definition, while the fifth and sixth included only sexual abuse, and the seventh and eighth looked only at sexual abuse in

Table 8.1 Studies of trauma and psychosis

Author	N	Population	Frequency of trauma
Mueser et al. (1998)	275	Serious mental illness (+ schizophrenic + manic depressive)	98%
Drayer and Langeland (1999)	135	Psychiatric hospital patients	95%
Jacobson and Richardson (1987)	100	Psychiatric hospital (29% psychotic)	87%
Goodman et al. (1995)	99	Homeless women (59% schizophrenic)	97%
Muenzenmaier et al. (1993)	78	Outpatients women (57% schizophrenic)	74%
Davies-Netzley et al. (1996)	105	Homeless women (47% schizophrenic)	77%
Craine et al. (1988)	105	Inpatients state hospital (41% schizophrenic)	51%
Carmen et al. (1984)	122	Psychiatric hospital (18% psychotic)	53%
Romme and Escher (1996)	50	Voice hearers (36% schizophrenic)	77%

childhood. In our own research we looked for the frequency of trauma related to the onset of hearing voices. We did this in three different studies, two with adults and one with children hearing voices. In all three studies we found a relationship between the experienced trauma and the voice hearing. In the first study we did not use a psychiatric diagnostic instrument, in the second study we used the DSM diagnosis, assessed with the CIDI (Robins et al. 1988). In the children's study we used the BPRS (Lukoff et al. 1986; Overall and Gorham 1962). We will first report the adult studies, and describe the study focusing on children separately.

First study

The first study was an experiment (Romme and Escher 1989; Romme et al. 1992) in which our aim was to get in touch with voice hearers who could cope with their voices. All the patients we knew in our community mental health centre were not able to cope with them. We looked for help from the media. In a popular TV talk show, one of my (MR) patients told how much she was hindered and overpowered by her voices and that she felt unable to resist their demands. As a psychiatrist, I explained on the talk show that psychiatry did not have much to offer, and therefore, we asked people who heard voices and could cope with them, to call by telephone after the broadcast. We also invited them to the first congress for voice hearers. About 750 people responded and 540 said they heard voices. There were more responses than we could handle. We then sent out a questionnaire, with 30 questions in 10 sections, about all kinds of aspects derived from the spontaneous information given by telephone. We sent out 450 questionnaires and received back 178 suitable for analysis. One of the sections in the questionnaire was about the personal history of hearing voices and we asked about what had happened to them when the voices started. From the answers it became clear that about 70 per cent indicated a relationship between their voices and traumatic events they had experienced.

We also invited those individuals who clearly explained their experiences to become speakers at the congress (Romme and Escher 1989). To our astonishment, a number of those voice hearers could cope well with their voices and functioned well socially, but could not be given a diagnosis and did not need any help with their voices. At that time (1987) we were more impressed by the fact that we met people hearing voices without involvement with the psychiatric services, than the fact that 70 per cent told us about a relationship with a traumatic event. Like most people working in mental healthcare, we were convinced that hearing voices (auditory hallucinations) were a sign of psychopathology and most probably a symptom of a psychiatric disorder. Meeting many people with whom this was not the case motivated us to start reading more differentiated literature and this informed our next study.

Second study

In the second study (Romme 1996; see also Pennings et al. 1996; Honig et al. 1998) we compared people hearing voices who became psychiatric patients, and people who had not become psychiatric patients. We selected voice hearers from two diagnostic categories, one group diagnosed with schizophrenia and one group diagnosed with a dissociative disorder. The third group were the non-patient voice hearers we had met. We assessed them all with a psychiatric diagnostic instrument (CIDI).

In this second study we were interested in the differences and similarities in the characteristics of the voice-hearing experience between patients and non-patients. Psychiatry has for a long time tried to differentiate real and pseudo-hallucinations. Real hallucinations were seen as a symptom of schizophrenia. They were characterised by being experienced as 'not-me', heard from outside their head (by the ears), speaking to them in the third person, giving comments on their thoughts and behaviour and the person would not be able to talk to the voices (Schneider 1959). From our second study, it became evident that the nature of the experience did not significantly differ between the two patient groups as well as between the patients and the non-patients group. In the three groups all individuals experienced their voices as 'not-me'. In all three groups there were people hearing their voices as coming from outside themselves, as well as hearing voices inside their head. All three groups could have a dialogue with them, were spoken to in the second and in the third person, and heard commenting voices. The only difference was that in the patient group diagnosed with schizophrenia, voices speaking to them in the third person were more frequent (see Table 8.2).

An important difference between the patients and the non-patients

Table 8.2 Characteristics of voices in the three groups

Characteristics of voices*	Schizophrenia (N = 18)	Dissociative (N = 15)	Non-patients (N = 15)
By the ears	13 (72%)	9 (60%)	7 (50%)
In the head	9 (50%)	11 (73%)	10 (67%)
Voices are me	2 (11%)	1 (7%)	3 (20%)
Voices are not me	18 (100%)	14 (93%)	14 (93%)
Can talk with voices	12 (67%)	5 (33%)	10 (67%)
Cannot talk with voices	6 (33%)	10 (67%)	5 (33%)
Spoken to in second person	17 (94%)	14 (93%)	15 (100%)
Spoken to in third person	7 (39%)	3 (23%)	4 (27%)
Commenting voices	13 (72%)	12 (80%)	7 (47%)

* The characteristics can be different for each voice.

concerned the attributions and the influence of the voices on the voice hearer. This is also accentuated by Chadwick and Birchwood (1994). All groups heard positive as well as negative voices. However, the patient groups experienced the voices as predominantly negative, while the overall experience of the non-patient group was predominantly positive. The most important difference was that nearly all the patients were afraid of their voices, while no one in the non-patient group was afraid of them. This possibly explains why cognitive therapy has a positive effect. It has an anxiety reducing result (Bentall et al. 1994). The anxiety might be one of the main reasons why people are hindered by the voices in daily life. From this study it shows that the patient groups were more hindered by their voices.

Personal history

We interviewed all respondents with an interview developed from the questionnaire we used in the first study. One of the ten sections of this interview is about the person's personal history. To explore the personal history we focus on the onset of voice hearing, starting with the question 'How old were you when you first heard voices?' To stimulate them to focus on that time we would say: 'Let us return to the time you first heard voices. Where did you live? What did you do? Did anything happen to you at that time?' In this section we have added life events, a list of twenty-five stressful situations categorised into four categories: 'stressful changes'; 'confrontations with illness and death'; 'troubles with love and sexuality'; 'religion, spirituality, mystic or cosmic experiences'. We first ask if this has happened to them independently of the voices in order to differentiate what is related to the voices and what is not related. We do this because everybody, not just voice hearers, has experienced stressful situations. We then ask if these experiences had anything to do with the onset or change in their voices.

The results showed that 70 per cent of voice hearers related their voices to traumatic events (77 per cent in the schizophrenia patients, 100 per cent in the dissociative disorder patients and 53 per cent in the non-patients). This last group showed more people hearing voices from childhood onwards, which might have influenced their memory about the events that triggered their voices (see Table 8.3). As far as the history of lifetime abuse is concerned, some differentiations are reported in Table 8.3.

It looks as if there are some discrepancies between the information about the frequency of trauma at the onset of the voices and the information about the experienced neglect or abuse. We have to keep in mind that abuse and neglect were not always the trigger at onset, and that other trauma may have triggered the voices. We also have to acknowledge that there are other kinds of trauma that might be of importance in the relationship with the voice-hearing experience.

Table 8.3 Comparison of three groups of voice hearers relating to trauma

	Schizophrenia (N = 18)	Dissociative (N = 15)	Non-patients (N = 15)
Emotional neglect	12 (67%)	13 (87%)	10 (67%)
Physical abuse	11 (61%)	10 (67%)	7 (47%)
Sexual abuse	3 (17%)	8 (57%)	5 (33%)
No abuse	3 (17%)	2 (14%)	4 (27%)

The history of trauma

In our studies patients as well as non-patients experienced trauma in relation to the onset of the voices. Similarities between the patients and the non-patients are the traumatic events that evoked the onset of the voices. They are perceived as threatening because the event is

- physically threatening to themselves, as in severe illness with the threat of dying
- socially threatening because it threatens the continuity of one's expectations of the future, in the case of losing one's job, a divorce or the death of a loved one
- emotionally threatening, because of an overwhelming emotional confrontation, like that of the death of a father by whom the person was abused, or the confrontation of a confused sexual identity in case of sexual abuse.

However, there are differences as well. The differences between patients and the non-patients are as follows:

- The difference in the consequences the traumatic event has on one's life, for instance, one can be cured of a life-threatening illness, but still remain seriously handicapped.
- The difference in the number of traumata. We explored this with children and saw that the cumulative trauma score was higher in patients than in non-patients. This was also highlighted by Ensink (1992) in her research about the consequences of sexual abuse in childhood.
- The differences in defensibility and identity formation build-up during upbringing, before the voice-triggering trauma happened. In the second study this difference between patients and non-patients seemed to be important in overcoming trauma. One might say the difference in vulnerability originates from the life history. This is understandable from the research of Bowlby (1951) where he states that feeling unsafe and

experiencing broken relationships in childhood are harmful for the capacity to cope with stress later in life.

- There seem to be differences in coping with traumatic events between patients and non-patients. We saw that non-patients do not deny the traumatic events and have been able to resolve them, or have changed their lives in such a way that the consequences did not harm them any longer. Patient voice hearers more often deny the events or the problems resulting from them. They often stick to a victim role, not being able to put the events in the past and take up their lives again. Neither are they supported with solving their problems, because the trauma is often denied by others. They are seen as a patient with an illness, instead of the victim of a trauma inflicted by others. The aggressor might even blackmail the voice hearer, threaten him or her with punishment or put all the guilt with the victim, like the priest who raped an 11-year-old boy and accused the boy of seducing him.

Further research

In a fourth study we have started to explore the trauma histories of patients who had recovered from their psychotic experiences. We found a number of similarities:

- The patients' traumatisation concerned a number of traumatic events or a long period.
- There is a second generation problem. For example, a woman told us that her grandfather lost a leg in the Second World War. He thereafter changed his character completely and started to beat up members of the family, including his son, who later became the father of the woman who told us the story. She was physically abused by her father over a longer period of time. She also told us that since she knew the history of her father and grandfather, she is better able to forgive her father's aggression towards her and her mother.
- Unsafe social situation in youth in which the trauma was often inflicted by a very aggressive male (father, uncle, brother, priest or boyfriend). This was not compensated by a supportive party (mother, friend or family member). They were isolated and powerless with their problem.
- Toxic factors. In the trauma history we saw a number of elements that complicated working through the trauma. One of these factors is the early age of the traumatic experience. Ensink (1992) finds in her study that the age of 7 is a turning point in people's coping possibilities. Another factor is the threat and aggression connected with the trauma and the blackmail associated with the trauma.
- In the children's study we found four factors that predicted the continuation of the voice-hearing experience: a high score on depression and

anxiety on the BPRS as well as a high score of dissociation on the DES, and a high frequency of the voices. These factors seem to make it more difficult to cope with the experience as well as with the underlying traumatic events.

Pathways from trauma to psychosis

From the trauma history it becomes understandable that in certain conditions traumatic experiences may lead to a psychosis for which the person feels a need for care. We have met quite a number of people with different psychoses who told us about the same traumatic events that ultimately led to the onset psychosis; we have also met people with similar psychotic reactions as a result of very different traumatic experiences. Therefore it is clear that there is no simple connection between cause and effect in the relationship between trauma and psychosis. From our comparison of voice hearers who became patients suffering from psychosis and those who heard voices but did not become patients, we had learned that the vulnerability to developing psychosis was related to the influences of the trauma on their ability to cope with problems and stress (Pennings et al. 1996; Romme 1996). We saw that in patients, this coping ability was much more harmed than in non-patients. This depended on the kind of trauma and the support experienced. This is in line with the stress-vulnerability model for psychosis (Zubin and Spring 1977). Vulnerability does not have to be biological, but can also originate from traumatic experiences. Our comparative study made us curious to explore the different pathways that were taken by different individuals, who suffered from psychosis. We therefore invited a few people who had suffered psychotic episodes and also had suffered from serious trauma, to describe their pathway from trauma to psychosis. They had more or less completely recovered and were able to look back at their experiences and were willing to do so.

From these descriptions we would like to present six pathways and these are partly also described in literature. The basic principle with psychosis is the impossibility for the person to accept the reality of the trauma and the involved emotions. Individuals differ in the kind of solutions they attempt. The kind of solution influences the person's development. Denial (see pathway 6) blocks the development more intensely than an active fantasy (delusion, see pathway 4).

1 The dissociative pathway

One of the dissociative pathways is to create a substitute. Another is the realisation of partial splits. For example, during the trauma of sexual abuse, the person is emotionally and psychically setting her/himself apart, and looks from a distance at what is going on. Alternatively, another person might take his/her place. This other person might become a voice that reminds the voice hearer what has happened. In this way, emotions are kept at bay or literally at a distance. This is often combined with an effort to deny what has happened. Mostly this dissociation is a survival strategy. Psychosis develops when the dissociation fails and the memory becomes intrusive with anxiety-provoking images. A psychosis, for example, might develop when there is an emotional reliving of the trauma following a reminder like the death of the perpetrator; the loss of protective life circumstances; anxiety-provoking circumstances; conditions that lower the self-esteem; stress or emotions that diminish the defence function of dissociation. This process of dissociation is very well described by Judith L. Herman (1992). Many others have studied dissociation, but few describe the relationship with psychotic disintegration.

2 Turning the suffered powerlessness and aggression towards oneself

Although this pathway is described in psychodynamic and psychoanalytic literature, it can be experienced differently by patients. For example, an aggressive father, who had great difficulty managing his firm, acted out his distress on his son, who had to work in the business from the age of 6. The father beat his son often. Over the years the son became deaf, quite possibly from being beaten up. When he was 15 years old, the son hit back at his father. The father reacted extremely badly to this event, walked away and threatened to kill himself. This provoked the family to react in a way that made the son feel guilty for his father's state of mind. This did not change when the father returned a few hours later unharmed. From that moment on, the son told us that he did not feel any anger any more. He was convinced that he himself was the source of the problem, and not the abusing father. His first mental health problems began when he left home and started living on his own. He was not used to making any kind of decisions and in this new situation he lacked sufficient emotional orientation. This situation led to psychotic episodes and delusions of guilt. He let voices make his decisions and had delusions centred around being worthless. One could say that he lacked a self-identity.

Physical abuse and intense verbal aggression over longer periods, we observed, can often result in an abolition of emotions of aggression. People don't feel those emotions any more or mix them up with other emotions. When this is combined with a negative self-image and guilt feelings, psychosis develops when the defence is attacked by circumstances such as in the first example. Aggression turns into negative hallucinations or delusions combined with anxiety-provoking intrusive images, and then guilt, which can result in suicidal ideation.

3 The abolition of all emotions or becoming like a robot

We observed this reaction a few times in individuals after being rejected in love, after suicide of a loved one, or confrontation of unresolved issues of sexual identity. Psychotic reactions can be postponed as long as there are compensatory possibilities in work or sport activities that take all the person's energy and promote the self-esteem. When the compensation fails, the lost lover might start speaking as a voice, or a compensatory delusion (e.g. a Christ delusion) might develop. When the person is not able to interpret the experience as a signal of an existing emotional problem, coping with these experiences is more difficult. Secondary reactions can mimic a full picture of schizophrenia, as we described earlier.

4 A flight reaction from the existing problems into a fantasy solution

When reality is too difficult to accept, people can try to prevent what is happening by doing their utmost best in all kinds of activities. Because what is going to happen does not so much depend on their own decisions (in the case of divorce, a friend dying from cancer, a critical attitude of someone else and so on), these activities are doomed to fail. When this occurs, or just before or after, the mind snaps and finds a mental way out in a delusional solution. This, combined with exhaustion because of all the activities done for the prevention of what was feared, can result in a manic reaction pattern. As an example, one woman's marital relationship was near divorce at the time her mother died. She also had difficulties at work because she worked at the same office as her husband. When it became clear that divorce could not be prevented, she heard the voice of her mother telling her that she should take an airplane to Iswahan, because she would find a new husband there. Another example is of a woman whose best friend had cancer and was near to death. This was problematic because she could not accept the loss of this friend, who had helped her so much in difficult situations. She spent all her energy trying to care for her, but at the same time also had her own job. In her mind she could not accept her friend's death and was afraid of being swept back into the difficult living conditions she had experienced once before. She became rather exhausted from all her activities. Then her mind snapped, and she developed a delusion in which the world all of a sudden turned backwards. As a consequence, time also ran backward. So everybody became younger, and her friend was not ill any more. These examples are from psychotic episodes diagnosed as bipolar psychosis in the manic phase. Exhaustion is part of the process that leads to the snapping of the mind into a psychotic experience that produces a magical solution for an unacceptable reality.

5 Trying to fulfil impossible expectations

This is also a pathway that might lead to manic-depressive episodes. There are examples in the literature described by Thomas Bock (2000). In these examples he accentuated the influence of the context as a pressure on the person's behaviour. Bock described a woman who annually developed a manic episode around her birthday. She was participating in a self-help group and together they analysed what happened in the time before she compensated. It became clear that in preparing her birthday party, she had to fulfil the expectations of her mother, who would come to the party and would have all kinds of critical comments. Every year she tried to prove that she could organise her party so well that her mother would find no reason for comment. But each year, just before the party, she would experience a manic episode. Together, in the self-help group, they came up with the idea that she would organise her party this year separately for friends, and for her parents. This appeared to help, because she did not have a manic episode.

6 Denial or transforming what has happened

The pathway of denial means that a person cannot accept what has happened. We saw this with being rejected in a love relationship or being misused in a love relationship and also in the case of a person struggling with a personally unacceptable sexual identity, like homosexuality. The denial of a sexual identity is very difficult because one is reminded often by the nature of one's sexual urges and the constant meeting of people. Isolation is only partly a solution. Another solution is the projection in the outer world of a critical voice talking about homosexuality. Creating conflict between you and the voice also functions as an obstacle to acceptance. This reaction pattern will be easily seen as a condition of schizophrenia, because of the voices and the avoidance, delusions of being followed etc. The stress of accepting a different sexual identity or being rejected in love is not seldom, thus will not commonly be a reason for a psychotic reaction but that depends upon the vulnerability. We saw this in the case of a family background in which a father, who was very critical of all the activities of the children and belittled them and the mother, was highly idealistic. Therefore what they did was hardly ever good enough. This resulted in constant efforts to satisfy the parents and to avoid failure. With this kind of vulnerability failure, being rejected in love or coming to terms with homosexuality takes on a different emotional value.

7 To surrender to a higher power

For this pathway a spiritual solution is sought to cope with an unsolvable contradiction. This might lead to a positive as well as a negative outcome. We observed this pathway in many healthy voice hearers. They see their voice as a higher power and use it as an adviser in making difficult choices. This has similarities, perhaps, with how many people in the general population use their religious beliefs in prayer. However, they do not deny their problems or conflicts. It works out negatively, however, when at the same time the original conflict is denied or transformed. Then the voices are no longer experienced as a helping power, but as threatening. Consequently the behavioural problems might expand because of the secondary reactions as described in pathway 1 and also referred to in pathway 3.

These great differences in the pathways people might take indicate that a personal approach is necessary to understand the psychotic experiences in relation to the trauma and context. Every time one has to explore the reaction that people develop, in relation to their psychosis, in coping with their life experiences. This is often a time-consuming procedure, because the individuals themselves have immersed themselves in their coping strategies. Denial and deformation of their reality takes place in the context of aggression, blackmail, induced guilt and broken down self-esteem. These elements hinder coping and working through the problems.

Psychological theories needed in understanding the process

Most research in psychology leads to or is derived from theories that explain only a small part of the process in the development of psychosis. We shall highlight some important theories to clarify this issue.

Psychoanalytic theory and the defence mechanism

We learned from this that an emotion is replaced by what we call a symptom. This means that the symptom has to be translated back into the involved emotion(s).

Psycho-trauma theory

When a trauma is not emotionally worked through, all kinds of symptoms show up on the level of psychotic symptoms. The most important research we know of is by Erich Lindemann (1944). Lindemann conducted a follow-up study on grief experienced by the family or partners who lost somebody in a fire in a discotheque in New York. He showed the development of a paranoid psychosis that resulted for one of the victims when they could not grieve. Also worth reading is Ensink (1992), who wrote about the psychiatric symptoms women developed after being sexually abused in childhood. John Read and colleagues highlight this process in Chapter 2 in this book. Furthermore Judith L. Herman (1992) wrote a detailed account of the process of trauma and their consequences, as well as how to treat these problems.

Attachment theory

From the research of Bowlby (1951; Bowlby et al. 1952) and others, it becomes clear that feeling unsafe and experiencing broken relationships in childhood are also harmful for the capacity to cope with stress later in life (psychological vulnerability).

Cognitive behavioural theory

Cognitive behavioural theory is concerned with how individuals acquire and apply knowledge about the world (cognition = knowledge). Psychologists worldwide, but mainly in Britain, have done much research into psychotic phenomena. They have developed interventions that teach patients to cope with those phenomena, and specifically to get more control over them (Chadwick et al. 1996; Kingdon and Turkington 1994; Morrison 2002; Morrison et al. 2003b).

Epidemiology

Various studies (Bijl 1998; Eaton et al. 1991; Romme 1996; Tien 1991; Van Os et al. 2001) show that in the general population, it is common for people to experience auditory hallucinations and delusions without involvement with psychiatric services. The studies referred to used a psychiatric diagnostic instrument. The consequence of these studies is that these phenomena cannot be interpreted as psychopathology or a symptom of a psychotic illness. This indicates that we might have to change our ideas profoundly. Mental health professionals tend to interpret these experiences as indicators of potential latent problems. By doing this they deny the implications of these epidemiological studies and base their ideas on research on a relatively small group of patients. A step forward would be the emancipation of these experiences, in a similar way to homosexuality in the 1950s and 1960s. This would free the individual and help would be oriented toward accepting and coping instead of treating an 'illness'.

Context analysis

There is now a small but growing body of knowledge relating to psychoses and the context in which they develop, for example Bock (2000), Bracken and Thomas (2004), Romme and Escher (1993, 1996, 2000), Watkins (1998) and White (1996). These studies suggest a mostly differentiated but sometimes simple relationship between the so-called psychotic phenomena and the context of people's lives who experience them.

Spirituality

Theories in this area concern themselves with the latest step in evolution, when out of life arose consciousness. They recognise the differences between matter, life and mind. Many individuals with spiritual experiences, and also those with psychotic experiences, relate them to a higher level of consciousness and to relationships between living humans and the deceased. In order to understand those ways of thinking and the experiences associated with it, some knowledge and openness to these concepts are necessary. A kind of bible in this field is Ken Wilber's (1995) book *Sex, Ecology, Spirituality*. There are less complex readings, and one way for therapists to inform themselves is to ask patients who share spiritual beliefs to bring with them some texts that particularly inspire them. Another way would be to befriend themselves with non-patients sharing the same frame of reference. I (MR) used to cooperate in some cases with a paranormal healer who heard voices and was recommended by other voice hearers as trustworthy. This was because for me, as a psychiatrist oriented in the physical world, it is difficult to be really able to believe in some people's spiritual experiences. When a patient believed that he was influenced by a deceased person, this healer talked about this influence in way that related to what the patient felt. At the same time I worked with the patient on his daily life conditions. So we split our focus and divided it into two fields in which we both had our understanding and most of the knowledge.

Normalising

In the area of hearing voices, Kingdon and Turkington (1994) have studied those situations in life that trigger the onset of hearing voices, for example, situations such as isolation, long-term threats, life-threatening stress, torture. It is part of the context analysis to see if the conditions a patient actually lives in, or has lived in, might have characteristics of those situations that might give rise to hearing voices.

User literature

There is a growing body of knowledge from people who have experienced psychosis as well as the traditional treatment for it. They give worthwhile insights into the way they have developed their psychosis and also give advice about interventions that are helpful. They generally accentuate the importance of the relationship in treatment, the support, the respect, the search together for coping strategies and solutions of problems, and the importance of safety in daily life etc. They also describe how they support each other. Worthwhile reading is Ron Coleman's (1999) *Recovery: An alien concept*, Judi Chamberlin's (1978) *On our own*, Read and Reynolds' (1996) *Speaking our mind* and furthermore, articles by Wilma Boevink (2002), Pat Deegan (1994), Campbell and Schraiber (1989) and Bock et al. (2002). Research accounts worth reading are from Topor (2001) and Tooth (1997).

Important elements in treatment

From these important fields of knowledge, there are also interventions for treatment that have been developed. From our experience with voice hearers, we learned that interventions should follow a certain system or order. When, for example, a person who feels very unsafe because of his or her voices is not able to cope with them, in that phase, that person is not open for working through the experienced trauma. The person then needs to have more control over the voices first. The interventions used to get more control, however, are again secondary to a relationship of trust and acceptance. Therefore we propose the following order in the therapeutic process:

1   Accept the reality of the experience for the voice hearer. Accepting the reality of the experience means acknowledging within yourself that the person hears voices. This means that you have to show this acknowledgement in your language by talking about the voices as separate from the person, as if the voices were neighbours, and possibily negative, troublesome neighbours. Acceptance means also being more interested in the message and the characteristic of the messenger (see also Beliefs About Voices Questionnaire (BAVQ): Chadwick and Birchwood 1995).

2   Build up a relationship in which the person feels safe. This means being accepted, respected and the feeling of genuine interest from the therapist in the experience of the person as an expert on their voices. Therapists should also show their experience or they should acknowledge that they do not know much about the voice-hearing experience. A genuine interest can be expressed with a systematic interview, like the Maastricht interview with voice hearers (Escher et al. 2000).

3   Exchange well-organised information in order to exclude misunderstandings. This can be reached by making a report from the interview and discussing this report with the voice hearer.

4   Inform oneself about issues in the person's daily life concerning safety. This should be done in the actual context of his/her life, and realistically help and support the person in making social conditions better (see also Kingdon and Turkington 1994). This should have priority above starting technical interventions aimed at reducing preoccupation with the voices.

5   Discuss coping strategies that the voice hearer has used and those others have used in order to get more control over the voices. Better control enables the person to spend his or her time better, and get more social control over his or her own life. Then start training sessions and accentuate the use of these strategies in a systematic way.

6 Support the voice hearer in addressing the influences of the voices that hinder them in daily life. This concerns family relationships, social interactions and triggers that provoke the voices. This is part of the exploration of existing problems (see Alanen 1997). It also might concern sleeping, medication, or encouraging the person to talk about the voices.

7 Use more specific cognitive interventions aimed at helping the individual to cope with the voices. For example, 'focusing', a method developed by Haddock et al. (1996), coping enhancement (Tarrier et al. 1996), or influencing the belief system (Chadwick and Birchwood 1996). For this part of the process, there is extensive literature.

8 Work through the traumatic experiences with their emotional and social consequences. These can include guilt and aggression problems, or shame and lack of support. In more classical ways this is described by Gail Hornstein (2000) in her biography of Frieda Fromm-Reichmann and more recently in a less theoretical way by Herman (1992) in her book *Trauma and recovery*.

9 Use social rehabilitation and recovery-oriented interventions in order to compensate for the most serious problems and to realise dreams and capacities. This is about taking up one's own life again and trying out choices, fulfilling roles in a wider society in concordance with ambitions, and overcoming discrimination by self and others. Literature on this subject is quite extensive, but is based on very different ideas about mental health difficulties. Worth reading are Alanen (1997), Boevink (2002), Coleman (1999), Deegan (1993) and Sayce (2000).

Children, hearing voices and trauma

Our interest in children hearing voices was stimulated by our studies on adults, where we found that about 10 per cent started to hear voices in childhood. In our studies on adults we also found in 70 per cent of cases a relationship between trauma and the onset of hallucinations. This made us wonder about the course of this experience in children.

We conducted a three-year follow-up study for which eighty children were recruited between 8 and 18 years of age; around half (53.8 per cent) were female. About 50 per cent of the children were in professional mental healthcare because of the voices. The other half were not receiving mental healthcare, which did not mean that the experience was unproblematic (Escher and Romme 1998). About 80 per cent of the children reported problems at home because of the voices.

For this follow-up study the children were interviewed four times, with about one year in between each interview.

In this research five instruments were used. The main instrument was the Maastricht Voices Interview for Children (MIC), a version of our adult interview (Romme 1996; Romme and Escher 1996) which we adapted for children with the aid of a clinical child psychologist. The MIC explores many elements of the experience of hearing voices, but does not measure psychopathology. To measure general and specific psychopathology, the Extended Brief Psychiatric Rating Scale (BPRS: Lukoff et al. 1986; Overall and Gorham 1962) was used. As dissociation might be a reaction to trauma, we also used the Dissociative Experience Scale (DES: Bernstein and Putman 1986). With the Youth Self Report 11–18 (YSR) we measured general problem behaviour expressed as the total score (Verhulst et al. 1996), and for the global level of functioning, the Children's Global Assessment Scale (CGAS: Shaffer et al. 1983) was used. (For extended information about this research, see Escher 2004; Escher and Romme 1998; Escher et al. 2002a, 2002b, 2003, 2004.)

Nearly all the children were interviewed at home. The baseline interview was conducted in the presence of at least one parent or grandparent. During the interviews, care was taken to elicit and record the child's experiences, rather than those of their parents.

One of the sections of the MIC concerns a total score of life events that might be related to the onset of the voices. In a structured way, about twenty-two childhood events/trauma, that in the pilot study children related to the onset of voice hearing, were scored 'present' or 'absent' (e.g. death, illness, accidents, friends moving away, changing school, first menstruation, pregnancy, unrequited love, arguments, parental divorce, repeating a school year and other life events). The last question was if the child thought there was a relationship between the onset of the voices and the life event mentioned.

One other topic in the MIC concerned the possible presence of childhood adversities. The child was also asked if the childhood was pleasant or unpleasant, if the child was feeling safe or unsafe at home, if the child was feeling safe or unsafe on the street, if the child was feeling safe or unsafe at school, if the child was being punished in strange ways, being beaten regularly, being scolded regularly, feeling unwanted, a witness of physical abuse, a witness of sexual abuse, molested or abused sexually (Escher 2004; Escher et al. 2002, 2002a, 2002b).

The course of voice hearing

From our study it became clear that hearing voices in children is not a continuous phenomenon. Over the three-year period 60 per cent of the children lost their voices. However, in 13 per cent of children whose voices disappeared on one occasion, the experience recurred at another time. Looking for factors that might influence the persistence of voice hearing, four predictors were found: a high level of anxiety, a high level of depression, a high frequency of the voices and a high level of dissociation (Escher et al. 2002, 2002a, 2002b, 2003, 2004). Professional healthcare was not related to the discontinuation of the voices (Escher et al. 2004).

Severity of voices as assessed by the BPRS, as well as associated anxiety and depression, influenced both receipt of care and voice persistence, confirming the possible role of cognitive processes regulating appraisals and frequency of experience of voices and the ensuing affective response (Escher et al. 2002, 2002a, 2002b, 2003).

A favourable course was associated with the child being able to identify triggers in time and place (for example, hearing voices only when at school or when alone in one's bedroom at night), suggesting that individuals whose voices are not omnipresent, but instead limited to a circumscribed situation, are more likely to overcome the experience (Escher et al. 2002, 2002a, 2002b, 2003).

Higher scores on the DES were associated with increased likelihood of voice persistence (Escher et al. 2003). High levels of dissociation measured with the DES are associated with higher levels of psychosis proneness, and the current findings suggest that the DES may be identifying those individuals who are most liable to develop enduring psychotic symptoms (Allen and Coyne 1995; Pope and Kwapil 2000; Spitzer et al. 1997). High scores on the DES in the context of psychosis may be associated with childhood adversity (Goff et al. 1991) and although reported childhood adversity did not predict voice persistence, it may be that part of the effect of the DES is mediated through its association with childhood adversity. Individuals with high DES scores represented the group most prone to enduring experiences of voices given exposure to early adversity.

Trauma

Childhood adversity was found in a small group of children, while in the whole group high scores on life events relating to the onset of the voice hearing were found. Of the children 86.3 per cent reported one or more traumas around the time of the onset of the voices. Most children experienced one trauma (48 per cent); two traumas were reported by 15.9 per cent and three by 7.3 per cent. We distinguished six groups of trauma: confrontation with death; problems in and around home; problems in and around school; physical condition interfering with development; trauma in relation to sexuality; other kinds of problems that did not fit into the other groups (see Table 8.4). Children who experienced more trauma more often looked for care.

Trauma and discontinuation of the voices

In the last year of the study we discussed with the children the trauma at the onset of the voices in relation to the emotions concerned. In the six distinguished groups we saw examples of the following.

Table 8.4 Trauma reported at or around the onset of the voice hearing

	N	Total N	%
Confrontation with death		18	22.5
Problems in and around home		19	23.7
Serious tension with parents and/or brothers/sisters	10		
Divorced parents	6		
Moving house	3		
Problems in and around school		19	23.7
Capability problems	9		
Changing schools	7		
Being bullied	3		
Physical condition interfering with development		7	8.7
Brain damage caused by traffic accident	1		
A physical health problem with long-term hospital admission	4		
Birth trauma	2		
Traumas in relation to sexuality		5	6.2
Sexual abuse*	4		
Rejection in love	1		
Abortion	1		
Other kinds of problems		4	5
Seeing something weird	3		
Anaesthesia	1		
No trauma	0	11	13.7

* The small percentage of reported sexual abuse might be related to the research context. Most children and adolescents came to participate in this research through their parents. The four girls who reported sexual abuse were not abused by parents or siblings, but by people they knew, for example the boy next door, classmates, a boyfriend and an uncle.

Confrontation with death

For eighteen of the children the onset of the voices was related to a period of grieving, for example, the death of a grandparent, the suicide of an uncle or the death of a friend or a classmate. When these deaths occurred, parents often tried to protect the child from the ensuing emotions. One example is that of a 4-year-old girl living next door to a grandmother who suddenly died. In the following days her mother, aunts and uncles were expressing their grief in the evenings at the house of the grandmother. As the girl was perceived to be too young to take part, she was put to bed instead. She started to hear voices.

In the last year of the study, fifteen out of eighteen children reported that they had learned to cope with the emotion of grief and no longer heard voices.

Problems in and around home

Nineteen of the children in the study related the voices to problems in the home situation, such as severe tension between the parents or problematic relationships with their siblings (ten children). For example, for one boy in the study the voices disappeared when he got his own bedroom and no longer had to share it with his younger brother. Moving house was felt to be a threat by three of the children and brought on the voices; also divorce was related to the onset of voice hearing for six of the children. In the last year of the study, the situation at home and the related emotions had changed for the better for sixteen of the children and the voices had disappeared. Three children whose voices were related to the divorce of their parents still heard voices.

Problems in and around school

School could become problematic for many reasons: peer bullying, problems with teachers, learning capacity problems. In total nineteen children reported voices that related to problems of this kind. In the last year of the study, four children, whose problems at school had not been solved, still heard voices. When care was provided, it was not oriented towards these problems.

Powerlessness and circumstances that cannot be changed

There were ten children who related the onset of the voices to circumstances that made them feel powerless, such as sexual abuse, birth trauma, long-term physical illness requiring hospitalisation and abortion. Four girls began to hear voices after they had been sexually abused, not by family members, but nevertheless by people they knew. Nowadays there is more literature about the relationship between sexual abuse and hearing voices (Ensink 1992; Herman 1992). This is a difficult problem and involves complex emotions. All four girls developed poorly. Three still hear voices and the one who does not receives long-term medication, which unfortunately also influences her development negatively.

The two children with birth traumas had difficulty accepting their disability and acted out with aggressiveness. Both were given neuroleptic medication. In one child the voices disappeared and in the other, an adolescent, the voices moved to the background when he accepted his disability and subsequently acquired a part-time job as a carpenter in the firm of his father and brother.

Four of the children related the voices to physical illnesses and long stays in hospital. One boy stayed on a ward where other children had died. Another boy started to hear voices after he had been operated on and had been given anaesthetics. In the last year of the study, all five children in this group still heard voices.

Relationship to problems

Although one or more traumatic experiences might have happened around the time of the onset, for most children (and parents) the possible relationship between trauma and the onset of their voices was not clear. Interviewers did not push a relationship, but followed a list and asked the children if events had happened and then if the event had evoked or changed the voices. Most children (62.6 per cent) had never thought about a relationship between trauma and the voices (no one ever mentioned it) and did not connect the voices to any traumatic experience, for 11.2 per cent of the children it was clear that there was no relationship at all and 26.2 per cent reported a possible relationship. It was striking that two girls who had been sexually abused said there was no relationship while the voice had all the characteristics of the abusers.

During the research period we noticed that parents and children started to talk about possible problems at the time the voices started, especially when the characteristics of the voices were indicative of the problems that lay at the root. For example, one boy heard the voice of his teacher, who he found very abusive, but he never dared to tell his mother about it; other children heard the voice of their grandparent who had died. Voices could be metaphorical in cases of capacity problems at school. In these cases we noticed that when the voices mixed up numbers, the child already had problems in following the educational level and the voices made it worse. When the children changed schools and the voices disappeared, parents and children then discussed the relationship between the voices and problems at school.

Some of the traumas were related to school or situations at home in which the child was not seen as a person with his/her own emotions and therefore the child's problems were not talked about openly in situations such as divorce, grieving, school bullying or sexual abuse. It might also be that the onset of the voices and the related trauma is not recognised or the trauma might be related to a secret or a shameful experience and therefore not talked about.

Some children did not mention any kind of trauma in the first interview, but disclosed in the second or third. For example, a girl of 18 had a total DES score of 60 at the first interview, but reported no trauma. At the second interview, after being admitted to a psychiatric hospital and diagnosed as schizophrenic, this girl told the interviewer about the sexual abuse she experienced when she was 12. At this point she had a boyfriend of 19. The boyfriend gave her drugs and let his friends sexually abuse her in this condition. She did not tell anyone and asked the interviewer not to tell her parents or therapist, as she felt ashamed and guilty about what had happened.

Voices and development

During the interviews, it became evident that quite a few children had experienced all kinds of changes. Their social network grew, they formed more friendships and life seemed to be broader than just the voices. As some children stated, 'There is more to life than my voices'. With other children, the initial problems often relating to the onset of the voices were not resolved and continued to influence their lives.

The changes we noticed seemed to concern the development of the children. It looked as if development had a positive influence on the discontinuation of the voices. We therefore became interested in development and the relationship between discontinuation, or continuation of voices.

To assess the importance of child development on voice hearing, we developed our own instrument (Escher et al. 2004). To avoid stigmatising statements about development, we documented changes that had been discussed during the three-year follow-up. We did not originally hypothesise the issues that might arise; they emerged during the follow-up period.

Prior to analysing any data, and blind to possible relationships, we specified our criteria for undisturbed development, based on discussion within the research team regarding what was observable and measurable in the developmental process:

1 Acquiring more friends at the peer group level.
2 Knowing better what they wanted to become in life.
3 Learning to cope better with emotions.
4 Having fewer conflicts within the family and at school.
5 Receiving a positive report on development reported by the child concerned and/or by the parents.

For each child an assessment was made in terms of a negative change, undisturbed development or disturbed development, or no change between baseline and last interview. When four out of five elements were positive, the positive development was marked.

In the analysis, we included only the sixty-seven children who participated throughout the whole research period. Outcome factors were the discontinuation of the voices as well as the development of the child. There was a significant association between discontinuation of the voices and positive development ($\chi^2_{(1)}$=18.56, P<0.001). However, discontinuation of the voices does not always result in a positive development. From the forty-five children with discontinuation, thirty-eight (84 per cent) had a positive and seven had a negative development. Equally so, continuation of the voices does not always result in a negative development (see Table 8.5). Out of the twenty-two children who still heard voices, a negative development was observed in seven children in professional care. Of the twenty-two children who continued to

Table 8.5 Continuation or discontinuation of the voices, development and received care

	N	Continuation of hearing voices		Discontinuation of hearing voices	
		Positive development	Negative development	Positive development	Negative development
Professional care	38	3	10	19	7
No care	29	4	5	19	1
Total	67	7	15	38	8

hear voices, a negative development was seen in fifteen (68 per cent) (Escher et al. 2004).

If professional mental healthcare is not related to discontinuation of voices, but development is, this suggests that development might be of a greater importance in overcoming the distress associated with voices. This suggests that voices should be seen as a signal of problems and not as a symptom of mental illness.

Conclusions

The traditional psychiatric system is to categorise psychotic disorders as a serious handicap in the mental healthcare of people with psychotic disorders (Van Os and McKenna 2003). It does not take into account the factors that lead to the disorder. It only promotes attention toward the behaviour and experiences of the person and neglects individual variation. It denies the interaction between the symptoms and interprets all the symptoms as a consequence of the disorder. It thereby neglects the relationship of the different symptoms to the life history. In this way it mystifies the causes and does not take into account the experienced traumatic events.

From our research it became clear that in about 70 per cent of the people hearing voices with a diagnosis of schizophrenia, hearing voices was triggered by traumatic events and a psychological vulnerability was present from childhood adversity. From our research and from epidemiological studies (Bijl et al. 1998; Eaton et al. 1991; Tien 1991), we learned that in itself hearing voices is not a psychopathological phenomenon. However, it leads to problems functioning and to being diagnosed with an 'illness' when the person is not able to cope with their voices and the problems in life that lie at the root of their voice-hearing experience. In these cases we see a variation of secondary reactions that can mimic the full picture of a schizophrenia disorder but can also lead to other mental health disorders like dissociative disorders. The pathways to psychosis demonstrate great variation.

The traumatic background of psychotic disorders means there is a great urgency to ensure that the treatment should not be based on a traditional psychiatric diagnosis but on a thorough analysis of the life history in relation to the different complaints (symptoms). The traumatic experiences at the onset of the voices are not indicators for the continuation of hearing them. In adults and in children we saw that voices might disappear when the trauma is worked through or the powerless situation has changed. However, some conditions handicap this process. In our research we were able to identify a number of factors that influence the coping possibilities. This became most clear in the children's study. In this study 60 per cent of the children lost their voices during the three-year follow-up research period. The factors related to continuation were high level of anxiety, high level of depression, high level of dissociation and a high frequency of hearing voices. These factors all indicate that the attributions associated with the voices are of more importance for the difficulties associated with them and the need for help because of them, than the experience of hearing voices itself.

From the analysis of the effectiveness or ineffectiveness of treatment, it is to be concluded that giving attention to the development of the person who hears voices might well be of greater importance for recovery than a reduction in preoccupation with the phenomenon itself (Escher et al. 2004).

References

Alanen, Y. (1997) *Schizophrenia: Its origin and need-adapted treatment*. London: Karnac.

Allen, J. G., and Coyne, L. (1995) Dissociation and vulnerability to psychotic experiences: The Dissociative Experience Scale and the MMP1–2. *Journal of Nervous and Mental Disease, 183*, 615–622.

American Psychiatric Association (1994) *Diagnostic and statistical manual of mental disorders* (4th edn). Washington, DC: APA.

Bentall, R. P., Haddock, G., and Slade, P. D. (1994) Cognitive behavior therapy for persistent auditory hallucinations: From theory to therapy. *Behavior Therapy, 25*, 51–66.

Bernstein, E. M., and Putman, F. W. (1986) Development, reliability and validity of a dissociation scale (DES). *Journal of Nervous and Mental Disease, 174*, 727–735.

Bijl, R. V., Ravelli, A., and van Zessen, G. (1998) Prevalence of psychiatric disorder in the general population: Results from the Netherlands mental health survey and incidence study. *Social Psychiatry, Psychiatric Epidemiology, 33*, 587–596.

Bock, T. (2000) *Lichtjahre, Psychose ohne Psychiatrie* (Psychosis without Psychiatry). Bonn, Germany: Psychiatrie Verlag.

Bock, T., Dorner, K., Heim, S., Kotulla, J., Schafer, C., Schmitt, E., and Stolz, P. (2002) It is normal to be different, Department of Psychiatry, University of Hamburg.

Boevink, W. (2002) Monsters from the past. In P. Lehmann (ed.) *Coming off psychiatric drugs*. Shrewsbury, UK: Peter Lehmann.

Bowlby, J. (1951) *Maternal care and mental health*. Geneva: WHO.

Bowlby, J., Robertson, J., and Rosenbluth, A. (1952) *A two-year-old goes to hospital: The psychoanalytic study of the child*, no. 7. London: Tavistock.

Bracken, P. and Thomas, P. (2004) Postpsychiatry: A new direction for mental health. *British Medical Journal, 322*, 724–727.

Campbell, J., and Schraiber, R. (1989) *The Well-Being Project: Mental health clients speak for themselves*. California Department of Mental Health: www. Pie.org/ mimhweb/database/getarticle.asp?value=1601

Carmen, E., Rieker, P. P., and Mills, T. (1984) Victims of violence and psychiatric illness. *American Journal of Psychiatry, 141*, 378–383.

Chadwick, P., and Birchwood, M. (1994) The omnipotence of voices: A cognitive approach to auditory hallucinations. *British Journal of Psychiatry, 164*, 190–201.

Chadwick, P., and Birchwood, M. (1995) The omnipotence of voices II: The Beliefs About Voices Questionnaire (BAVQ). *British Journal of Psychiatry, 166*, 773–776.

Chadwick, P., and Birchwood, M. (1996) Cognitive therapy for voices. In G. Haddock and P. Slade (eds) *Cognitive-behavioural interventions with psychotic disorders* (pp. 71–86). London: Routledge.

Chadwick, P., Birchwood, M., and Trower, P. (1996) *Cognitive therapy for delusions, voices and paranoia*. Chichester: John Wiley.

Chamberlin, J. (1978) *On our own: Patient-controlled alternatives to the mental health system*. New York: Hawthorn, McGraw-Hill paperback edition 1979.

Coleman, R. (1999) *Recovery: An alien concept*. Gloucester: Handsell.

Craine, L. S., Henson, C. E., Colliver, J. A., and MacLean, D. G. (1988) Prevalence of a history of sexual abuse among female psychiatric patients in a state hospital system. *Hospital and Community Psychiatry, 39*, 300–304.

Davies-Netzley, S., Hurlburt, M. S., and Hough, R. (1996) Childhood abuse as a precursor to homelessness for homeless women with severe mental illness. *Violence and Victims, 11*, 129–142.

Deegan, P. (1993) Recovering our sense of value after being labeled mentally ill. *Journal of Psychosocial Nursing and Mental Health Services, 31*, 7–11.

Drayer, N., and Langeland, M. A. (1999) Childhood trauma and perceived parental dysfunction in the etiology of dissociative symptoms in psychiatric inpatients. *American Journal of Psychiatry, 156*, 379–385.

Eaton, W., Romanoski, A., Anthony, J. C., and Nestadt, G. (1991) Screening for psychosis in the general population with a self report interview. *Journal of Nervous and Mental Disease, 179*, 689–693.

Ensink, B. (1992) *Confusing realities: A study on child sexual abuse and psychiatric symptoms*. Amsterdam: Free University Press.

Escher, S. (2004) An exploration of auditory hallucinations in children and adolescents. MPhil. thesis, University of Central England, Birmingham.

Escher, S., and Romme, M. (1998) Small talk: Voice-hearing in children. *Open Mind, 92*, 12–14.

Escher, S., Hage, P., and Romme, M. (2000) Interview with a person who hears voices. In M. Romme and S. Escher (eds) *Making sense of voices*. London: Mind.

Escher, S., Romme, M., Buiks, A., Delespaul, P., and Van Os, J. (2002a) Independent course of childhood auditory hallucinations: A sequential 3-year follow-up study. *British Journal of Psychiatry, 181* (suppl. 43), s10–s18.

Escher, S., Romme, M., Buiks, A., Delespaul, P., and Van Os, J. (2002b) Formation of delusional ideation in adolescents hearing voices: A prospective study. *American Journal of Medical Genetics, 114*, 913–920.

Escher, S., Delespaul, P., Romme, M., Buiks, A., and Van Os, J. (2003) Coping defence and depression in adolescents hearing voices. *Journal of Mental Health, 12*, 91–99.

Escher, S., Morris, M., Buiks, A., Delespaul, P., Van Os, J., and Romme, M. (2004) Determinants of outcome in the pathways through care for children hearing voices. *International Journal of Social Welfare, 13*, 208–222.

Goff, D. C., Brotman, A. W., Kindlon, D., Waites, M., and Amico, E. (1991) Self-reports of childhood abuse in chronically psychotic patients. *Psychiatry Research, 37*, 73–80.

Goodman, L. A., Dutton, M. A., and Harris, M. (1995) Physical and sexual assault prevalence among episodically homeless, women with serious mental illness. *American Journal of Orthopsychiatry, 65*, 468–478.

Haddock, G., Bentall, R., and Slade, P. (1996) Treatment of auditory hallucinations. In G. Haddock and P. Slade (eds) *Cognitive-behavioural interventions with psychotic disorders* (pp. 45–71). London: Routledge.

Hamner, M. B., Frueh, B. C., Ulmer, H. G., Huber, M. G., Twomey, T. J., Tyson, C., and Arana, G. W. (2000) Psychotic features in chronic posttraumatic stress disorder and schizophrenia. *Journal of Nervous and Mental Disease, 188*, 217–221.

Herman, J. L. (1992) *Trauma and recovery*. London: Pandora.

Honig, A., Romme, M., Ensink, B., Escher, S., Pennings, M., and de Vries, M. (1998) Auditory hallucinations: A comparison between patients and non-patients. *Journal of Nervous and Mental Disease, 186*, 646–651.

Hornstein, G. (2000) *To redeem one person is to redeem the world: The life of Frieda Fromm-Reichmann*. London: The Free Press.

Jacobson, A., and Richardson, B. (1987) Assault experience of 100 psychiatric inpatients: Evidence of need for routine inquiry. *American Journal of Psychiatry, 144*, 908–913.

Kingdon, D. G., and Turkington, D. (1994) *Cognitive behavioural therapy of schizophrenia*. Hove: Lawrence Erlbaum.

Lindemann, E. (1944) Symptomatology and management of acute grief. *American Journal of Psychiatry, 101*, 141–148.

Lukoff, D., Neuchterlein, K. H., and Ventura, J. (1986) Manual for expanded Brief Psychiatric Rating Scale. *Schizophrenia Bulletin, 12*, 594–602.

Morrison, A. P. (ed.) (2002) *A casebook of cognitive therapy for psychosis*. London: Routledge.

Morrison, A. P., Frame, L., and Larkin, W. (2003a) Relationships between trauma and psychosis: A review and integration. *British Journal of Clinical Psychology, 42*, 331–353.

Morrison, A. P., Renton, J., Dunn, H., Williams, S., and Bentall, R. (2003b) *Cognitive therapy for psychosis: A formulation-based approach*. London: Routledge.

Muenzenmaier, K., Meyer, I., Struening, E., and Ferber, J. (1993) Childhood abuse and neglect among women outpatients with chronic mental illness. *Hospital and Community Psychiatry, 44*, 666–670.

Mueser, K. T., Goodman, L. B., Trumbetta, S. L., Rosenberg, S. D., Osher, F. C., Vidaver, R., et al. (1998) Trauma and posttraumatic stress disorder in severe mental illness. *Journal of Consulting and Clinical Psychology, 66*, 493–499.

Overall, J. E., and Gorham, D. (1962) The Brief Psychiatric Rating Scale. *Psychological Reports, 10*, 799–812.

Pennings, M., Romme, M., and Buiks, A. (1996) Auditieve hallucinaties bij patienten en niet-patienten. *Tijdschrift voor Psychiatrie, 38*, 648–660.

Pope, C. A., and Kwapil, T. R. (2000) Dissociative experiences in hypothetically psychosis-prone college students. *Journal of Nervous and Mental Disease, 188*, 530–536.

Read, J., and Reynolds, J. (1996) *Speaking our minds: An anthology of personal experiences of mental distress and its consequences*. London: Macmillan.

Robins, L. N., Wing, J., Wittchen, H. U., Helzer, J. E., Babor, T. F., Burke, J., et al. (1988) The Composite International Diagnostic Interview: An epidemiologic instrument suitable for use in conjunction with different diagnostic systems and in different cultures. *Archives of General Psychiatry, 45*, 1069–1077.

Romme, M. (1996) *Understanding voices*. Gloucester: Handsell.

Romme, M., and Escher, S. (1989) Hearing voices. *Schizophrenia Bulletin, 15*, 209–216.

Romme, M., and Escher, S. (1993) *Accepting voices*. London: Mind.

Romme, M., and Escher, S. (1996) Empowering people who hear voices. In G. Haddock and P. Slade (eds) *Cognitive-behavioural interventions with psychotic disorders* (pp. 137–151). London: Routledge.

Romme, M., and Escher, S. (2000) *Making sense of voices*. London: Mind.

Romme, M., Honig, A., Noordhoorn, O., and Escher, S. (1992) Coping with voices: An emancipatory approach. *British Journal of Psychiatry, 161*, 99–103.

Sayce, L. (2000) *From psychiatric patient to citizen*. Basingstoke: Palgrave.

Schneider, K. (1959) *Clinical psychopathology* (5th edn). New York: Grune and Stratton.

Shaffer, D., Gould, M. S., Brasic, J., Ambrosini, P., Fisher, P., Bird, H., and Aluwahlie, S. (1983) A Children's Global Assessment Scale (CGAS). *Archives of General Psychiatry, 40*, 1228–1231.

Spitzer, C., Haug, H. J., and Freyberger, H. J. (1997) Dissociative symptoms in schizophrenic patients with positive and negative symptoms. *Psychopathology, 30*, 67–75.

Tien, A. Y. (1991) Distributions of hallucination in the population. *Social Psychiatry and Psychiatric Epidemiology, 26*, 287–292.

Tooth, B. (1997) Recovery from schizophrenia: A consumer perspective. Final report to Health and Human Services Research, Australia. Unpublished.

Topor, A. (2001) *Managing the contradictions: Recovery from serious mental disorders*. Stockholm: Department of Social Work, Stockholm University.

Van Os, J., and McKenna, P. (2003) Does schizophrenia exists? Maudsley discussion paper no. 12. Institute of Psychiatry, King's College London.

Van Os, J., Hanssen, M., Bijl, R. V., and Vollebergh, W. (2001) Prevalence of psychotic disorder and community level of psychotic symptoms. *Archives of General Psychiatry, 58*, 663–668.

Verhulst, F. C., Van der Ende, J., Koot, H. M. H., et al. (1996) Handleiding voor de CBCL 4–18. *Sopia Kinderziekenhuis/Academisch Ziekenhuis, Erasmus Universiteit*.

Watkins, J. (1998) *Hearing voices: A common human experience*. Melbourne: Hill of Content.

White, M. (1996) Power to our journeys. *American Family Therapy Academy Newsletter*, summer, 11–16.

Wilber, K. (1995) *Sex; ecology; spirituality: The spirit of evolution*. Boston, MA: Shambhala.

Yusupoff, Y., and Tarrier, N. (1996) Coping strategy enhancement for persistent hallucinations and delusions. In G. Haddock and P. Slade (eds) *Cognitive-behavioural interventions with psychotic disorders* (pp. 86–103). London: Routledge.

Zubin, J., and Spring, B. (1977) Vulnerability: A new view of schizophrenia. *Journal of Abnormal Psychology, 86*, 103–126.

Part III

From theory to therapy

Chapter 9

Breaking the silence

Learning why, when and how to ask about trauma, and how to respond to disclosures

John Read

'You know, there were so many doctors and registrars and nurses and social workers and psychiatric district nurses in your life asking you about the same thing, mental, mental, mental, but not asking you why.'

'It took ten years, many admissions, a lot of different medication, ECTs. No-one was able to draw out any abuse issues until my very last admission when a psychologist asked me "have you been abused?"'

(Users of mental health services, quoted in
Lothian and Read 2002: 101)

The relationship between adverse life events and the probability of using mental health services is now established beyond reasonable contention. In 2004 a review of forty studies of female inpatients and samples of predominantly psychotic female outpatients between 1984 and 2003 (N = 2396) calculated that 50 per cent had been subjected to childhood sexual abuse (CSA) and 48 per cent to childhood physical abuse (CPA). The majority (69 per cent) had been subjected to either CSA or CPA. The figures for men were CSA 28 per cent, CPA 51 per cent, CSA or CPA 60 per cent (Read et al. 2004a).

Child abuse has been shown to have a causal role in depression, anxiety disorders, PTSD, eating disorders, substance abuse, sexual dysfunction, personality disorders and dissociative disorders (Boney-McCoy and Finkelhor 1996; Fergusson et al. 1996; Kendler et al. 2000) (most of which are common in people who experience hallucinations and delusions). The more severe the abuse, the greater the probability of these problems in adulthood (Mullen et al. 1993). Psychiatric patients subjected to CSA or CPA have earlier first admissions, longer and more frequent hospitalisations, spend longer in seclusion, receive more medication, are more likely to self-mutilate, and have higher global symptom severity (Beck and van der Kolk 1987; Briere et al. 1997; Goff et al. 1991; Lipschitz et al. 1996; Mullen et al. 1993; Read et al. 2001a; Rose et al. 1991; Sansonnet-Hayden, et al. 1987). The high rate of suicide in people diagnosed schizophrenic can be partially explained by findings that psychiatric patients who have suffered CPA or CSA try to kill themselves more often than non-abused psychiatric patients (Briere et al. 1997;

Lanktree et al. 1991; Lipschitz et al. 1996; Read 1998). One study, of 200 adult outpatients, found that suicidality was better predicted by child-hood abuse than by a current diagnosis of depression. This finding led to the recommendation that child abuse be considered an integral part of suicide assessments for all clients, psychotic or not (Read et al. 2001a).

The more specific relationship between childhood abuse and psychotic symptoms has only been on the research agenda for a few years, having been ignored or denied for decades. The relationship has now been well docu-mented (see Chapter 2; see also Bebbington et al. 2004; Briere et al. 1997; Friedman and Harrison 1984; Hammersley et al. 2003; Janssen et al. 2004; Read 1997; Read and Argyle 1999; Read et al. 2001b; Read et al. 2003; Read et al. 2004a; Ross et al. 1994).

Users of mental health services are also more likely than the general popu-lation to be exposed to violence in adulthood (Goodman et al. 1997). One study, of chronically mentally ill people, found the following rates: men – adult physical assault (APA) 71 per cent, adult sexual assault (ASA) 17 per cent; women – APA 90 per cent, ASA 79 per cent (Goodman et al. 1999).

A New Zealand study of 200 outpatients found that both child abuse (particularly CSA) and ASA were correlated with hallucinations, delusions and thought disorder, but not the negative symptoms of 'schizophrenia' (Read et al. 2003). For example hallucinations were experienced by 18.5 per cent of the non-abused clients, 55 per cent of those who had suffered CSA, 60 per cent of those who had suffered ASA, and 86 per cent of those who had suffered both CSA and ASA.

These bodies of research literature might suggest that interpersonal vio-lence would be a primary focus when mental health professionals assess their clients, formulate the causes of their difficulties and make treatment plans. One might reasonably expect mental health professionals to be well trained in when and how to take trauma histories and how to respond to clients' disclosures of abuse. Indeed, since the mid 1980s, countless researchers and clinicians have been recommending the routine taking of trauma histories in mental health services (e.g. Dill et al. 1991; Jacobson and Richardson 1987; Mitchell et al. 1996; Read and Fraser 1998a; Sansonnet-Hayden et al. 1987; Swett et al. 1990).

This chapter will summarise the research concerning current clinical prac-tice and beliefs relating to taking, and responding to, trauma histories – focusing on childhood abuse. It will then go on to suggest avenues towards improving clinical practice. This will include a list of principles to guide the development of training programmes and the description of a training pro-gramme currently operating in New Zealand based on those principles. The literature summarised above, on the prevalence and sequelae of trauma, as well as the literature that now follows, about current practice and barriers to good practice, are both important parts of what needs to be presented in training programmes.

Current practice

Asking

There has not been much research examining the frequency with which mental health professionals ask about trauma. What there has been does not paint a picture of which we can be proud.

In the mid 1990s a questionnaire about practices relating to assessment of sexual abuse was sent to nurse managers at all general hospitals in the United States offering psychiatric inpatient services. Of the 466 who responded, 69 per cent believed that admission assessments should always include sexual abuse history, but only 43 per cent reported that such histories were already included in admission assessments (Mitchell et al. 1996).

Inpatient studies in the United States and the United Kingdom have found that clinicians fail to identify the majority of the abuse cases reported to researchers. The percentages identified by clinicians were 48 per cent (Craine et al. 1988); 30 per cent (Wurr and Partridge 1996); 29 per cent (Lipschitz et al. 1996); 20–32 per cent (Muenzenmaier et al. 1993) and 20 per cent (Goodwin et al. 1988). Another inpatient study found even lower rates: CPA 15 per cent, CSA 0 per cent, APA 10 per cent, ASA 0 per cent (Jacobson et al. 1987). A chart review of female users of a psychiatric emergency room revealed only a 6 per cent rate of sexual abuse. When clinicians were asked to take abuse histories, the rate rose to 70 per cent (Briere and Zaidi 1989). The majority of men attending a British outpatient clinic had not been asked about sexual abuse (Mills 1993). Many people having extensive contact with mental health services never reveal their victimisation to clinicians (Elliott 1997; Finkelhor 1990). A study of thirty 'heavy users of acute inpatient and emergency services' who disclosed CSA or CPA to the researchers found that none had ever been asked about abuse before (Rose et al. 1991). In 2003 a survey of New Zealand women who had suffered CSA and were later treated by mental health services found that 63 per cent had never been asked about CSA by mental health staff, 22 per cent had been asked and 15 per cent were unsure (McGregor 2003). These studies focus on CSA and CPA. However, childhood emotional abuse may be similarly unrecognised by mental health services (Thompson and Kaplan 1999). Three other New Zealand studies, summarised next, also found low levels of abuse identification.

Some research opportunities come about more by luck than planning. After nearly twenty years of working as a clinical psychologist and manager of mental health services in which I rarely saw a clinician ask about trauma (including, for years, myself), I entered academia in 1994. In my final year in the real world I had been working in the psychiatric unit of an urban general hospital in New Zealand. A multidisciplinary committee (including the consultant psychiatrist and the unit manager) had spent a year developing an abuse policy, which included the principle that all patients should be asked about trauma, including past or recent sexual and physical abuse. At the last minute the psychiatrist in charge of psychiatric registrar training wrote to the unit manager decreeing that the policy must not be implemented. He argued that psychiatrists were not bound by unit policies (imagine a nurse taking such a stance in writing!) and must be allowed to deploy their 'clinical judgement'. Second, he thought it pointless asking disturbed people about their pasts as they were likely to imagine things that hadn't happened.

As a result the policy was not introduced. Just before I left, however, the consultant psychiatrist and I decided the best we could do was to add an abuse section to the admission form. A year or so later I returned in my new guise as researcher to see what had happened (Read and Fraser 1998a). I read, in their entirety, the charts of a hundred consecutively admitted patients. My first discovery was that the new admission form, with the abuse section, had been used in only fifty-three cases. This allowed an evaluation of whether simply adding questions to forms improves identification of abuse.

It did not. The new and old forms both produced a combined rate of 32 per cent for childhood or adulthood sexual or physical abuse. The main reason was obvious. In thirty-six of the fifty-three cases (68 per cent) where our new form had been used, the abuse section had been avoided.

This disappointing finding provided, however, a chance to compare abuse rates when abuse questions are asked on admission and when they are not asked (and therefore abuse identification relies on either spontaneous disclosure or staff asking later during the hospital stay). Significant differences were found for all four abuse categories: CSA – if asked 47 per cent, if not asked 6 per cent; CPA – 30 per cent versus 0 per cent; adult sexual assault – 12 per cent versus 0 per cent; adult physical assault – 35 per cent versus 3 per cent. At least one of the four types of abuse was reported by 82 per cent of those asked, but only 8 per cent of those not asked. It had been unrealistic to expect well-engrained attitudes and habits to change just because a few words had suddenly appeared on a form. Training was necessary.

Even where a policy of asking all inpatients about abuse on admission was already in place, leaving it up to psychiatrists to decide whether and how to ask, led to their failing to identify 44 per cent of CSA cases and 59 per cent of CPA cases later identified by researchers (Dill et al. 1991). Policies and inclusion of trauma sections on forms are, in the absence of training, not very effective.

We wondered whether another partial explanation for the low level of inquiry in our inpatient study was the setting. Inpatient units traditionally deal with stabilisation of crises and short-term symptom reduction (predominantly with drugs) rather than exploration of psychosocial causes and solutions. Therefore we replicated the study with 200 consecutive clients of a New Zealand community mental health centre (CMHC) (Agar et al. 2002). We also wondered whether having a broader range of professions involved in the initial assessments might impact upon abuse disclosure rates. (In the inpatient unit all admissions had been conducted by psychiatrists; in the

CMHC only 54 per cent of the initial assessments were conducted by psychiatrists.)

In this outpatient study the use of a new form with an abuse section did make a difference, leading to a rate, for one or more of the four types of abuse (CSA, CPA, ASA, APA), of 46 per cent compared to 22 per cent when the form was not used. This time the abuse questions were avoided in only 23 per cent of cases. Again there was a different outcome depending on whether or not the questions were asked, with 60 per cent of those who were asked identifying at least one form of abuse compared to 15 per cent of those who were not asked. An additional important finding, however, was that fifty-eight cases of abuse were recorded in records of previous contacts with mental health services attached to the current file but were not mentioned at all anywhere in the notes of the current contact with the CMHC (the average length of which was twenty-one weeks).

In the third New Zealand study seventy-four members of mental health consumer groups were asked about their initial assessment (most common diagnoses: schizophrenia 45 per cent, bipolar disorder 40 per cent). The majority (64 per cent) had experienced some form of abuse. However, 78 per cent had not been asked about abuse at initial assessment. The majority of the abused participants (66 per cent) felt that the assessment situation was not comfortable enough for them to discuss their abuse. Those reporting abuse to the researchers were significantly less satisfied with their treatment, and less likely to believe their diagnosis was an accurate description of their problems, than the non-abused participants (Lothian and Read 2002).

Interestingly, 69 per cent of the abused participants believed there was a connection between their having been abused and their mental health problems (with 15 per cent unsure) but only 17 per cent of them believed that the mental health staff believed there was a connection (with 60 per cent unsure).

Mental health staff are not unique among health professionals in their reluctance to ask about interpersonal violence. A similar body of research literature exists for physicians in medical settings (Acierno et al. 1997; Friedman et al. 1992), even sexual health clinics (Hurst et al. 2003).

Responding

There is even less research on what staff do when a client tells them that they have been abused. Again we see a disparity between perceived and actual practice. In the survey of US managers of inpatient units (Mitchell et al. 1996), 43 per cent thought patients who disclosed sexual abuse received inpatient therapy specifically related to the abuse, and the same percentage believed that abused patients were referred for outpatient therapy on discharge. In a survey of British mental health staff, only 5 per cent of nurses, 10 per cent of psychologists and 24 per cent of psychiatrists reported that they take no action when a male client discloses CSA (Lab et al. 2000).

A chart review of seventy-two US outpatients with trauma recorded in their chart was conducted at a New York teaching hospital (Eilenberg et al. 1996). The frequency of the trauma was recorded in only 15 per cent of the charts. Similarly the severity of the trauma was recorded in 15 per cent. Information on symptoms commonly associated with trauma was rarely documented. A suicide assessment was reported in all of the seventy-two cases, but in only one case was it related to a trauma history. Only 10 per cent of formulations incorporated the trauma history appropriately, with 28 per cent making no mention of the trauma and a further 38 per cent mentioning the trauma without making any linkage at all to the patient's problems. More than half the treatment plans (56 per cent) made no mention of the trauma. In a further 35 per cent the trauma was mentioned without relevant treatment recommendations. Appropriate treatment recommendations were found in only 10 per cent of the charts. The researchers concluded: 'eliciting histories of abuse does not necessarily lead to improved treatment for trauma-related symptoms' (Eilenberg et al. 1996: 169).

A New Zealand inpatient study found that only eleven of the thirty-two files (34 per cent) in which CSA, CPA, ASA or APA was documented had any mention of whether previous disclosure or treatment had occurred. (This is crucial information in terms of treatment planning.) There was no evidence of any of the thirty-two having received any support, counselling or abuse-related information while in hospital. None of the fifty-two separate instances of abuse were reported to any legal authorities. This was the case despite there being eight ASA cases and fifteen APA cases, several of which were ongoing. A referral for post-discharge referral for abuse-related therapy was considered for 25 per cent of the clients and actually happened for just 9 per cent (all of which were a continuation of pre-existing, interrupted therapy) (Read and Fraser 1998b). One of the charts included: 'X was most dissatisfied that the general staff in the unit had not been trained to deal with sexual abuse issues' (Read and Fraser 1998b: 209).

In a New Zealand CMHC study, of the ninety-two charts in which CSA, CPA, ASA or APA had been recorded, only thirty (33 per cent) included documentation of previous disclosure or treatment. In only about one-third of the files the abuse was mentioned in either the formulation (36 per cent) or the treatment plan (33 per cent), while 22 per cent either received abuse-related therapy at the CMHC or were referred on for such therapy (Agar and Read 2002). None of the 128 separate alleged crimes were reported to legal authorities, and there was no evidence of any discussion with any of the ninety-two clients about that possibility.

Reasons for inadequate clinical practice

People in general are often reluctant to spontaneously tell anyone, including health and mental health professionals, about the abuse they have suffered

(Acierno et al. 1997). The average time it takes women who have suffered CSA to tell anyone is sixteen years (McGregor 2003). It is therefore essential that we don't wait for spontaneous disclosures but, instead, develop the confidence and skills to ask. In designing training programmes to accomplish this goal, we should understand the barriers to taking trauma histories.

A survey of clinicians' reasons for not asking

In a questionnaire survey of 114 New Zealand psychologists and psychiatrists, the majority reported that their workplace encouraged inquiry about abuse. The clinicians also believed that in the majority of cases they knew whether or not the client had suffered child abuse (psychiatrists – 73 per cent of their cases, psychologists – 82 per cent) (Young et al. 2001).

When asked to rate the relevance of fifteen possible reasons for sometimes not asking about child abuse, the two most endorsed items (for both professions) were external to the clinician: 'There are too many more immediate needs and concerns' and 'Clients may find the issue too disturbing, or it may cause a deterioration of their psychological state.' This is consistent with studies of why physicians don't ask (Acierno et al. 1997; Sugg and Inui 1992). Few of the New Zealand clinicians endorsed items internal to the clinician, such as lack of training or skills.

Other things are more important

There are certainly times when there are more urgent needs and concerns to address. These include acute suicidality, extreme emotional distress or flagrant current psychosis. The presence of family members is another reason for delaying a trauma history (Young et al. 2001). Training programmes should stress the importance of recording that a trauma history has not been taken and of ensuring that there is a system in place that guarantees this will happen later when the person is less distressed. As we have seen earlier, it is easy for the taking of a trauma history to be deferred indefinitely.

Upsetting the client

Fear of disturbing the client is not a good reason for not asking. It is a very good reason, however, for learning how to ask sensitively and how to respond therapeutically to disclosures. Clinicians need reassuring that when done appropriately, most users of health services do not mind being asked about abuse (Shew and Hurst 1993). For example 85 per cent of assault victims and 64 per cent of non-victims welcome physician inquiries about assault (Friedman et al. 1992). The same study found that 78 per cent of primary care patients favoured routine assessment of physical assault, and 68 per cent favoured routine assessment of sexual assault. When 138 female psychiatric inpatients were asked to participate in a survey of 'current symptoms and past life experiences, including possible experiences of abuse', 103 (75 per cent) consented (Dill et al. 1991).

Of course trauma assessment, especially if done insensitively, can be stressful for some people. However, the minority who do find trauma questions stressful also describe positive impacts of such inquiry (Brabin and Berah 1995). Even a brief discussion of previous trauma can significantly reduce psychological symptoms (Briere 1999; Murray and Segal 1994). 'Thus the examiner may be most successful to the extent that he or she approaches the trauma identification process with due care and sensitivity, yet also views conversations about traumatic events as potentially helpful' (Briere 1999: 47).

In fact many users of mental health services are more disturbed by *not* being asked about childhood abuse than by being asked (Lothian and Read 2002). A large survey of British users of mental health services found that they expected their life experiences to be considered at length and thought this was crucial in diagnosing and treating them. Their experience, however, was that clinicians frequently conducted relatively cursory interviews in the belief that their problems were 'illnesses' requiring physical treatments. That is, 'the patient's communications are only of interest to doctors in revealing symptoms, not in terms of them being personally meaningful and the basis for shared exploration in a therapeutic relationship' (Rogers et al. 1993: 53).

Client characteristics

Demographics

Some of the few studies focusing on gender have found that male clients are less likely to be asked about abuse than female clients (Holmes and Offen 1996; Holmes et al. 1997). A survey of 121 British mental health staff found that only 15 per cent thought that male clients should always be asked about childhood sexual abuse, and that 33 per cent (50 per cent of psychologists) never actually ask (Lab et al. 2000).

The New Zealand inpatient study found that when an abuse section was included in the admission form, 43 per cent of women but only 25 per cent of men were asked the abuse questions (Read and Fraser 1998a). The outpatient study found no gender difference (Agar et al. 2002). The New Zealand survey of clinicians, about reasons for not asking, presented an identical vignette, with different genders, and found no difference in self-reported probability of abuse inquiry (Young et al. 2001). However, an evaluation of the New Zealand training programme (presented later) found that, prior to the training, 49 per cent reported that the probability of their asking about abuse was influenced by either the gender or age of the client, while 24 per cent of the staff reported that the probability of their asking increased if the client was female (Cavanagh et al. 2004). For 20 per cent the reported probability of asking about child abuse increased if the client was aged between 20 and 40, and for 16 per cent it decreased if the client was over 60. The New Zealand inpatient study found no differences according to age (Read and Fraser 1998a).

Men and older people may also have a smaller chance of receiving appropriate responses when they disclose abuse. In the inpatient study 17 per cent of the women but none of the men were referred for abuse-related therapy. The mean age of those considered for referral was 32 years, compared to 39 years for those not considered (Read and Fraser 1998b). The figures for the CMHC study were: Documentation of previous disclosure or treatment – women 42 per cent, men 13 per cent; Abuse included in formulation – women 41 per cent, men 27 per cent; Abuse included in treatment plan – women 39 per cent, men 20 per cent; Abuse-related therapy – women 24 per cent, men 17 per cent (Agar and Read 2002). Age was unrelated to responses in this study.

Ethnicity was not significantly related to asking or responding in any of the New Zealand studies reported above.

Diagnosis

Another client variable (beyond being male or older) related to low levels of inquiry and response is of particular importance in the context of this book. Despite the high levels of abuse found in people who experience psychosis, having a diagnosis indicative of psychosis seems to lower your chances of being asked, and also of having your needs met if you disclose. In the New Zealand inpatient study 23 per cent of clients with a diagnosis of 'schizophrenia' were asked about abuse, compared to 39 per cent of those with other diagnoses (Read and Fraser 1998a). Documentation of previous disclosure or treatment occurred in only 13 per cent of the abused people diagnosed 'schizophrenic' but 42 per cent of the other abused patients. Referral for abuse-related therapy was considered for 67 per cent of the abused inpatients with non-psychotic diagnoses, but only 5 per cent of those with psychotic diagnoses and for none of those diagnosed 'schizophrenic' (Read and Fraser 1998b). Actual referrals occurred for 25 per cent of the abused non-psychotic cases, 5 per cent of the psychotic diagnoses and for none of those diagnosed 'schizophrenic'.

In the New Zealand CMHC study schizophrenia spectrum clients (SCZ) were compared to other patients (OTH): Documentation of previous disclosure or treatment – SCZ 13 per cent, OTH 38 per cent; Abuse included in formulation – SCZ 0 per cent, OTH 48 per cent; Abuse included in treatment plan – SCZ 0 per cent, OTH 44 per cent; Abuse-related therapy – SCZ 6 per cent, OTH 25 per cent (Agar and Read 2002). In the evaluation of the New Zealand training programme (Cavanagh et al. 2004), 53 per cent of the mental health professionals acknowledged, prior to the training, that the probability of their asking about abuse was influenced by diagnosis. Psychosis was the diagnosis cited most often in relation to decreased probability.

Staff characteristics

Gender

The New Zealand studies found no differences in terms of the gender of the clinician in relation to self-reported, or actual, overall probability of asking about abuse (Agar et al. 2002; Young et al. 2001). However, some New Zealand clinicians (male and female), report being particularly unlikely to ask clients of the opposite gender (Cavanagh et al. 2004). In a US study female clinicians were more likely than male colleagues to identify sexual (but not physical) violence (Currier and Briere 2000). Interestingly, however, one study found that clinician gender has no impact on clients' willingness to disclose (Dill et al. 1991).

Following disclosures, female staff in a New Zealand study were more likely to offer appropriate responses, especially documenting previous disclosure or treatment, incorporating the abuse into treatment plans, and providing (or referring for) abuse-related therapy (Agar and Read 2002).

Profession

Similarly, profession was unrelated to overall probability of asking but was related to response. Psychiatrists had lower response rates than the other three professions combined (psychologists, nurses and social workers) in all categories: Documentation of previous disclosure or treatment – PSY 25 per cent, OTH 50 per cent; Abuse included in formulation – PSY 26 per cent, OTH 60 per cent; Abuse included in treatment plan – PSY 21 per cent, OTH 47 per cent; Abuse-related therapy – PSY12.5 per cent, OTH 33 per cent (Agar and Read 2002). This is consistent with the British self-report study mentioned earlier (Lab et al. 2000).

Beliefs about veracity of disclosures

The survey of New Zealand psychiatrists and psychologists asked 'What percentage of disclosures do you think are probably false allegations of childhood abuse?' The average response was 4.9 per cent, with no difference between professions. Only 11 per cent reported that 'My inquiring could be suggestive and therefore possibly induce false memories' was relevant to their decisions to sometimes not ask about abuse. Nevertheless, out of fifteen possible reasons for not asking about abuse, this item was most strongly correlated with self-reported probability of failing to ask about abuse. Similarly, the percentage of disclosures thought to be false was correlated with low probability of asking about abuse (Young et al. 2001). So although the majority of these mental health professionals seem immune to the frequently made public claims about epidemics of false allegations of child abuse and the 'implanting' of abuse memories by mental health staff, a minority may be believing the media stories and failing to do their job as a consequence.

The evaluation of the training programme found that the participants believed, on average, that 16 per cent of disclosures were not true (Cavanagh et al. 2004). The percentage considered untrue was negatively correlated with believing that all clients should be asked about abuse, with the percentage of disclosures documented in files and with the percentage of clients for whom the participant knew whether or not they had been abused. Thus, our biases about disclosure veracity may be impacting our performance.

Of the disclosures the participants believed were untrue, nearly half (46 per cent) were considered to be 'the result of psychotic delusions'. This introduces the second type of belief of relevance to clinical practice and which, like attitudes about veracity, must be addressed in training programmes.

Causal beliefs

The failure of researchers and clinicians to acknowledge, and act on, the well-documented relationship between trauma and psychosis can be explained by a number of factors (Read 1997), including fear of being accused of 'family-blaming' (Aderhold and Gottwalz 2004; Read et al. 2004c). Another related factor is the dominance of the biomedical model. This paradigm is particularly dominant, and especially unhelpful, in relation to psychosis (Bentall 2003; Read et al. 2004b).

We have seen that psychiatrists seem less likely to respond appropriately to abuse disclosures than other professionals. However, this is obviously not true of all psychiatrists. Causal beliefs may be more important than professional affiliation. Although surveys in numerous countries show that the general public understands that 'mental illnesses' like 'schizophrenia' are caused predominantly by psychosocial factors – such as adversity in childhood, trauma and poverty (Read and Haslam 2004), some mental health staff subscribe to a more bio-genetic ideology. In the New Zealand survey of professionals about abuse inquiry, 42 per cent of the psychiatrists, and 9 per cent of the psychologists, scored on the 'Endogenous' (bio-genetic) side of the mid-point of the Mental Health Locus of Origin (MHLO) scale measuring causal beliefs (Young et al. 2001). Those endorsing more 'Interactional' (psychosocial) items were more likely to ask about abuse. Furthermore there was a three-way interaction between profession (psychiatrist), MHLO ('Endogenous' causal beliefs) and diagnosis (schizophrenia). Thus psychiatrists with particularly strong bio-genetic causal beliefs were less likely to ask about abuse if clients were 'schizophrenic' than if they were depressed. So rigid causal beliefs must be a focus of training programmes.

The particular belief on which the controller of psychiatric training in Auckland some years ago blocked the introduction of our abuse policy is pervasive and damaging. The notion that mad people should not be believed when they tell of bad things happening to them has prevented countless distressed people from being heard, understood and offered appropriate help. Training programmes need to counter such myths with research-based facts. Reports of trauma by psychiatric patients, including those diagnosed psychotic, are actually highly reliable (Dill et al. 1991; Goodman et al. 1999; Meyer et al. 1996). Corroborating evidence for CSA reports by psychiatric patients have been found in 74 per cent (Herman and Schatzow 1987) and 82 per cent (Read et al. 2003) of cases. As seen earlier, psychiatric patients under-report rather than over-report abuse to mental health professionals. An important study, in the context of this book, found that 'The problem of incorrect allegations of sexual assaults was no different for schizophrenics than the general population' (Darves-Bornoz et al. 1995: 82).

Lack of training

In the New Zealand survey psychologists and psychiatrists reported that 76 per cent had received some training in how to ask about trauma, and 72 per cent had received training in how to respond to disclosures (psychologists 81 per cent, psychiatrists 61 per cent). Having received training was positively correlated to self-reported probability of taking a trauma history (Young et al. 2001). In another New Zealand study, of a variety of mental health professions, only 33 per cent reported having had training in trauma inquiry (medical staff 26 per cent, non-medical 52 per cent) and only 39 per cent had received training in responding to disclosures (medical 34 per cent, non-medical 52 per cent). Again, those with inquiry training were more likely to report that they knew how to ask, and to know whether their clients had been abused (Cavanagh et al. 2004).

A British study found that only 30 per cent of mental health staff had received training in the 'assessment and/or treatment of sexual abuse' (nurses 13 per cent, psychiatrists 33 per cent, psychologists 46 per cent). Of the psychiatrists who had received no training, 44 per cent stated that they had received 'sufficient training' (Lab et al. 2000). A US study of psychiatric residents found that only 28 per cent had received training in recognising or treating traumatic events such as domestic violence. Previous training was the best predictor of case identification and initiation of appropriate care (Currier et al. 1996).

Where training is voluntary, which is often the case, the fact that those who had been trained were those with the best clinical practice may reflect nothing more than the fact that individuals with enlightened attitudes and good information about abuse are more likely to seek out training. It seems, however, that training *can* increase the identification of trauma. A randomly selected group of US mental health staff received just a one-hour 'trauma orientation' lecture covering prevalence, impacts and issues around sensitive assessment. Those who received the training subsequently identified significantly higher levels of sexual and physical violence, including CSA (37 per cent versus 14 per cent), than those who did not receive the lecture, even though both groups were given the same structured interview tool (Currier and Briere 2000).

When asked what they would like included in an abuse training programme (Young et al. 2001), New Zealand clinicians most frequently suggested:

- what questions to ask
- when to ask
- how to ask so as not to distress clients
- how to ask specific client groups
- the effects of child abuse
- issues relating to false allegations.

Lack of policy or guidelines

In the New Zealand survey of psychologists and psychiatrists, only 15 per cent reported that their workplace had a policy addressing abuse inquiry (Young et al. 2001). However, there is a happy ending to the story which had begun with the blocking of an inpatient unit's attempt to introduce an abuse policy. For over a year clinicians, managers, service users and university staff later met to develop a policy for the whole of the District Health Board (DHB). As a result, in 2000 Auckland DHB added to its *Mental Health Service Policy and Procedure Manual* a 'Recommended Best Practice' document for 'Trauma and Sexual Abuse'. Its stated purpose was 'to ensure that routine mental health assessments include appropriate questions about sexual abuse/trauma, and that disclosure is sensitively managed'. Its two guiding principles are

1   Assessment of mental health clients must include questions about possible trauma/sexual abuse to ensure that appropriate support and therapy is made available.
2   Clinicians should routinely ask about history of trauma, especially occurring during the client's childhood.

It includes the crucially important statement: 'Clinical staff are required to undertake a one day skill based training to ensure that questioning techniques are appropriate' and mandates that the training covers

- prevalence and effects of abuse
- cultural and consumer perspectives

- learning to ask about abuse
- how to respond to a disclosure of abuse
- notetaking
- legal obligations
- resources available within Auckland DHB mental health services
- resources available in the community
- vicarious traumatisation/staff safety.

This training programme, based on the research summarised thus far, will be summarised later.

Policies without training may not be effective (and probably vice versa). Evidence of this is that of the first few cohorts of staff to receive the training, only 51 per cent had heard of the policy and only 22 per cent had read it (Cavanagh et al. 2004). Written policies need to be monitored by managers and senior clinicians. I know, from years of clinical experience, that reading policy manuals is not usually a clinician's top priority. (Or was it just me?)

Principles of training in abuse inquiry and response

Three overarching principles come before the eight specific principles listed below.

- Training should be mandatory either for all mental health staff within an agency or (less desirable but in some situations more practical) for all those conducting initial assessments.
- The training needs to be both skill and knowledge-based. All the prevalence and effects data in the world can leave an untrained staff member just as unconfident about how to actually 'do the job'. Skills training, such as role-plays, without using the available research to explain why it is so important to ask, can leave staff unmotivated to use their new skills.
- Any new training programme needs to take account of local circumstances and resources. Users of mental health services, who are slowly beginning to be included in service planning (Chamberlin 2004; Happell et al. 2003; Kent and Read 1998), should definitely be involved in developing policy, best practice guidelines, and training programmes in a given locality or service. Surveys of current practice and attitudes may be a useful component of the planning process, as there may be different barriers in, say, a non-government community-based agency than in a highly medicalised inpatient service.

I All clients must be asked

This is necessary because of the very high prevalence of abuse, across nearly all diagnostic categories (including psychosis). Therefore the current practice among some clinicians, of asking only those clients with certain symptoms (e.g. of PTSD) is inadequate. Particular emphasis must be placed, in training, on the need to ask those groups known to be less likely to be asked, namely men, older people and people with diagnoses of psychosis. To overcome ideological barriers it can be stressed that regardless of the causal beliefs one employs to explain the high numbers of abused patients in psychotic samples (causal, contributory or coincidental) the high numbers themselves mandate inquiry so that the trauma can be addressed if necessary.

The second reason for routine inquiry of all clients is the very low spontaneous disclosure rate documented above. Waiting for clients to tell you just doesn't work.

2 Ask specific/objective/behavioural questions

Training programmes should stress that asking 'Were you sexually [or physically] abused?' is an ineffective form of inquiry. Many clients will not have used that term in relation to their experiences. Questions should be about specific behavioural events. For example, 'As a child, did an adult ever hurt or punish you in a way that left a bruise, cut or scratches?' and 'As a child, did anyone ever do something sexual that made you feel uncomfortable?'

Trainees can be informed of the relevant research. Dill et al. (1991) found that general questions about abuse elicited only about half of the abuse identified by specific behavioural questions. Structured questionnaires (e.g. Bryer et al. 1987) or interview schedules (e.g. Briere 1999; Currier and Briere 2000) may be helpful. See Briere (1997) for a review of such instruments.

Obviously such questions should not be asked near the outset of an assessment, nor should they come 'out of the blue' with no preface or understandable context. The obvious context is a comprehensive psychosocial history, which naturally includes childhood. The abuse questions can be approached using a funnel from broad questions such as 'Tell me about your childhood' and 'What's your best memory of your childhood?' and 'And the worst memory?', via more focused questions, such as, 'How was discipline dealt with in your family?' to the specific questions described above. After covering childhood, similarly specific questions should be asked covering adulthood.

3 Ask at initial assessment

In our New Zealand survey, 62 per cent chose 'Once rapport has been established' as the most appropriate time to ask, but 47 per cent chose 'Usually on admission/initial assessment unless the client is too distressed' (participants could select more than one response). The reason for training staff to ask at initial assessment is that when this does not occur, it all too often never occurs later on (Read and Fraser 1998a). Training should stress that there are indeed good reasons for delaying inquiry, such as acute suicidality and current fla-grant psychosis, but in these circumstances the clinician conducting the initial assessment should clearly record that a trauma history has not been taken (and why) and take responsibility for following up when the client is less distressed. The tendency of some clinicians to wait for an imagined magic moment when rapport is just right should be challenged, not least with the point that for some clients the act of asking may be crucial in establishing rapport.

4 Awareness of types and prevalence of abuse

The research presented in this chapter should be summarised, to ensure sufficient motivation to ask.

5 Awareness of effects of abuse

One of the reasons for summarising this body of research is to discourage staff from playing the diagnostic-odds game in which they ask only if PTSD-type symptoms are present. It should be stressed that trauma and abuse have multiple sequelae which cross diagnostic boundaries.

6 Awareness of current clinical practice

Again the reason for briefly summarising the research presented above on this topic is to challenge complacency and thereby provide motivation for change.

7 Know how to respond to disclosures

Not knowing how to respond may be a reason for not asking in the first place. This is an understandable reason but not an acceptable one for a mental health professional. A one-day training programme should obviously not set out to train people to do therapy with abused clients; see Briere (2000) and McGregor (2001) for research-based guidelines for therapy. Training should be focused, instead, on how to respond at the moment the client discloses. Suggestions for this are summarised in the New Zealand training programme below.

8 Awareness of vicarious traumatisation

Another reason for not asking is fear (conscious or otherwise) of being dis-tressed by what you might hear. This may especially be the case for clinicians who have experienced trauma themselves. Training programmes must acknowledge this and encourage staff to use supervision and peer support groups (and, where necessary, personal therapy) to address the inevitable emotional consequences of being a competent mental health professional who does not shy away from trauma issues in their clients.

A New Zealand training programme

The programme described below takes the form of a one-day session. A two-day structure, allowing for follow-up and consolidation of learning, is probably preferable but it was anticipated that many staff would not be able to attend two sessions (because of rostering, high staff turnover etc.). Cost was another factor.

The session is conducted by a staff member of Auckland Rape Crisis and myself, with contributions from a consumer consultant and a Maori mental health clinician. It is offered four times a year and is attended, on average, by fourteen clinicians. Participants work in different units (inpatient, outpatient etc.) and belong to a range of professions (including relatively untrained support workers). The morning focuses on asking about trauma and the afternoon on responding to disclosures.

Asking

9.00–9.30 Introductions, groundrules and questionnaires

Participants introduce themselves, say where they work and what they are hoping to get out of the day (and anything they strongly want not to happen). Groundrules, such as confidentiality regarding personal information (but not about skills/knowledge acquired) and respectful listening to other participants etc., are generated by the group. A brief questionnaire may be administered at this point to obtain pre-training measures as part of evaluating the training.

9.30–10.00 'Setting the scene' brainstorm

Four small groups generate answers (on flipchart sheets) to one of the following questions:

- Why is it important to ask about abuse?
- What can happen if we don't ask about abuse?
- When is the best time to ask about abuse?
- Why do clinicians sometimes not ask about abuse?

The small groups summarise their answers to the larger group, who can add to the lists. These are then posted up as a backdrop for the next session.

10.00–10.30 Research summary (responding to brainstorm)

Summaries of three bodies of research literature are presented, linking the summaries to the answers already provided by the participants, and allowing a brief discussion period:

- Prevalence of sexual and physical abuse.
- Long-term effects of sexual and physical abuse (including psychosis). The need to ask all clients is stressed here, in the context of the broad range of symptoms and diagnoses associated with trauma.
- Current clinical practice in relation to abuse (covering low inquiry rates and reasons for that – including inappropriate fear of being accused of 'planting memories' as a result of media coverage of the 'recovered memory' debate). The findings that men and people diagnosed psychotic are particularly unlikely to be asked is emphasised. The timing issue is addressed here, including the research finding that if not asked about at admission, abuse usually never gets asked about later. Fear of upsetting clients is also addressed as a reason for sometimes not asking, and this leads into the next session.

10.30–10.50 Break

10.50–11.20 Consumer perspectives

This component can obviously vary in content and structure – but we believe it is essential to have a user perspective represented in person.

A user of mental health services summarises her interviews with other users about best ways to ask about, and respond to disclosures of, sexual abuse. The emphasis is on variability of clients' views about trauma and, therefore, the need for flexibility of response from clinicians, with the 'take home' message being 'throw away your text books and be a human being'. It is stressed that people attending a mental health service *expect* to be asked about adverse events in their lives.

11.20–11.40 Cultural perspectives

A Maori mental health practitioner summarises Maori perspectives on trauma, with a focus on similarities with European perspectives as well as differences – such as the need to offer Maori services/clinicians. (Again this component will vary according to locality.)

11.40–1.00 Role-plays: asking

An experienced clinician summarises the principles of when and how to ask (see above). This includes asking routinely as part of the childhood part of a psychosocial history, and 'funnelling' towards specific, behavioural questions (see above). The clinician then role-plays (for about ten minutes) asking about abuse, with one of the participants taking the part of a client. The role-play ends at the point where the client answers 'yes' to a specific question (the 'client' is asked not to disclose abuse to one of the more general – funnelling –

questions). The group then critiques the role-play, offering suggestions as to how they might have done it differently etc.

Participants then try out the task in pairs (simultaneously, without being observed). The group then re-forms to discuss the exercise.

1.00–2.00 Lunch break

Responding

2.00–2.15 Resources and procedures

The need to know about resources for staff and clients, within the DHB and in the community, is stressed as a prerequisite for effective responding. These include trained trauma/abuse clinicians/units within the DHB and agencies and services in the community. This information is provided for all participants to take back to their workplaces and disseminate. The DHB policy (see above) and procedures (e.g. regarding notetaking, issues about reporting to legal/protection agencies, etc.) are outlined.

2.15–2.30 Research summary: current responding practice

A summary of the research on low levels of adequate clinician response is presented.

2.30–2.50 Brainstorm: best and worst ways to respond

Participants are asked to write on a flipchart one good and one appalling way to respond to a disclosure of trauma. This is usually a humorous time (akin to the 'World's Worst' game in the *Whose Line is it Anyway?* TV show), but trainers sometimes have to come up with something awful first to 'give permission' to the participants. (Some participants offer actual things they have heard other clinicians say. This can temporarily remove the humour from the room!)

2.50–3.10 Principles of responding to disclosures

The clinician-trainer summarises six principles of effective responding, as follows.

1 Not necessary to gather lots of detailed information

It is not necessary, or desirable, on first being told by a client that they have been abused, to immediately gather details of that abuse.

2 Affirm that it was a positive thing that they told you

It *is* important that the client feels that the staff member has understood the importance of what has been disclosed and that this will, if the client wishes, be returned to later.

People have a range of responses to disclosing abuse. They might feel anger, shame, self-blame, fear, relief, a lack of connection with their feelings, appear numb, or feel ambivalent about the abuse. For the survivor, what is important at this point is that the fact they have disclosed is met with an immediate and positive response from the staff member.

Acknowledge that abuse can sometimes be difficult to talk about but that it is a positive thing to talk about it. It is also important to gauge how the person is feeling about disclosing rather than making judgements about what they should be feeling. It is important to normalise the disclosure by using statements like:

> 'In my experience talking with people about this, people often find that although it is difficult, it can often be really helpful to talk about it. How has it been / is it for you talking about this now?'

Acknowledge how the client is reacting.

Survivors of abuse often experience self-blame. If self-blame does occur it is important to affirm that self-blame is a common reaction, and, if appropriate, to state that any abuse they have experienced is not their fault.

3 Offer support

It is important to discuss possible treatment/support for effects of the disclosed abuse. Ask about previous disclosure and support/treatment. Examples of ways of asking if the client wishes to have counselling include: 'Do you have any support for how you feel about what has happened? Some people find talking to a counsellor to be very supportive. If you are interested we can find a counsellor for your support' or 'Would you like to talk to someone about how you feel about it all now?' or (if you are trained and able to offer counselling yourself) 'Would you like us to talk about that at some point?'

4 Check current safety

Ask about any ongoing abuse. Ask, also, about any possible ongoing risk to others from the same perpetrator. For example, if the child abuse was perpetrated by a teacher, priest, etc., ask if that person is still in contact with children.

5 Check emotional state at end of session

6 Offer immediate follow-up/check in

Before ending the session, ask the person how they feel after talking about the abuse: 'Telling someone about what happened can sometimes bring up a lot of feelings. How are you feeling about having told me?' or 'If you feel upset about what we have talked about today, later this evening you can talk to [staff member's name/crisis phone line] about how you are feeling'.

Assist clients to identify their own support systems: 'Do you have someone that is a real support person that you could talk to or call if you needed to?'

3.10–4.10 Role-plays: responding

The clinician again goes first followed by practice in pairs and then discussion in the large group. The clinician role-play for responding involves several pauses in which the trainees are asked for suggestions about what to do next. (This acknowledges that there are judgements to be made based on the state of the person, and involves the group in the process.)

4.10–4.20 Vicarious traumatisation

The possible emotional effects of being a competent mental health professional who asks about abuse and trauma are named. These include being distressed about individual stories, depressed about hearing so many, and becoming emotionally numb when hearing disclosures as an understandable defence to being emotionally overwhelmed. Participants are encouraged to seek out supervision, peer supervision or to form support groups with other staff.

Finally, participants are thanked for choosing to take part in the training and for choosing to undertake work that is so emotionally demanding and so important to so many people.

4.20–4.30 Wrap-up and evaluation

Participants complete a brief questionnaire about what they found helpful/unhelpful about the content and process of the training programme.

For a more detailed description of this training programme, please email me: j.read@auckland.ac.nz

Programme evaluation

On the evaluation sheet completed at the end of the training day 94 per cent of the first eighty-five participants responded 'Yes' to 'Did you benefit from the training today?' On a Likert scale (1 = 'strongly agree', 6 = 'strongly disagree') the mean response to 'The training programme increased my confidence in my ability to inquire about sexual abuse' was 1.7. The mean response to the item about confidence in ability to respond was 1.6; 97 per cent agreed to some extent (1, 2 or 3) with both of these items (Cavanagh et al. 2004).

There was no significant variation in the extent to which participants found each of the programme's components useful. On a Likert scale (1 = 'very useful', 4 = 'not at all useful') all components elicited a mean score below 2. The consumer perspectives session produced a mean score of 1.3, as did the written take-home material about referral resources and procedures (e.g. how to ask/respond, when to refer, when to report to legal authourities).

A two-month follow-up revealed significant ($p<0.001$) increases in the beliefs: 'I have the knowledge and skills to inquire about sexual abuse in a sensitive and effective manner' and 'I have the knowledge and skills to respond appropriately to disclosures of sexual abuse'. The percentage stating that diagnosis influences whether they ask fell from 53 per cent to 37 per cent (not statistically significant) and the percentage of CSA disclosures thought to be psychotic delusions fell from 6 per cent to 3 per cent ($p<0.05$). Even after this relatively short follow-up period one-third were already able to cite specific examples of improvements in actual clinical practice (Cavanagh et al. 2004).

Conclusion

The relationship between childhood trauma and psychosis has been ignored by too many clinicians for too long. The public, that is to say our clients, believe there is a relationship. They expect to be asked what has happened to them in their lives. We should ask. We should know how to do so sensitively and confidently. We should know how to respond calmly and helpfully. We have a professional and ethical responsibility to seek out training.

Not asking colludes with broader societal forces that operate to deny or minimise the frequency and importance of child abuse, and also with an ideology within mental health services (reductionistic biological psychiatry) that promotes the silly idea that the problems of people diagnosed psychotic have nothing to do with what happened to them as children. Asking will save huge amounts of money via the provision of appropriate treatment that can curtail a lifetime of expensive readmissions (Newmann et al. 1998). Asking meets the expectations, and needs, of the people we are employed to assist.

'I think there was an assumption that I had a mental illness and you know because I wasn't saying anything about my abuse I'd suffered no-one knew.'

'My life went haywire from thereon in [after being abused]. I went into a spiral of ... I just can't describe it. I just wish they would have said "What happened to you? What happened?" But they didn't.'

(Lothian and Read 2002: 101)

Acknowledgements

I would like to acknowledge Rachel Harrison and Sheryl Maung of Auckland Rape Crisis, Debra Lampshire of Mind and Body Consultants, and Ainsleigh Cribb, a Maori mental health practitioner. It has been a privilege, and lots of fun, to work with you all in the training programme described in this chapter. I must also thank the managers and staff of Auckland DHB mental health services for having the wisdom and courage to introduce the policy guidelines and training progamme.

References

Acierno, R., Resnick, H., and Kilpatrick, G. (1997) Prevalence rates, case identification, and risk factors for sexual assault, physical assault and domestic violence in men and women. *Behavioural Medicine, 23*, 53–76.

Aderhold, V., and Gottwalz, E. (2004) Family therapy and schizophrenia: Replacing ideology with openness. In J. Read, L. Mosher and R. Bentall (eds), *Models of madness: Psychological, social and biological approaches to schizophrenia* (pp. 335–348). London: Brunner-Routledge.

Agar, K., and Read, J. (2002) What happens when people disclose sexual or physical abuse to staff at a community mental health centre? *International Journal of Mental Health Nursing, 11*, 70–79.

Agar, K., Read, J., and Bush, J.-M. (2002) Identification of abuse histories in a community mental health centre. *Journal of Mental Health, 11*, 533–543.

Bebbington, P., Bhugra, D., Brugha, T., Singleton, N., Farrell, M., Jenkins, R., et al. (2004) Psychosis, victimization and childhood disadvantage: Evidence from the second British national survey on psychiatric morbidity. *British Journal of Psychiatry, 185*, 220–226.

Beck, J., and van der Kolk, B. (1987) Reports of childhood incest and current behavior of chronically hospitalized psychotic women. *American Journal of Psychiatry, 144*, 1474–1476.

Bentall, R. (2003) *Madness explained: Psychosis and human nature*. London: Penguin.

Boney-McCoy, S., and Finkelhor, D. (1996) Is youth victimization related to trauma symptoms and depression after controlling for prior symptoms and family relationships? *Journal of Consulting and Clinical Psychology, 64*, 1406–1416.

Brabin, P., and Berah, E. (1995) Dredging up past traumas: Harmful or helpful? *Psychiatry, Psychology, and the Law, 2*, 165–171.

Briere, J. (1997) *Psychological assessment of adult posttraumatic states.* Washington, DC: American Psychological Association.

Briere, J. (1999) Psychological trauma and the psychiatric emergency room. In G. Currier (ed.) *Recent developments in emergency psychiatry. New directions for mental health services* series (pp. 43–51). San Francisco, CA: Jossey-Bass.

Briere, J. (2000) Treating adult survivors of severe childhood abuse and neglect: Further developments of an integrative model. In J. Myers, L Berliner, J. Briere, C. Hendrix, C. Jenny and T. Reids (eds), *The APSAC handbook on child maltreatment* (2nd edn, pp. 175–204). Newbury Park, CA: Sage.

Briere, J., and Zaidi, L. (1989) Sexual abuse histories and sequelae in female psychiatric emergency room patients. *American Journal of Psychiatry, 146,* 1602–1606.

Briere, J., Woo, R., McRae, B., Foltz, J., and Sitzman, R. (1997) Lifetime victimization history, demographics, and clinical status in female psychiatric emergency room patients. *Journal of Nervous and Mental Disease, 185,* 95–101.

Bryer, J., Nelson, B., Miller, J., and Krol, P. (1987) Childhood sexual and physical abuse as factors in psychiatric illness. *American Journal Psychiatry, 144,* 1426–1430.

Cavanagh, M., Read, J., and New, B. (2004) Childhood abuse inquiry and response: A New Zealand training programme. *New Zealand Journal of Psychology, 33,* 137–144.

Chamberlin, J. (2004) User-run services. In J. Read, L. Mosher and R. Bentall (eds), *Models of madness: Psychological, social and biological approaches to schizophrenia* (pp. 283–290). Hove: Brunner-Routledge.

Craine, L., Henson, C., Colliver, J., and MacLean, D. (1988) Prevalence of a history of sexual abuse among female psychiatric patients in a state hospital system. *Hospital and Community Psychiatry, 39,* 300–304.

Currier, G., and Briere, J. (2000) Trauma orientation and detection of violence histories in the psychiatric emergency service. *Journal of Nervous and Mental Disease, 188,* 622–624.

Currier, G., Barthauer, L., Begier, E., and Bruce, M. (1996) Training and experience of psychiatric residents in identifying domestic violence. *Psychiatric Services, 47,* 529–530.

Darves-Bornoz, J.-M., Lempérière, T., Degiovanni, A., and Gaillard, P. (1995) Sexual victimization in women with schizophrenia and bipolar disorder. *Social Psychiatry and Psychiatric Epidemiology, 30,* 78–84.

Dill, D., Chu, J., Grob, M., and Eisen, S. (1991) The reliability of abuse history reports: A comparison of two inquiry formats. *Comprehensive Psychiatry, 32,* 166–169.

Eilenberg, J., Fullilove, M., Goldman, R., and Mellman, L. (1996) Quality and use of trauma histories obtained from psychiatric outpatients through mandated inquiry. *Psychiatric Services, 47,* 165–169.

Elliott, D. (1997) Traumatic events: Prevalence and delayed recall in the general population. *Journal of Consulting and Clinical Psychology, 65,* 811–820.

Fergusson, D., Horwood, J., and Lynskey, M. (1996) Childhood sexual abuse and psychiatric disorder in young adulthood: II. Psychiatric outcomes of childhood sexual abuse. *Journal of the American Academy of Child and Adolescent Psychiatry, 34,* 1365–1374.

Finkelhor, D. (1990) Early and long-term effects of child sexual abuse: An update. *Professional Psychology: Research and Practice, 21*, 325–350.

Friedman, L., Samet, J., Roberts, M., Hudlin, M., and Hans, P. (1992) Inquiry about victimization experiences: A survey of patient preferences and physician practices. *Archives of Internal Medicine, 152*, 1186–1190.

Friedman, S., and Harrison, G. (1984) Sexual histories, attitudes and behavior of schizophrenic and normal women. *Archives of Sexual Behaviour, 13*, 555–567.

Goff, D., Brotman, W., Kindlon, D., Waites, M., and Amico, E. (1991) Self-reports of child abuse in chronically psychotic patients. *Psychiatry Research, 37*, 73–80.

Goodman, L., Rosenberg, S., Mueser, K., and Drake, R. (1997) Physical and sexual assault history in women with serious mental illness: Prevalence, correlates, treatment and future directions. *Schizophrenia Bulletin, 23*, 685–686.

Goodman, L., Thompson, K., Weinfurt, K., Corl, S., Acker, P., Mueser, K., et al. (1999) Reliability of reports of violent victimization and PTSD among men and women with serious mental illness. *Journal of Traumatic Stress, 12*, 587–599.

Goodwin, J., Attias, R., McCarty, T., Chandler, S., and Romanik, R. (1988) Reporting by adult psychiatric patients of childhood sexual abuse. *American Journal of Psychiatry, 145*, 1183.

Hammersley, P., Dias, A., Todd, G., Bowen-Jones, K., Reilly, B., and Bentall, R. (2003) Childhood traumas and hallucinations in bipolar affective disorder. *British Journal of Psychiatry, 182*, 543–547.

Happell, B., Pinikahana, J., and Roper, C. (2003) Changing attitudes: The role of a consumer advocate in the education of postgraduate psychiatric nursing students. *Archives of Psychiatric Nursing, 17*, 67–76.

Herman, J., and Schatzow, E. (1987) Recovery and verification of childhood sexual trauma. *Psychoanalytic Psychology, 4*, 1–14.

Holmes, G., and Offen, L. (1996) Clinicians' hypotheses regarding clients' problems: Are they less likely to hypothesise sexual abuse in male clients compared to female clients? *Child Abuse and Neglect, 20*, 493–501.

Holmes, G., Offen, L., and Waller, G. (1997) See no evil, hear no evil, speak no evil: Why do relatively few male victims of childhood sexual abuse receive help for abuse-related issues in adulthood? *Clinical Psychology Review, 17*, 69–88.

Hurst, C., MacDonald, J., Say, J., and Read, J. (2003) Routine questioning about non-consenting sex: A survey of practice in Australasian sexual health clinics. *International Journal of STD and AIDS, 14*, 32–36.

Jacobson, A., and Richardson, B. (1987) Assault experiences of 100 psychiatric inpatients: Evidence of the need for routine inquiry. *American Journal of Psychiatry, 144*, 508–513.

Jacobson, A., Koehler, J., and Jones-Brown, C. (1987) The failure of routine assessment to detect histories of assault experienced by psychiatric patients. *Hospital and Community Psychiatry, 38*, 386–389.

Janssen, I., Krabbendam, L., Bak, M., Hanssen, M., Vollebergh, W., de Graaf, R., and Van Os, J. (2004). Childhood abuse as a risk factor for psychotic experiences. *Acta Psychiatrica Scandinavica, 109*, 38–45.

Kendler, K., Bulik, S., Silberg, J., Hettema, J., Myers, J., and Prescott, C. (2000) Childhood sexual abuse and adult psychiatric and substance use disorders in women. *Archives of General Psychiatry, 57*, 953–959.

Kent, H., and Read, J. (1998) Measuring consumer participation in mental health services: Are attitudes related to professional orientation? *International Journal of Social Psychiatry, 44*, 295–310.

Lab, D., Feigenbaum, J., and De Silva, P. (2000) Mental health professionals' attitudes and practices towards male childhood sexual abuse. *Child Abuse and Neglect, 24*, 391–409.

Lanktree, C., Briere, J., and Zaidi, L. (1991) Incidence and impact of sexual abuse in a child outpatient sample: The role of direct inquiry. *Child Abuse and Neglect, 15*, 447–453.

Lipschitz, D., Kaplan, M., Sorkenn, J., Faedda, G., Chorney, P., and Asnis, G. (1996) Prevalence and characteristics of physical and sexual abuse among psychiatric outpatients. *Psychiatric Services, 47*, 189–191.

Lothian, J., and Read, J. (2002) Asking about abuse during mental health assessments: Clients' views and experiences. *New Zealand Journal of Psychology, 31*, 98–103.

McGregor, K. (2001) *Therapy guidelines: Adult survivors of sexual abuse.* Wellington, New Zealand: Accident Compensation Corporation.

McGregor, K. (2003) It's a two-way thing: Women survivors of child sexual abuse describe their therapy experiences. Unpublished doctoral dissertation. University of Auckland, New Zealand.

Meyer, I., Muenzenmaier, K., Cancienne, J., and Struening, E. (1996) Reliability and validity of a measure of sexual and physical abuse among women with serious mental illness. *Child Abuse and Neglect, 20*, 213–219.

Mills, A. (1993) Helping male victims of sexual abuse. *Nursing Standard, 7*, 36–39.

Mitchell, D., Grindel, C., and Laurenzano, C. (1996) Sexual abuse assessment on admission by nursing staff in general hospital psychiatric settings. *Psychiatric Services, 47*, 159–164.

Muenzenmaier, K., Meyer, I., Struening, E., and Ferber, J. (1993) Childhood abuse and neglect among women outpatients with chronic mental illness. *Hospital and Community Psychiatry, 44*, 666–670.

Mullen, P., Martin, J., Anderson, J., Romans, S., and Herbison, G. (1993) Childhood sexual abuse and mental health in adult life. *British Journal of Psychiatry, 163*, 721–732.

Murray, E., and Siegal, D. (1994) Emotional processing in vocal and written expression of feelings about traumatic experiences. *Journal of Traumatic Stress, 7*, 391–405.

Newmann, J., Greenley, D., Sweeney, G., and Van Dien, G. (2000) Abuse histories, severe mental illness, and the cost of care. In B. Levin, A. Blanch and A. Jennings (eds) *Women's mental health services: A public health perspective* (pp. 279–308). Thousand Oaks, CA: Sage.

Read, J. (1997) Child abuse and psychosis: A literature review and implications for professional practice. *Professional Psychology: Research and Practice, 28*, 448–456.

Read, J. (1998) Child abuse and severity of disturbance among adult psychiatric inpatients. *Child Abuse and Neglect, 22*, 359–368.

Read, J., and Argyle, N. (1999) Hallucinations, delusions and thought disorders among adult psychiatric inpatients with a history of child abuse. *Psychiatric Services, 50*, 1467–1472.

Read, J., and Fraser, A. (1998a) Abuse histories of psychiatric inpatients: To ask or not to ask? *Psychiatric Services, 49*, 355–359.

Read, J., and Fraser, A. (1998b) Staff response to abuse histories of psychiatric inpatients. *Australian and New Zealand Journal of Psychiatry, 32*, 206–213.

Read, J., and Haslam, N. (2004) Public opinion: Bad things happen and can drive you crazy. In J. Read, L. Mosher and R. Bentall (eds), *Models of madness: Psychological, social and biological approaches to schizophrenia* (pp. 133–146). Hove: Brunner-Routledge.

Read, J., Agar, K., Barker-Collo, S., Davies, E., and Moskowitz, A. (2001a) Assessing suicidality in adults: Integrating childhood trauma as a major risk factor. *Professional Psychology: Research and Practice, 32*, 367–372.

Read, J., Perry, B., Moskowitz, A., and Connolly, J. (2001b) The contribution of early traumatic events to schizophrenia in some patients: A traumagenic neurodevelopmental model. *Psychiatry, 64*, 319–345.

Read, J., Agar, K., Argyle, N., and Aderhold, V. (2003) Sexual and physical abuse during childhood and adulthood as predictors of hallucinations, delusions and thought disorder. *Psychology and Psychotherapy: Theory, Research and Practice, 76*, 1–22.

Read, J., Goodman, L., Morrison, A., Ross, C., and Aderhold, V. (2004a) Childhood trauma, loss and stress. In J. Read, L. Mosher and R. Bentall (eds), *Models of madness: Psychological, social and biological approaches to schizophrenia* (pp. 223–252). Hove: Brunner-Routledge.

Read, J., Mosher, L., and Bentall, R. (eds) (2004b). *Models of madness: Psychological, social and biological approaches to schizophrenia.* Hove: Brunner-Routledge.

Read, J., Seymour, F., and Mosher, L. (2004c) Unhappy families. In J. Read, L. Mosher and R. Bentall (eds), *Models of madness: Psychological, social and biological approaches to schizophrenia* (pp. 253–268). Hove: Brunner-Routledge.

Rogers, A., Pilgrim, D., and Lacey, R. (1993) *Issues in mental health: Experiencing psychiatry, users' views of services.* London: Macmillan.

Rose, S., Peabody, C., and Stratigeas, B. (1991) Undetected abuse among intensive case management clients. *Hospital Community Psychiatry, 42*, 499–503.

Ross, C., Anderson, G., and Clark, P. (1994) Childhood abuse and positive symptoms of schizophrenia. *Hospital and Community Psychiatry, 45*, 489–491.

Sansonnet-Hayden, H., Haley, G., Marriage, K., and Fine, S. (1987) Sexual abuse and psychopathology in hospitalized adolescents. *Journal of the American Academy of Child and Adolescent Psychiatry, 26*, 753–757.

Shew, R., and Hurst, C. (1993) Should the question 'Have you been sexually abused?' be asked routinely when taking a sexual health history? *Venerology, 6*, 19–20.

Sugg, N., and Inui, T. (1992) Primary care physicians' response to domestic violence. *Journal of the American Medical Association, 267*, 157–160.

Swett, C., Surrey, J., and Cohen, C. (1990) Sexual and physical abuse histories and psychiatric symptoms among male psychiatric outpatients. *American Journal of Psychiatry, 147*, 632–636.

Thompson, A., and Kaplan, C. (1999) Emotionally abused children presenting to child psychiatry clinics. *Child Abuse Neglect, 23*, 191–196.

Wurr, C., and Partridge, I. (1996) The prevalence of a history of childhood sexual abuse in an acute adult inpatient population. *Child Abuse and Neglect, 20*, 867–872.

Young, M., Read, J., Barker-Collo, S., and Harrison, R. (2001) Evaluating and overcoming barriers to taking abuse histories. *Professional Psychology: Research and Practice, 32*, 407–414.

Chapter 10

CBT for traumatic psychosis

Pauline Callcott and Douglas Turkington

Introduction

Kingdon and Turkington (1999) noted the diverse nature of the phenomenology of schizophrenia and argued for the existence of separate syndromes within the schizophrenia spectrum. They suggested five subgroups based on a review of cognitive behavioural therapy (CBT) notes and case formulations. These postulated subgroups included sensitivity disorder, catatonia, anxiety psychosis, drug-induced psychosis and traumatic psychosis (see Table 10.1). It was suggested by Kingdon and Turkington (1999) that the basic CBT for psychosis manuals would have to be adapted with new techniques to work with each subgroup.

This chapter will draw together the elements of the traumatic psychosis subtype with clinical case examples that cover different aspects of the presentations. There will be an attempt to provide recommendations for CBT interventions on a formulation-based approach. Models from CBT in PTSD as well as in psychosis are blended to produce some new directions in the psychological treatment of this group of clients whose psychotic symptoms are often resistant to conventional treatments.

A rationale for using CBT for traumatic psychosis

Mueser et al. (1998) noted high levels of PTSD symptoms among individuals with severe mental illness. They reported that 98 per cent of those people with a diagnosis of illness had a history of trauma with 48 per cent of these meeting criteria for PTSD. Romme and Escher (1989) found that 70 per cent of people who heard voices developed their hallucinations following a traumatic event. It is well established that CBT for PTSD has good efficacy (Department of Health (DOH) 2001; Ehlers and Clark 2000; Roth and Fonagy 1999). CBT for individuals with a diagnosis of schizophrenia is also well established as an effective treatment modality. Reviews of the efficacy of CBT in schizophrenia have been positive (Pilling et al. 2002; Rector and Beck 2001) with the effect size in residual positive symptoms being large at end of therapy (ES = 0.65)

Table 10.1 Characteristics of traumatic psychosis

- Content of hallucinations – abusive, violent or sexual.
- In the second person.
- Commanding – e.g. kill yourself/kill your children.
- Perpetuated by increased arousal and avoidance.
- Repetitive and distressing with fluctuating insight.
- Association with PTSD e.g. sexual abuse or assault.
- Depression linked to suicidal and depressive thoughts.
- Response to antipsychotic medication is less than in other subgroups, often resulting in high-dose treatment and polypharmacy.

with more gains over time (ES = 0.93) (Gould et al. 2001). The positive results in research settings are cost-effective (Healy et al. 1998) and also appear to translate to clinical practice (Turkington et al. 2002). Treatment resistant schizophrenia is relatively common with between 20 and 30 per cent of people with a diagnosis of chronic schizophrenia demonstrating very little symptomatic response to adequate trials of conventional or atypical antipsy-chotic medications (Conley and Buchanan 1997). Of that group, those people whose psychotic symptoms linked to trauma appear to have a particularly poor response to medication alone. In addition Williams-Keeler et al. (1994) described a higher suicide rate when the conditions of PTSD and psychosis coexisted. Epidemiological research supports the hypothesis of a clear link between psychotic symptoms and earlier trauma (McGorry et al. 1991; Meuser et al. 1998). The prevalence rates using DSM-III-R criteria (American Psychiatric Association 1987) for PTSD in these studies are 52 per cent and 98 per cent, leading one of the authors to conclude that psychosis may be indeed a response to trauma (McGorry et al. 1991). Work by Holmes and Steel (2004) on schizotypy and by Allen et al. (1997) on dissociation has explored particular vulnerabilities to developing psychosis as a response to trauma. In a combination of patient and analogue studies, Morrison and colleagues are exploring this link further (Frame and Morrison 2001). Trauma can effect the psychotic presentation in three ways. First, is by the influence of early childhood trauma (Ross et al. 1994). The second is by the trauma entailed in receiving a diagnosis of psychosis and subsequent invasive treatments (Jackson and Birchwood 1996). The third instance is of trauma experienced as a result of increased vulnerability to victimisation (Walsh et al. 2003). One of the main problems in traumatic psychosis presentations is that PTSD is often undiagnosed (Read et al. 2001), untreated and the indi-vidual and professionals involved do not always make a link between trauma and the presenting symptoms (Morrison et al. 2003; Young et al. 2001). Ellason and Ross (1997) suggest that a type of schizophrenia characterised by positive symptoms is trauma induced. The literature suggests there is much to be learned about the relationship between the symptoms of PTSD and psychosis and that formulating those links with the individual can lead to sustained therapeutic gains (Morrison et al. 2003).

The aim of this chapter is to describe detailed investigations of symptom change in PTSD and psychosis as well as adapting appropriate therapeutic interventions to individualised formulations. This could enable us to optimise the delivery of future CBT to maximise the likelihood of sustained effects to a group who do not normally respond to antipsychotics alone. There are a number of personal factors that could mediate or moderate successful outcomes at the cognitive, behavioural and relationship levels, and these case studies will offer detailed scrutiny at each level, as well as investigating how the levels interact.

Whether the trauma can be seen as a factor in the development of psychosis, or whether it is seen as a factor to be treated as a separate diagnosis, is in many cases unclear. It would make sense to develop a formulation-based approach that will increase understanding, aid collaboration and reduce symptoms. In relation to working clinically with individuals with chronic PTSD, Ehlers and Clark (2000) emphasised other emotional 'hotspots', such as guilt. This has helped to refine reliving techniques to more than just exposure to fear and to develop specific cognitive approaches. In survivors of child sexual abuse (CSA) and early trauma, Smucker et al. (1999) hypothesised that exposure would not be enough and schema change models would need to be used because of the earlier nature of the trauma. He developed a method of imaginal exposure and rescripting. Rusch et al. (2000) have demonstrated that it is an effective treatment in PTSD.

Client examples

CBT techniques for psychosis and PTSD are described below in relation to the individuals presenting with characteristics of traumatic psychosis.

CSA and schizophrenia

Tom, 28, had a history of psychotic symptoms from the age of 12 and was referred for CBT. He reported experiencing command hallucinations instructing him to engage in ritualistic behaviour. Tom was diagnosed as suffering from schizophrenia with delusions. He attributed the origin of these voices to demons and believed that if he did not engage in rituals, a member of his family would be sent to hell.

These experiences continued throughout adolescence and he became obsessed with books on the occult. He had many admissions to hospital. Tom was sexually abused throughout his teenage years and was also bullied at school. Tom did not tell anyone that he had been sexually abused from the age of 5 by his father until he began experiencing visual hallucinations. At the beginning of therapy his problem list included paranoid feelings when outside the home, avoidance of social settings and compulsive rituals both within and outside the home. He heard commanding voices and coped with the anxiety of these by undertaking rituals.

Initial CBT sessions focused on reformulating symptoms as being explained by the experience of abuse and PTSD symptomatology was discussed. Normalising of the voices as being linked in tone and content to the abuse helped Tom to occasionally respond less by excessive checking.

Neutralising behaviours, including excessive checking, were conceptualised as maintaining paranoid feelings and flashbacks. 'Visual hallucinations' were reframed as 'flashbacks' to his father's face. 'Safety behaviours' such as repeatedly checking the clock were explained as being a factor in anxiety maintenance and a possible trigger for recurring flashbacks.

Three sessions of 'reliving' helped to place the sexual abuse in the past and changed the degree of belief in the thought 'I was to blame' from 80 per cent to 10 per cent.

In the second phase of therapy, improvement in chronic sleep disturbance also led to a reduction in alcohol intake. Tom reduced the amount of times he checked the clock at night and stopped sleeping so much into the day by setting the alarm then turning the clock to the wall. A subsequent focus of treatment involved weighing the evidence around automatic thoughts when outside of the home. This decreased paranoia and consequently reduced some of the ritualistic behaviour that, Tom began to notice, drew attention to him. Gangs around the local shop were seen as 'just hanging around' rather than being 'out to get him'.

In the third phase of therapy we looked at the impact of the bullying relationships that Tom had experienced throughout his life. This began with his father but also occurred at school and in psychiatric care. Tom was able to practise assertiveness techniques within our sessions via role-play and that helped him to regain aspects of his social life that he had been avoiding. The formulation revealed an extreme curtailment of many activities because of the fear of bumping into a particular former resident of a care home, where they had both been resident some years before. We set up some behavioural experiments around initiating social contacts and rehearsed in session what could be said to this person should he come into contact with him.

Here the targets of therapy involved a reduction in flashbacks as well as psychotic symptoms as a means of reducing symptomatology. Consolidation of the therapy also led to a further regaining of life activities. Tom had very much accepted that he experienced these symptoms because of the illness of schizophrenia, and that he could do very little about it apart from take medication. A CBT formulation offered an alternative explanation (within the PTSD model) for many of his symptoms and he was able to make gains in improving the quality of his life. Symptomatically he reduced the distressing impact of his voices and eradicated flashbacks and visual hallucinations. Negative symptoms were also improved.

In summary, therapy for this client was influenced by PTSD models described by Ehlers and Clark (2000) as well as using a normalising rationale around auditory and visual hallucinations. Behavioural experiments were particularly effective, drawn from knowledge of other anxiety models. Crucially, the therapy was tailored to the individual via a formulation rather than a DSM diagnosis. The issue of 'when to ask' is a matter for debate because it could be argued that if the right questions had been asked when Tom was first seen, the history and treatment would have looked a lot different. This is pertinent to early intervention diagnosis, but with this individual the time seemed right for him later, once the visual hallucinations started. The link to the effects of being sexually abused as a child was then much easier for Tom to accept.

Delusions and 'false memories'

With this next client a different approach was taken, involving a long process of developing a formulation that was continuously helping to draw links between symptoms and trauma history (Fowler 1997).

Harriet is a 28-year-old woman with a six-year history of delusional disorder. She managed her day-to-day life fairly well and played in a folk band. She was studying gender studies at university and had a live-in partner. However, she had a complex paranoid delusional system, which had led to several hospital admissions. She specifically requested CBT for her psychotic symptoms, which were exacerbated by binge drinking. A review of specific situations showed that the paranoid beliefs were a consequence of strong emotion in social situations, in particular playing at the folk group. Harriet would begin to notice thoughts such as 'They know about my father and the IRA'. As paranoia increased, drinking escalated to the point that Harriet was continuing to make connections in a complex delusional system involving her father, the IRA and Margaret Thatcher. She would leave the club in a very distressed state with her paranoia increased and return home.

We approached this pattern of emotional distress and increased delusional thought in two ways. We explored the cycle and made interventions at a thought-challenging level. Eventually, as she became more skilled at stepping back from situations using mood diary work, Harriet made the link that these thoughts were given a strength of meaning by the associated increase in emotion. We also tried several behavioural experiments to provide immediate symptom relief.

As Harriet became more engaged in the CBT process, we were able to track back to some of the origins of her delusional beliefs by using a time line. This proved a useful method of testing the validity of her memories, particularly as she had come to therapy wondering, because of what seemed like real memories, if her father had sexually abused her. As we built up the memory of situations and attaching them to episodes in time, she started to make sense of some of the origins of her delusions. Being abused by her father in a cave while Margaret Thatcher stood by seemed like a real and graphic memory. We traced it back to being in a cave by the sea; she had been lost from her mother but her father couldn't have been there. We were able to do this with several instances. We likened her delusional system to a strong tree with many interconnecting branches; we needed to get back to the root of these to understand the seed from which the 'memory' had grown.

The therapy process and therapeutic alliance were extremely important. The strong emotion Harriet experienced in relation to her parents stemmed from their divorce and the subsequent change in her lifestyle as a young child of 3. As she grew older she became increasingly angry with her father for treating her less favourably than her half-sibling and we talked about many instances of this occurring. Harriet's relationship with her father deteriorated completely after a babysitter employed by her father raped her and he apparently did not believe her.

The therapy process uncovered and explored anger towards her mother for having her sectioned under the Mental Health Act 1983 (MHA), and to her father for not believing her. This strong emotion, we hypothesised, seemed to be maintaining the memories and delusional system. Memory fragments were therefore pieced together to work out their origin. This coupled with changing the meaning and attribution of thoughts and behavioural experiments provided real symptomatic relief. This approach shares much in common with the approach adopted by Fowler et al. (1995) where the relationship and the formulation draw links that have not been previously made by the patient to the trauma experience and the origins of the delusional system.

A combination of voices and delusions

Jake had a complex delusional system that was grandiose in nature. Although thinking about these beliefs could be pleasant, it interfered with daily functioning, particularly sleep. He suffered daily from what he described as 'mental pain' from voices. This is illustrated in Figure 10.1.

The voices were described as various people that he had known in the past. Some could be critical, some were experienced as mental images of unpleasant past events, such as his very first experience of hearing voices after a hypnotherapy session, or his memories of hospital admissions. He had been sectioned several times and had attempted suicide on a couple

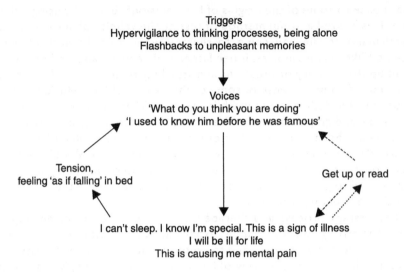

Figure 10.1 Formulation diagram: Based on Morrison's (1998) model of auditory hallucination.
Source: British Journal of Clinical Psychology, 42: 343. © The British Psychological Society.

of occasions. These we reframed as flashbacks to traumatic experiences in relation to his experience. The therapy approach for Jake was to continue to make connections with his experience of psychiatric care in his late teens and early twenties, the flashbacks and the content of his voices. We did not focus on the delusional system specifically, but on rating these beliefs using the Psychotic Symptoms Rating Scales (PSYRATS) (Haddock et al. 1999) his strength of belief in this reduced. He started to describe thoughts relating to this delusional system as a way of escaping from the unpleasant voices and flashbacks and could separate himself from the thoughts involved in it. 'I know I'm not really a famous actor but sometimes I think I must be.' He even conducted his own behavioural experiment unprompted by the therapy and checked for his namesake on the internet to check for a likeness. There was an immediate experience of low mood, which shifted when Jake began to think he might be another actor.

The next phase of therapy focused on Jake's self-esteem. He began to write poetry again and to take it to poetry meetings. This helped build up the creative aspect of Jake's self-concept that he had found in the delusional system to some extent. Work in this area was aimed at promoting some alternative positive self-beliefs. This work, which focuses on the experience of low self-esteem, and targets the development of more positive self-esteem, has been usefully developed as a CBT model and group of interventions by Fennell (1999).

This therapy relationship needed not only to focus on the specific traumatic incidents experienced as flashbacks, but also to look for links between voice content and episodes of bullying at school as well as in the psychiatric system. The issue of the trauma that is experienced as a result of being detained against your will, and in Jake's case as a result of his first experience of hearing voices, has implications for the current psychiatric system. Staff should not feel necessarily threatened if they are asked to explain the reasons for their actions, to someone experiencing flashbacks relating to when they were experiencing psychosis and subsequently detained. This has parallels in treating PTSD. An example from clinical practice when treating PTSD is when paramedics are asked to explain their actions to accident victims to assist the development of a more comprehensive memory and understanding and to move the memory beyond the 'flashback' or 'worst point' moment.

CSA and rescripting

In working with visual hallucinations that are linked to flashbacks, it has become apparent that there is often a catastrophic misinterpretation of the image that transforms it into an hallucination. The misattribution that a catastrophic or distorted image is in fact really there in front of the person, rather than being a flashback to a real event, or a flashback to the strong distress experienced at the time of trauma.

For Tanya, her experience of being sexually abused was described in a matter-of-fact way, with no anger being expressed to either the perpetrator (her stepfather) or other adults involved (her mother, who knew about the abuse but apparently did nothing). Indeed she described feeling sorry for both of them, particularly her mother, who she saw as weak and in need of protection.

Instead Tanya experienced graphic visual hallucinations where, for example, after an argument with a neighbour, she saw herself stabbing the neighbour and ran screaming into the house believing herself to be covered in blood. Work with Tanya focused on altering and changing the image in imaginal exposure, with the purpose of reducing the distress associated with the hallucinatory experience.

She described the hallucinatory experience as distressing, rather than the experience of abuse which she remembered without strong emotion. This process of imagery transformation drew on Smucker et al. (1999) and was been described in previous case descriptions (Callcott and Turkington 2001; Callcott et al. 2003).

Tanya's response to her earlier experience of sexual abuse was explained by dissociation during the traumatic events. Dissociation is characterised by a sense of derealisation, depersonalisation, explicit memory loss and emotional numbing (Foa and Hearst-Ikeda 1996). It is also considered to be a defensive response that may serve a functional role during intense distress (van der Kolk et al. 1996). Alternatively, Tanya's response to the abuse may be accounted for by protective factors such as being in a good relationship and having children to care for, which may explain a more balanced view of her experience.

Indeed, she may have 'come to terms' with what happened to her. In fact she associated some instances of being abused with pleasant emotions such as feeling cared for and needed. Potentially her psychosis could have developed as result of the dissociation experienced during the more unpleasant and coercive experiences of being sexually abused.

The therapeutic approach the most helpful for the client, and the one which fitted with the collaborative formulation, seemed appropriate because the client was able to link trauma with the presenting symptoms.

Another client, who was not able to connect her experience of being raped with her voices, was willing to participate in coping strategies work to reduce the distress associated with the voices. Her recurrent self-harm episodes changed the focus of the intervention to strategies ensuring her safety and engagement with services. At the same time offering a chance to engage in a psychological approach based more on 'grounding' techniques to monitor and prevent periods of self-harm occurring during periods of dissociation (Kennerley 2000).

Which therapeutic approach for whom?

Randomised controlled trials have demonstrated the value of psychological interventions. For instance, CBT for psychosis reduces symptoms and rates of relapse in comparison to those people receiving supportive counselling, befriending or waiting list control. In essence the RCT is a hypothesis testing approach that investigates the degree of change between groups. The RCT is limited in explaining what works for whom, why or how. An alternative has been proposed, whereby a hybrid single-case methodology can be used to effectively combine pre- and post-standard measures with the repeated measurement of individualised personal variables.

It will initially be important to assess to what extent the trauma has impacted on the course of the psychosis. The following factors will need to be considered:

- The assessment and diagnosis of PTSD in psychosis, in particular the potential role of trauma in the history and whether the client makes any links between the trauma they have experienced and their symptoms. Mueser et al. (2002) describe a model in which PTSD and schizophrenia have a circular role in exacerbating each other.

- A distinction needs to be made between stressful life events (Zubin and Spring 1977) and type I and type II trauma (DSM-IV: American Psychiatric Association 1994) experienced either before, as part of, or after a diagnosis of psychosis.
- In relation to chronic PTSD, Ehlers and Clark (2000) emphasised emotional 'hotspots', such as guilt. This may have parallels with the shame and stigma associated with a diagnosis of schizophrenia.
- These notions have helped to refine reliving techniques to more than just exposure to fear and to develop specific cognitive approaches.
- In survivors of child sexual abuse (CSA) and early trauma, Smucker et al. (1999) hypothesised that exposure would be inadequate, suggesting that schema change models would be needed because of the earlier nature of the trauma.

The particular CBT treatment modality chosen will depend on the problem list generated, as well as the individualised formulation. The focus of the second intervention phase (after a period of monitoring) will take into account the following areas and will be led by individual formulation and collaboration.

Cognitive change

The self-monitoring diaries used in the research will track, rather like a modified thought diary, the changes and fluctuations in strength of belief regarding the nature of voices and intrusions, as well as form and content. Thus, reattribution of psychotic experiences to an internal source may reduce distress and impairment. The links will be made to the origin of these beliefs by use of standard psychosis assessment measures such as time line and standard CBT thought challenging. Fowler (1997) has also suggested that helping a client to clarify whether a psychotic symptom is a memory or not, and if so, assisting them in moving from externalising to internalising that memory, can be useful. Changes in imagery, including transformation, will target visual hallucinations and 'flashbacks'. For some clients this approach may not be appropriate and there is evidence that changing the attribution of symptoms in itself can achieve symptomatic improvement (Goodman et al. 1997, 2001).

Coping strategy enhancement

An alternative conceptualisation of CBT's effectiveness concerns the development of skills that help to combat psychotic symptoms when clients experience them. Under this model, clients learn more effective ways of responding to psychosis, and this is the primary therapeutic mechanism. So rather than benefiting from sustained changes in their view of their voices or delusional beliefs, they learn to reduce distress by using coping strategies. It is further recognised that many individuals with severe mental health difficulties have very poorly developed coping strategies (Tarrier et al. 1993). Many individuals who begin to hallucinate tend to withdraw socially and tend not engage in a positive therapeutic style with their auditory hallucinations. Effective coping strategies can be collaboratively developed within CBT leading to symptomatic improvement (Tarrier et al. 1993).

Behavioural change techniques

The use of behavioural experiments in reducing and eliminating safety behaviours is well developed in anxiety disorders and the psychological treatment of PTSD. Some therapeutic approaches advocate the link between safety behaviours and the continuation of 'voices' (Morrison and Renton 2001). Behavioural activation and assertiveness responses have been found to be useful in 'reclaiming life' marred by PTSD and psychosis respectively (Ehlers and Clark 2000; Pilling et al. 2002).

Moderators of change

Moderating variables are not responsible for producing therapeutic change, but different levels of a moderator influence the likely outcome. In other words, moderators interact with mediating processes, but are not themselves the mechanisms of change. They are, therefore, important to measure within this case series in order to identify possible points of interaction.

Therapeutic relationship

CBT for psychosis manuals (Fowler et al. 1995; Kingdon and Turkington 1999) stressed the importance of spending increased time with individuals experiencing psychosis, building trust and starting to test out the reality of their symptoms. There is a consistent finding across a range of psychological therapies, that the strength or quality of the therapeutic alliance offers a moderate prediction of therapy outcome (e.g. Martin et al. 2000).

External events

Apart from a distinct trauma, it is well known that high-impact negative life events can be precipitators of psychosis (Zubin and Spring 1977). Rather than view these as contaminating influences on the therapy process, one of the goals of CBT is to activate psychotic patients towards more satisfying social interactions outside of therapy. These might lead to high-impact events, or they might activate specific experiences between therapy sessions. These can be measured using diary and other experience sampling methods. To explore possible interactions between therapy and extra-therapy events, the patient will record external events prior, during and subsequent to the acute phase of therapy.

Client and therapist characteristics

Psychotherapy research has identified the potential moderating roles of various client and therapist characteristics, such as age, sex, social class and education. In addition, specific patient characteristics such as severity of psychotic symptoms prior to intervention might be influential, as might the number of previous psychotic episodes and prior treatment history. By similar reasoning, therapist adherence, competence and capability may be important factors. Established research in the CBT for psychosis field suggests there are not many main effects of these variables, with the exception that those diagnosed with chronic schizophrenia tend to respond quickly and gains are maintained longer with CBT as opposed to befriending (Sensky et al. 2000).

Conclusion

The approach discussed in this chapter does not provide a definitive answer to the preferred therapy modality for traumatic psychosis. Rather, we present a case series where knowledge of differing treatment modalities from PTSD, anxiety disorders as well as psychosis have helped to develop an individual formulation-based approach.

For some, reliving has been appropriate, for others rescripting and for others formulation work that helps the client draw links between their experience of psychosis and trauma has been enough to relieve distress. However, what they all share is the collaborative, guided discovery stance inherent in all CBT. Some clients need help normalising their experiences and their understanding of them, sometimes after years of a purely medical approach. If these last principles are used to guide therapy, there will be less chance of destabilising the client by retraumatisation. It may be that when more detailed histories of trauma are taken, or even asked about at first contact with psychiatric services, the client will receive an appropriate gold standard treatment for their PTSD that might completely alter their psychiatric diagnosis and consequent psychiatric experience.

The CBT for psychosis literature has only recently been able to get the message across to psychiatric services about the need to consider stress-vulnerability models in relation to psychotic symptoms. This message may need to move on and assessing clinicians will first of all need to ask questions about history of trauma, and then consider the meaning given to stressful life events by the client. There seems the need for a move in assessment by clinicians to differentiating stress from trauma by looking at the meaning of stressful events to the individual and comparing those with diagnostic criteria for PTSD. There is also a responsibility on the part of clinicians to consider the impact of a change in diagnosis with regards to stigma and different expectations in diagnosis. Clients with chronic PTSD can have as many serious and disabling problems as those clients with psychosis. The impact of change on symptoms may reduce distress but still leave residual symptoms such as voices and delusions.

Why not dispense with dual diagnosis and make sense of an individual's experience as a subtype of schizophrenia? This helps to guide a formulation approach that incorporates CBT approaches for psychosis as well as PTSD. 'Reliving' is seen as the gold standard approach for treating PTSD (Ehlers and Clark 2000). There is concern and caution around adopting this approach for PTSD in psychosis. However, this approach does seem to have utility where an individual is clearly making links between their traumatic experiences and their symptoms. Pure exposure principles are not advised because of the risk of retraumatising already vulnerable adults. Some form of modified reliving that incorporates imagery rescripting and change in the meaning of thoughts and beliefs will ensure a safe application of this therapy technique modified to suit individuals with traumatic psychosis.

This therapy appears to be best delivered after a period of engagement with good support in place and the cooperation of relatives and professional carers. Another issue is the choice of mode of delivery of therapy depending on whether there are multiple incidents of trauma or one specific event. This also relates to perception of trauma and whether ongoing psychological threat counts as trauma in itself. Life events previously described as just stressful can be given a new meaning and potency for the patient who has experience of mental health difficulties.

The study by Holmes and Steel (2004) on schizotypy gives some preliminary evidence indicating that individuals scoring high on positive symptom scales, and consequently exhibiting positive symptom schizotypy information processing styles, may be vulnerable to experiencing an increased number of trauma-related intrusions following exposure to trauma. This study is analogue but appears to be of relevance in understanding what might predispose individuals to either PTSD or psychosis. In summary, the types of treatment modalities used need to be built around an individual formulation. A possible flow chart with choice points is proposed as a possible guide (see Figure 10.2).

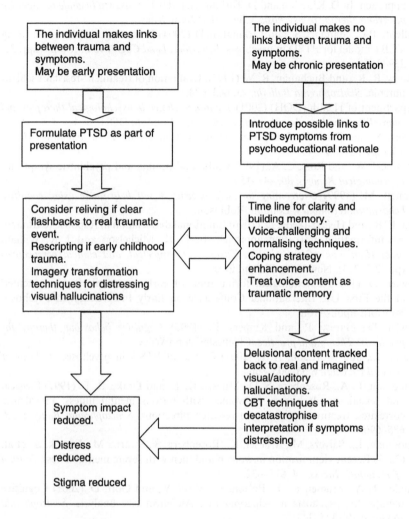

Figure 10.2 A possible therapeutic guide for CBT in trauma and psychosis

References

Allen, J. G., Coyne, L., and Console, D. A. (1997) Dissociative detachment relates to psychotic symptoms and personality decompensation. *Comprehensive Psychiatry, 38*, 327–334.

American Psychiatric Association (1987) *Diagnostic and statistical manual of mental disorders* (3rd edn revised) (DSM-III-R). Washington, DC: APA.

American Psychiatric Association (1994) *Diagnostic and statistical manual of mental disorders* (4th edn) (DSM-IV). Washington, DC: APA.

Callcott, P. C., and Turkington, D. (2002) Traumatic psychosis: A formulation approach. In D. Kingdon and D. Turkington (eds) *The case study guide to cognitive behaviour therapy of psychosis*. Chichester: John Wiley.

Callcott, P. C., Standart, S., and Turkington, D. (2004) Trauma within psychosis: Using a CBT model for PTSD in psychosis. *Behavioural and Cognitive Psychotherapy, 32*, 239–245.

Conley, R. R., and Buchanan, R. W. (1997). Evaluation of treatment-resistant schizophrenia. *Schizophrenia Bulletin, 23*, 663–674.

Department of Health (DOH) (2001) *Treatment choice in psychological therapies and counselling: Evidence based practice guidelines*. London: DOH.

Ehlers, A., and Clark, D. (2000) A model of persistent PTSD. *Behaviour Research and Therapy, 38*, 319–345.

Ellason, J. W., and Ross, C. A. (1997) Childhood trauma and psychiatric symptoms. *Psychological Reports, 80*, 447–450.

Fennell, M. (1999) *Overcoming low self esteem: A self help guide using cognitive behavioural techniques*. London: Robinson.

Foa, E. B., and Hearst-Ikeda, D. (1996) Emotional dissociation in response to trauma: An information-processing approach. In L. K. Michelson and J. R. William (eds) *Handbook of dissociation: Theoretical, empirical, and clinical perspectives* (pp. 207–224). New York: Plenum Press.

Fowler, D. (1997) Psychological formulation of early psychosis. Paper presented at the First UK International Conference on Early Intervention in Psychosis, Stratford-upon-Avon.

Fowler, D., Garety, P., and Kuipers, E. (1995) *Cognitive behaviour therapy for psychosis: Theory and practice*. Chichester: John Wiley.

Frame, L., and Morrison, A. P. (2001) Causes of PTSD in psychosis. *Archives of General Psychiatry, 58*, 305–306.

Goodman, L. A., Rosenberg, S. D., Mueser, K. T., and Drake, R. E. (1997) Physical and sexual assault history in women with serious mental illness: Prevalence, correlates, treatment, and future research directions. *Schizophrenia Bulletin, 23*, 685–696.

Goodman, L., Salyers, M., Mueser, K., Rosenberg, S., Swartz, M., Essock, S., et al. (2001) Recent victimization in women and men with severe mental illness. *Journal of Traumatic Stress, 14*, 615–632.

Gould, R. A., Mueser, K. T., Bolton, E., Mays, V., and Goff, D. (2001) Cognitive therapy for psychosis in schizophrenia: An effect size analysis. *Schizophrenia Research, 48*, 335–342.

Haddock, G., McCarron, J., and Tarrier, N. (1999) Scales to measure dimensions of hallucinations and delusions: The psychotic symptoms rating scales (PSYRATS). *Psychological Medicine, 29*, 879–889.

Healy, A., Knapp, M., Astin, J., Beecham, J., Kemp, R., Kirov, G., and David, A. (1998) Cost-effectiveness evaluation of compliance therapy for people with psychosis. *British Journal of Psychiatry, 172*, 420–424.

Holmes, E., and Steel, C. (2004) Schizotypy: A vulnerability factor for traumatic intrusions. *Journal of Nervous and Mental Disease, 192*, 28–34.

Jackson, C., and Birchwood, M. (1996) Early intervention in psychosis: Opportunities for secondary prevention. *British Journal of Clinical Psychology, 35*, 487–503.

Kennerley, H. (2000) *Overcoming childhood trauma: A self help guide using cognitive behavioural techniques*. London: Robinson.

Kingdon, D., and Turkington, D. (1999) Cognitive-behavioural therapy of schizo-phrenia. In T. Wykes, N. Tarrier and S. Lewis (eds) *Outcome and innovation in the psychological treatment of schizophrenia.* Chichester: John Wiley.

McGorry, P. D., Chanen, A., McCarthy, E., Van Riel, R., McKenzie, D., and Singh, B. S. (1991) Posttraumatic stress disorder following recent-onset psychosis: An unrecognized postpsychotic syndrome. *Journal of Nervous and Mental Disease, 179,* 253–258.

Martin, D. J., Garske, J. P., and Davis, M. K. (2000) Relation of the therapeutic alliance with outcome and other variables: A meta-analytic review. *Journal of Consulting and Clinical Psychology, 68,* 438–450.

Morrison, A. P. (1998) A cognitive analysis of the maintenance of auditory hallucin-ations: Are voices to schizophrenia, what bodily sensations are to panic?' *Behavioural and Cognitive Psychotherapy, 26,* 289–302.

Morrison, A. P., and Renton, J. C. (2001) Cognitive therapy for auditory hallucin-ations: A theory-based approach. *Cognitive and Behavioral Practice, 8,* 147–160.

Morrison, A. P., Frame, L., and Larkin, W. (2003) Relationships between trauma and psychosis: A review and integration. *British Journal of Clinical Psychology, 42,* 331–353.

Mueser, K. T., Trumbetta, S. L., Rosenborg, S. D., Vivader, R., Goodman, L. B., Osher, F., et al. (1998) Trauma and post-traumatic stress disorder in severe mental illness. *Journal of Consulting Clinical Psychology, 66,* 493–499.

Mueser, K. T., Rosenberg, S. D., Goodman, L. A., and Trumbetta, S. L. (2002) Trauma, PTSD and the course of severe mental illness: An interactive model. *Schizophrenia Research, 53,* 123–143.

Pilling, S., Bebbington, P., Kuipers, E., Garety, P., Geddes, J., Orbach, G., and Morgan, C. (2002) Psychological treatments in schizophrenia: I. Meta-analysis of family intervention and cognitive behaviour therapy. *Psychological Medicine, 32,* 763–782.

Read, J., Perry, B. D., Moskowitz, A., and Connolly, J. (2001) The contribution of early traumatic events to schizophrenia in some patients: A traumagenic neurodevelopmental model. *Psychiatry: Interpersonal and Biological Processes, 64,* 319–345.

Rector, N. A., and Beck, A. T. (2001) Cognitive behavioural therapy for schizo-phrenia: an empirical review. *Journal of Nervous and Mental Disease, 189,* 278–287.

Romme, M. A. J., and Escher, S. D. M. (1989) Hearing voices. *Schizophrenia Bulletin, 15,* 209–216.

Ross, C. A., Anderson, G., and Clark, P. (1994) Childhood abuse and the positive symptoms of schizophrenia. *Hospital and Community Psychiatry, 45,* 489–491.

Roth, A., and Fonagy, P. (1999) *What works for whom? A critical review of psycho-therapy research.* New York: Guilford Press.

Rusch, M., Grunert, B., Mendelsohn, R., and Smucker, M. (2000) Imagery rescripting for recurrent distressing images. *Cognitive and Behavioral Practice, 7,* 173–182.

Sensky, T., Turkington, D., Kingdon, D., Scott, J. L., Scott, J., Siddle, R., et al. (2000) A randomised controlled trial of cognitive-behavioural therapy for persistent symptoms in schizophrenia resistant to medication. *Archives of General Psychiatry, 57,* 165–172.

Smucker, M., Dancu, C. and Foa, E. (1999) *Cognitive behavioral treatment for adult survivors of childhood trauma: Imagery rescripting and reprocessing.* Northvale, NJ: Jason-Aronson.

Tarrier, N., Beckett, R., Harwood, S., Baker, A., Yusupoff, L., and Ugarteburu, I. (1993) A trial of two cognitive-behavioural methods of treating drug resistant residual psychotic symptoms in schizophrenic patients I. Outcome. *British Journal of Psychiatry, 162*, 524–532.

Turkington, D., Kingdon, D., and Turner, T. (2002) Effectiveness of a brief cognitive-behavioural therapy intervention in the treatment of schizophrenia. *British Journal of Psychiatry, 180*, 523–527.

Van der Kolk, B. A., van der Hart, O., and Marmar, C. R. (1996) Dissociation and information-processing in posttraumatic stress disorder. In B. A. Van der Kolk, A. C. McFarlane and L. Weisaeth (eds) *Traumatic stress: The effects of overwhelming experience on mind, body, and society.* New York: Guilford Press.

Walsh, E., Moran, P., Scott, K., McKenzie, K., Burns, T., Creed, F., et al. (2003) Prevalence of violent victimisation in severe mental illness. *British Journal of Psychiatry, 183*, 233–238.

Williams-Keeler, L., Milliken, H., and Jones, B. (1994) Psychosis as a precipitating trauma for PTSD: A treatment strategy. *American Journal of Orthopsychiatry, 64*, 493–498.

Young, M., Read, J., Barker-Collo, S., and Harrison, R. (2001) Evaluating and overcoming barriers to taking abuse histories. *Professional Psychology: Research and Practice, 32*, 367–372.

Zubin, J., and Spring, B. (1977) Vulnerability: A new view of schizophrenia. *Journal of Abnormal Psychology, 86*, 103–126.

Chapter 11

The importance of traumatic events in formulation and intervention in cognitive behavioural therapy for psychosis

Three case examples

Ben Smith, Craig Steel, Rebecca Rollinson, Daniel Freeman, Amy Hardy, Elizabeth Kuipers, Paul Bebbington, Philippa Garety and David Fowler

Introduction

Psychosis is often a confusing and terrifying experience to those who experience it. Sometimes strong emotions, images, memories and thoughts connected to past traumatic experience can become caught up in the turmoil of the experience of psychotic symptoms. In such circumstances cognitive behavioural therapy (CBT) for psychosis can help an individual make sense of psychotic experiences by making links between emotional states, thoughts, beliefs, traumatic life events and their sequelae and psychotic symptoms. Assisting people to make sense of psychotic and emotional experience by discussing psychological formulations can help them make connections between seemingly unconnected events or beliefs and disabling and distressing psychotic symptoms. In this chapter we describe how understanding and validating people's experiences of traumatic events, and incorporating them into individualised formulations of psychosis, can shape CBT interventions. We illustrate how understanding the relationship between trauma and psychosis influences clinical intervention in CBT. Three individual cases are described and formulated using cognitive conceptualisations of psychosis (Garety et al. 2001; Morrison 2001; see also Fowler et al., Chapter 5 in this volume). Interventions are driven by the Fowler et al. (1995) manual of CBT for psychosis. Clinically the emphasis is on formulating psychosis but in these selected cases traumatic events are understood as key to the development and maintenance of psychotic symptoms. The cases show how CBT techniques developed for posttraumatic stress disorder can be adapted for work in psychosis. We argue that drawing on CBT for PTSD without adaptation would fail to consider the other important factors that are clearly implicated in the development of psychotic beliefs and experiences. Thus, the case illustrations are considered in the context of cognitive behavioural theories of the relationship between trauma and psychosis.

Associations between trauma and psychosis

There is evidence that significant life events are common in the three months before psychotic symptom onset (e.g. Bebbington et al. 1996). Mueser et al. (1998) found that a lifetime history of traumatic events is very common in individuals with serious mental illness and McGorry et al. (1991) suggest that psychosis itself can be traumatising. Romme and Esher (1989) found that 70 per cent of voice hearers developed their hallucinations following a traumatic event, a result supported by Honig et al. (1998). Read (1997) proposes that many individuals with psychosis have endured specific and cumulative experiences of sexual trauma prior to the onset of psychosis. Bebbington et al. (2004) have found that events such as bullying are likely to precede a later diagnosis of psychosis. It seems that trauma is a common occurrence for individuals with psychosis.

Cognitive theories of PTSD and psychosis

Nevertheless our understanding of how traumatic life events impact on psychosis remains poor. Historically, traumatic life events have been conceptualised as triggers for increased arousal in vulnerable individuals, which somehow led to the emergence of psychotic symptoms. It was easy to see traumatic events as faceless, contentless and meaningless stressors that simply act as the 'straw that breaks the camel's back'. Some cognitive models of PTSD and of psychosis indicate that such a relationship is simplistic. Cognitive theories of PTSD show that specific personally relevant traumatic events, memories and idiosyncratic appraisals are fundamental to the persistence of maladaptive posttraumatic stress reactions (e.g. Ehlers and Clark 2000). The same may be true when trying to understand the impact of trauma on individuals who develop psychosis.

Consistent with cognitive models of persistent PTSD, recent cognitive conceptualisations of psychosis describe a multifactorial model of the positive symptoms of psychosis (e.g. Garety et al. 2001). In this model it is proposed that in a social-cognitive context, emotional changes occur in response to intrusive anomalous experiences and triggering events, which then feed back influencing the content of intrusions. Biased conscious appraisal processes (e.g. externalisation and jumping to conclusions biases) contribute to an individual's judging the experiences as externally (rather than internally) caused. Social isolation contributes to the acceptance of the psychotic appraisal by reducing access to alternative, more normalising explanations. Symptoms are then maintained by biased appraisal processes, emotional distress, safety behaviours, negative schematic beliefs and aversive social environments (e.g. social marginalisation, traumatic experiences and unsupportive family environments).

Explanations of associations between trauma and psychosis

A history of traumatic experience can be hypothesised to impact upon individuals' schematic beliefs about themselves, the world and other people (e.g. Beck et al. 1979; Young 1990). Birchwood (2003) suggests that traumatic early experience can lead to negative schematic beliefs and that these may fuel both voices and paranoia. Morrison (2001) proposes that traumatic events can influence self and social knowledge and the interpretation of intrusions. Fowler et al. (Chapter 5 in this volume) also review the evidence that critical or threatening voices may relate to ongoing self-critical thinking, concerning interpersonal relationships with abusive figures. Extreme negative beliefs about self and others might be common among people with psychosis (Fowler et al. in press) and the moment to moment synthesising of such beliefs might relate to paranoia. Hence, understanding individuals' trauma history and the impact of this on their beliefs, assumptions and thoughts may be important when conceptualising their psychotic symptoms. Similar types of formulation are frequently considered in CBT formulations for neurotic disorders (Beck et al. 1979).

Morrison et al. (2003) note the symptomatic similarities between PTSD and psychosis. Both disorders are characterised by intrusive phenomena, high arousal, hypervigilance, sleep disturbance, avoidance and emotional numbing. Cognitive conceptualisations of psychosis (Garety et al. 2001; Morrison 2001) and PTSD (Ehlers and Clark 2000) all emphasise the role of the interpretation of experiences and symptoms in the development and maintenance of disorder. It is argued that the sense individuals make of their experiences is central to their emotional and behavioural response. Morrison (2001) argues that many psychotic symptoms can be conceptualised as intrusions and culturally unacceptable interpretations of these intrusions.

Steel et al. (2005) propose that individuals with schizotypal personality traits have an information-processing style characterised by a 'weakened contextual integration'. That is, a weakened ability to integrate new information into a spatial and temporal context. In PTSD theory such weakened contextual integration is thought to occur temporarily during trauma (Brewin et al. 1996). This then leads to poorly integrated memories that involuntarily intrude into consciousness (flashbacks in PTSD). Steel et al. (2005) assert that individuals high on schizotypy may routinely process information in this way and may therefore experience intrusions from memory. These intrusions are then open to the information-processing biases implicated by Morrison

(2001) and Garety et al. (2001) in the development of the positive symptoms of psychosis.

Evidence for associations between trauma and psychosis

Read et al. (2003) found in a sample of 200 community patients that hallucinations were significantly related to sexual abuse and childhood physical abuse, although results were only based on case notes review. Raune et al. (1999) report associations between themes expressed in positive symptoms and the characteristics of traumatic life events prior to first onset.

Hardy et al. (2005) investigated trauma–psychosis links in a sample (N = 75) of individuals diagnosed with non-affective psychosis; 53 per cent reported a traumatic event that still impacted upon them negatively. Of that group, 12.5 per cent experienced hallucinations that had a similar theme and content to their traumatic event. A further 45 per cent of the group experienced hallucinations that were thematically similar to their trauma but where specific content links were absent. Hardy et al. (2005) conclude that in many cases where trauma and psychosis coexist trauma is unlikely to impact on hallucinations via the same direct, associative memory processes that are thought to underlie the re-experiencing symptoms of PTSD (see Brewin et al. 1996). Given the consistency in thematic links it may be more likely that trauma induces emotion and that this emotional disturbance triggers information-processing abnormalities. The most common link between trauma and voices may therefore be their direct links with emotion. The ways in which trauma manifests itself in psychotic symptoms may therefore be many and varied.

Fowler et al. (Chapter 5 in this volume) building on Steel et al. (2005) suggest that following a traumatic event, it is normal for any individual to experience intrusions and ruminations. It may be that in psychosis this natural process is disrupted and exaggerated leading to frequent and distressing intrusions that are trauma related but experienced subjectively as perceptual abnormalities. It can be hypothesised that information-processing abnormalities in psychosis and traumatic emotional experiences might interact catastrophically, having the effect of exaggerating both phenomena. Potentially, then, there are a variety of ways in which processes linked to psychosis may be exaggerated or worsened by processes linked to the sequelae of trauma. Further investigations are needed to determine exact causal paths, but the evidence already supports the notion that processes associated with the sequelae of trauma can make psychosis worse, thus providing a credible basis for taking trauma seriously and targeting trauma processes in intervention.

Clinical implications

There are few accounts of how to use the developing understanding of trauma–psychosis links in CBT. There is a need for clinical case examples illustrating the varied manifestations of trauma in psychosis. On that basis this case series aims to describe how CBT can be used in psychosis where trauma is a key part of the formulation.

Methodology

The CBT interventions described formed part of the Psychological Prevention of Relapse in Psychosis Trial (PRP). Interventions are formulation driven and adherent to the Fowler et al. (1995) CBT for psychosis treatment manual and the Garety et al. (2001) cognitive model. The interventions described are characterised by the collaborative investigation of thematic links between traumatic life events and psychotic symptoms.

Fowler et al. (1995) suggest that CBT starts with a comprehensive engagement and assessment phase. This establishes a working collaborative therapeutic relationship, and allows for the collection of information that will inform cognitive-behavioural formulation. When individuals have experienced traumatic events it is important to allocate time early on in CBT for a discussion of these events at their own pace. Therapists should be mindful of sensitively assessing trauma-related intrusions (e.g. intrusive memories, dreams), arousal (e.g. heightened startle response, hypervigilance) and avoidance symptoms (e.g. specific behavioural avoidance of reminders, thought and memory suppression). Also, therapists should assess the meaning of trauma to an individual and any trauma-related secondary appraisals (e.g. 'I will never get over this' or 'I just can't trust myself any more').

Sometimes individuals will understandably and deliberately avoid discussion of their trauma. Trauma memories might be accompanied by extreme emotional responses and therapists need to take extreme care. A gentle approach in the assessment stage, assisting and facilitating feelings of safety when disclosing information about traumatic experience, can become a systematic strategy to help to overcome avoidance and manage the processing of strong emotion and extreme negative thinking which can accompany disclosure. Sometimes it may be appropriate for the therapist to directly address the client's negative thinking about what the therapist may think of the client after the disclosure. Often trauma disclosure can be accompanied by thoughts that the therapist will regard the person as bad, dirty, unworthy or to blame. Reality testing of such views within sessions using careful and systematic cognitive therapy approaches, where the therapist's opinions can be regarded as a test, can be useful in starting work on addressing extreme negative views of self ('I am bad, dirty, unclean, disgusting') and others ('Others will view me as bad, dirty, and reject me').

The Fowler et al. (1995) manual centres on developing and sharing with clients an individualised cognitive-behavioural formulation of their difficulties. In trauma-psychosis this remains the same but the impact of trauma on underlying beliefs, symptoms of psychosis and coping strategies is often particularly important to understand, highlight and share with the client. Specific aspects of management of trauma can then arise from the formulation. This can include gentle discussions of the traumatic event (exposure and overcoming avoidance) and promoting an awareness of links between past events and emotions and present experiences and symptoms. This can assist in decentring from current delusional thinking and distress. Specific CBT work on delusions and hallucinations will follow from the formulation and may incorporate work on underlying assumptions, coping strategies or relapse prevention. Where trauma has been repetitive or early it may be critical to conduct work on underlying assumptions or beliefs and to promote positive views of self and to help with coping, empowerment and self-efficacy. If voices are ongoing and trauma related it is important to formulate the relationships individuals have with their voices (e.g. submissive, in-control) and through the formulation to foster an understanding that although voices are an ongoing trauma that they may be related to past events. It is important to stress that all CBT interventions are highly individualised and therapists must be sensitive to issues of mental state and specific delusional beliefs when engaging, assessing, sharing formulations and conducting interventions.

Case examples

Three individual cases were chosen to illustrate a range of trauma-psychosis presentations. All therapists were clinical psychologists trained in CBT for psychosis. Simon was seen by BS, James by RR and David by CS. Simon, James and David all gave their consent for their cases to be written up. All therapists received a combination of regular peer supervision and expert supervision in groups as well as individual audiotape supervision (four tapes per case) by an identified peer.

All participants in the PRP trial were assessed by research workers at baseline and at three-, six-, twelve- and twenty-four-month follow-up intervals. Assessments comprise a comprehensive range of interview and self-report measures. PRP data collection is ongoing and the research methodology does not allow for analysis of any outcome data during this period. Hence, outcome data cannot accompany and supplement this clinical report at this time. The focus of this chapter is to describe the therapy in detail and to address trauma-psychosis issues.

Simon: a case of shattered assumptions

Presentation and background information

Simon was a 35-year-old white-British man. He had had no contact with mental health services before the age of 30, when he was diagnosed with paranoid schizophrenia. He reported a number of relapses during the previous five years when he would be admitted to hospital, usually following a period of intense distress, alcohol misuse and a suicide attempt. He entered CBT motivated to understand his difficulties better and to stop hospital admissions.

Simon believed very strongly (reported as 90 per cent sure in Session 1) that there was a higher alien power in control of human beings and that many people were in fact aliens. He described how this alien force intended to harm him and his family, and was able to provide multiple examples of how he had come to, and maintained this conclusion. The examples were typically incidents over the previous six years, which Simon understood to be aimed at or in reference to him and his family. He described how car number plates would carry warnings in code and many interactions with friends, colleagues and acquaintances which had been characterised by overt or covert bullying, threat or humiliation. Simon also described some odd perceptual experiences and low-level murmuring voices, which he also understood to be the alien force trying to make him out to be mad.

Simon reported that he often felt depressed and said that 'I have always been vulnerable and weak – the weak one in the family'. It was also clear that he had had a very optimistic view of the world and other people prior to the onset of his difficulties. He reported having had strong, unconditional beliefs that 'others are good, trustworthy, fair and honest' and an important assumption that 'others will treat you as you treat them'. It seemed that Simon's positive beliefs about others were at least in part due to a relatively protected family life. He had never left home and was an only child. Simon had also always had a keen interest in science-fiction; he believed in aliens and continued to be an avid fan of various sci-fi television programmes.

Traumatic events

One year prior to diagnosis Simon changed jobs. He described how he became the victim of systematic bullying in his new workplace, an experience that he reported as 'traumatising and impossible to understand'. It seems that Simon's enthusiastic attitude to his work went down badly with his new workmates, who had got used to a slow work-rate. His work was damaged and sabotaged and he was threatened with violence, excluded from conversation, verbally abused and teased and on one occasion beaten up. In response Simon began drinking heavily and did not discuss any of his experiences with his parents for fear of worrying them. He worked in this new job six days a week, for over nine months. Simon reported that the bullying had 'trampled all over my expectations' and he had suffered intrusive memories, images and thoughts of this bullying ever since. Simon believed that the bullying had caused him to have a nervous breakdown.

Formulation

The psychological formulation was collaboratively developed with Simon. It built upon his own idea that the bullying had stressed him out so much that he had had a breakdown. We formulated that in the context of pre-existing and firmly held beliefs regarding the positive nature of other people Simon had experienced a very traumatising, personal and protracted attack. He had had to make sense of this experience while coping with the arousal, distress and anxiety of the attacks and drinking large quantities of alcohol. He had chosen to try to work out what was going on at work on his own, without the input of others. He understandably became hypervigilant to the ongoing bullying. He began to draw a conclusion that did not require a distressing reconsideration of his beliefs about others; that what was happening could not possibly be the actions of humans, but may be due to some other force. As these beliefs developed (in the context of his positive beliefs about sci-fi) they tended to be confirmed and maintained by his appraisal of subsequent events and experiences. He was afraid that he would be exposed as too vulnerable to withstand the attacks from what he now saw as an alien force and that he would go mad, leaving his family endangered. The bullying was formulated as integral to Simon's deterioration in mental health. It was also identified as the trigger for his specific beliefs in the alien force. It also seemed that this intense period of stress led to the low-level perceptual abnormalities reported by Simon. These were subsequently interpreted as further evidence of alien aggression.

Intervention

CBT revolved around slowly and tentatively developing a shared formulation of what had happened. We developed a shared understanding of how Simon had learnt to see himself, others and the world. We established that his positive beliefs about others were, in his words, 'trampled all over' by the traumatic bullying. As a result we agreed that he had lost his ability to trust people and often felt under threat. The process of therapy itself was able to review his lack of trust in *all* other people and he began to see that he had almost completely rejected his prior positive beliefs in others. We looked at the impact that this change in perspective had had on his experiences since the bullying. He began to see the role of his perception of events, rather than events per se and to reappraise his interpretation of certain incidents in the light of this new information. In particular, he started to consider that his low-level voices and mutterings could be the result of the 'mental strain' rather than alien threats to his mental state.

During CBT Simon's mood oscillated, and he retained high levels of belief conviction at times. Talking through his trauma in detail led to hyperarousal and suspiciousness. On one occasion he became very worried that the therapist was involved with the higher force of aliens. This was dealt with straightforwardly by the therapist reassuring him that the therapist's intentions were only to try to help him. Intervention did not involve prolonged exposure to traumatic memories (as would occur in CBT for PTSD), but was instead limited to labelling traumatic events as schema and assumption incongruent and as events that had led to him losing his trust in others. We also highlighted that, once Simon had 'worked out' what was going on with the aliens (his delusional explanation) he had felt relieved, pleased with himself and quite excited as well as scared, all factors likely to maintain the belief and discourage disconfirmation.

Simon spontaneously decided to revisit his place of work midway through CBT. He spent enough time with his ex-colleagues to conclude that they were, in his words, 'idiots'. We were then able to use this new information to develop an alternative explanation of their actions in support of the rest of the formulation. Simon became aware that the labelling of them as 'idiots' was not an option open to him at the time of the bullying, given his pre-existing positive expectations of others. At the time he needed to come up with another explanation of what was happening to him. He was able to see this in retrospect and use it to reappraise his decision-making.

The role of avoidance was discussed. Simon had coped with the bullying alone and continued, for the most part, to keep incidents that confirmed his beliefs to himself and ruminate about them. Through discussion we concluded that this coping style meant he was overly reliant on just his opinion alone, and although we had no reason to doubt his abilities, as his trust in others was returning he would do well to use others for support. Simon could see that CBT was opening up new explanations of events that were plausible and, importantly, less distressing than his original explanations. He began to value the opportunity of gaining other's opinions and started intentionally seeking out other's explanations for events when he found himself ruminating.

The influence of his mood upon his interpretation of events was highlighted. Simon could see that on a bad day his belief conviction and distress was greater than on a good day. This link was emphasised and related specifically to his tendency to infer meaning and to say to himself 'It is as if they are saying . . .'. He became much more aware of the role of this particular reasoning bias in his belief development and maintenance.

Relapse prevention strategies were developed. These were based on Simon being able to access a version of our new formulation of events when in a vulnerable state. We produced a detailed booklet of the new conclusions we had come to which he could refer to when needed. We identified behavioural and cognitive factors (e.g. inactivity, alcohol misuse, negative thinking, and rumination about trauma) as those likely to make him vulnerable and applied standard CBT techniques to address them.

CBT outcome

Simon's belief conviction at the end of therapy was down to 20 per cent. Through CBT he had developed a new version of events that was more explanatory and in his words, 'plausible' than his original version. He also reported that his distress and preoccupation were significantly reduced and that he was becoming more confident about a slow return to work. At the end of CBT (twenty sessions) he still remained vulnerable to low mood and occasional alcohol misuse, and was still unemployed. Simon has not relapsed in the twelve months following CBT.

David: indirect links between trauma and voices

Presentation and background information

David was an unemployed 39-year-old white male who lived with his sister. Wherever possible he would avoid interactions with other people, though he would make shopping trips or attend meetings almost every day. His only social contacts were with his sister and his mother, both of whom he cared for. He stated that he believed people he didn't know were untrustworthy and had harmful intentions towards him. He was particularly anxious when around men, whom he feared might sexually assault him. He was also anxious around children, whom he thought might attack or humiliate him.

David also reported hearing voices, which he believed to be the voice of Jesus. While the voices would sometimes be comforting and reassuring, at other times they would sound angry and aggressive and say that he should hurt children. He found the aggressive voices confusing but not particularly upsetting.

David reported having had a good relationship with his mother when growing up, but stated that his father was occasionally violent and largely absent during his childhood. He was bullied at primary school, and his mother sought to protect him by helping him avoid having to attend. He developed beliefs that others were dangerous and that he was weak and powerless. His father died when he was 17. He had begun factory work at 16, and became increasingly anxious that other workers were talking about him and conspiring against him. He engaged in a high level of scanning for danger, and interpreted a wide range of ambiguous social interactions as personally threatening. These experiences led to a conflict with a colleague and his subsequent dismissal. Around this time he was experiencing increasingly violent and aggressive thoughts, often in relation to getting revenge on people he considered to have harmed him. These would include people he was at school or at work with. When these thoughts reached a certain level of aggression and intensity, he decided that they could not be his own. At this time, he concluded that Jesus was communicating with him in order to advise him with his difficulties.

An increase in David's level of perceived threat, both from strangers and people he had known in his past, combined with an increase in hearing voices with violent content led to his being sectioned for the first time, aged 19. This type of presentation led to a 'revolving door' situation for around ten years, during which he had many stays in hospital. The subsequent ten years prior to therapy starting had been relatively stable, the only admission being prior to CBT starting. David still heard aggressive voices around once or twice a week, and these usually occurred when he was outside.

Traumatic events

Clearly there were a number of traumas that David had experienced during his childhood. These included being bullied at school and experiencing physical abuse from his father. During his adult life, David had been raped by another male inpatient during an admission to a psychiatric hospital. While he felt angry towards the perpetrator, he also felt that he must have been somehow responsible for it happening.

Formulation

Early aversive events contributed towards David developing negative beliefs about himself and others. Specifically being bullied at school, and physically abused by his father, resulted in his beliefs that others are dangerous and that he, himself is weak and powerless. These beliefs about himself and others were maintained through the avoidance of school, which was encouraged by his mother. While his sister and mother would have become the only people he trusted, he would have felt particularly threatened by men and other children.

Starting work was particularly difficult for David, given his previous social avoidance and his beliefs about others. At this time it seems that he engaged in a high level of scanning for danger, and interpreted a wide range of ambiguous social interactions as personally threatening. The consequent high level of arousal contributed to a vicious cycle of increasingly anxious thoughts, behaviours and safety behaviours. David is likely to have felt particularly vulnerable in terms of direct conflict with others. Given the amount of threat he perceived, it is likely that he thought some kind of conflict was inevitable. Around this time he seems to have started to experience a lot of angry, violent and vengeful thoughts that may have provided him some comfort, in relation to his experience of being weak and powerless. However, when these thoughts reached a certain level of aggression, they made David feel even more vulnerable, due to his fear of acting on them, or making conflict seem even more likely. The high state of anxiety, and intensity of these thoughts contributed to David experiencing them in a somewhat perceptually unusual manner. This made him wonder if they were in fact not his own thoughts.

When David began to consider that these mental events might be Jesus speaking to him, this possibility allowed him to feel less vulnerable and threatened. Externalising his thoughts to originate from Jesus may have served to validate his anger towards others, and to reassure him regarding his self-belief as weak. Being raped in hospital would have confirmed his beliefs about others as threatening, and himself as weak and powerless. Given that David felt most vulnerable around men and children, it is likely that these would be the situations in which he found himself thinking angry thoughts and consequently hearing voices. David felt too scared to tackle a grown man, but may have been more tempted by the possibility of attacking a weak target, such as a child. Therefore, he may have been particularly bothered by the thoughts, and the associated voices that occurred when he was around children.

Intervention

Early sessions were spent slowly establishing engagement and gathering David's history. Once David had revealed his anxiety about men, and that he had been raped as an inpatient, particular emphasis was placed on how he felt during sessions with the (male) therapist. A basic formulation was shared, based on how, given his experiences, it was understandable that he considered others to be threatening and that he had consequently developed strategies to protect himself. David acknowledged the formulation, and the therapeutic relationship was discussed as an example of how he was prepared to challenge his previously learnt strategies in order to try and increase the quality of his life.

In relation to the voices, the therapist spent many sessions empathising with the confusion over the origin and content of the voices. A formulation was shared as to how the voices made him feel powerful, a feeling he had lacked in his life, and how they seemed to be aimed at revenge for his being bullied as a child. A voice diary was implemented, and it was noted that he was experiencing less frequent voices within the second half of therapy. David stated that he missed having Jesus in his life and efforts were made to facilitate Jesus being part of his life without the necessity of hearing his voice. In the last few sessions of therapy (twenty sessions in total) efforts focused on basic CBT techniques for tackling anxiety in relation to his attempting new activities.

CBT outcome

The main aim of the therapy was to develop a shared formulation that allowed David to put his current experiences of paranoia and hearing voices within an understandable context. This approach was relatively successful in relation to paranoia, in that David could understand how he had come to develop certain beliefs, due to his traumatic experiences. He also acknowledged that his current protective strategies may no longer be necessary to such a degree.

David continued to hear voices, which he considered to come from Jesus, and which caused him both comfort and confusion. That the voices had decreased during therapy may have been due to an overall lower level of arousal, which might have been a trigger for the voices. This decrease in arousal might have been associated with a slight shift in terms of feeling weak and powerless, and consequently a decrease in need for the reassurance the voice provided. It is of note that therapy was not aimed at directly challenging the beliefs regarding the origin of the voice. In summary, while David developed an understanding of his formulation, in terms of linking his past experiences with his current problems, there was a limited shift in his beliefs about himself and others. Thus, David maintained a view of himself as weak and others as generally dangerous.

James: direct links between trauma, voices and paranoia

Presentation and background information

James was a 40-year-old, intelligent and lucid man who lived alone. He had a history of depression from his teens and had experienced episodes of psychosis since his mid twenties. He had previously managed to return to work between episodes. Over the previous four years, however, since the loss of a parent, these episodes had increased in frequency to two or three a year and James had had to leave his job. He entered therapy motivated to change this pattern and re-establish an independent lifestyle.

James reported that his relapses typically started 'out of the blue'. He identified altered perceptual experiences as the early signs of a relapse that typically then triggered catastrophic beliefs about the inevitability and consequences of relapse. These early signs would then quickly escalate so that within a week he was hearing constant critical voices (e.g. 'You're useless', 'You're a failure') and feeling paranoid. His specific paranoid belief was that someone was attacking him by 'messing with my brain' through telepathy and trying to get him admitted to a psychiatric hospital.

A critical feature of James' relapse profile was that while he was able to intellectually formulate a relapse, he was unable to implement relapse prevention strategies due to strong negative self-beliefs that he deserved to relapse and wasn't worth taking care of. Once a clear relapse formulation was established, subsequent assessment and intervention focused upon these negative self-beliefs.

Assessment of James' early emotional environment indicated a family that strongly suppressed any emotional expression. He also reported specific childhood experiences that left him feeling unprotected and vulnerable to being abused or abandoned. In accordance with this, the Young Schema Questionnaire identified the following schemas of 'vulnerability to harm', 'unrelenting standards' and 'emotional suppression'. James had an understandable tendency to feel that he was vulnerable to threat and had to look after himself as nobody else would be available. The consequence of this and his unrelenting standards meant, however, that when anything did go wrong, he was highly likely to interpret it as his fault. This tendency toward self-blame had led to the development and maintenance of strong negative self-beliefs (e.g. 'I'm a failure', 'I'm useless', 'I'm worthless').

Traumatic events

James experienced a number of significantly threatening events throughout his life, including the loss of close family members, several physical attacks and a sexual assault. These events, his appraisal of them and the unfortunate responses of others around him, served to maintain his early maladaptive schemas.

Formulation

Although a wider formulation was shared with James, particular attention is paid here to the role of James' traumatic experiences in the development and maintenance of his psychosis.

Given James' family history of emotional suppression, it is perhaps not surprising that he had an extreme tendency to avoid trauma-related memories. He therefore had little opportunity to integrate this information and remained highly sensitive to reminders of previous traumatic experiences. By developing a broad narrative of these traumatic experiences and examining antecedents of changes in mood state during the course of therapy, James was able to identify reminders of previous traumas as typical triggers for the 'early signs' of relapse that he experienced. These reminders would also elicit the unprocessed, 'raw' emotional memory associated with the event. In addition at these times, he would hear his attacker's voice as an auditory hallucination. This was heard both as a direct memory of derogatory comments made at the time of the attack, as well as general schema-congruent derogatory remarks (e.g. 'You're useless', 'You're a failure').

James did not interpret these emotional and perceptual changes as the consequence of intrusive trauma memories, however: to him they appeared to occur 'out of the blue' leaving him with sudden, overwhelming feelings that he had to try to make sense of.

The interpretations he came to were strongly influenced both by his heightened emotional state and by his underlying schemas relating to his own worthlessness, his vulnerability to harm and lack of protection. He interpreted the emotional and perceptual changes as an indication of imminent threat that he needed protection from. His specific interpretation was that someone was attacking him through telepathy.

Intervention

We initially looked at the childhood origins of James' schemas and worked on developing alternative explanations for some of his key experiences. Most commonly, this involved explicitly labelling and reappraising his childhood tendency to view himself as the primary cause of any situation over which he actually had little, if any control. We went on to review later life events in a similar manner, reflecting upon and reviewing the distorted appraisals of self-blame that were central to his distress.

Although this review of traumatic events did not involve explicit exposure and reliving work, it was nonetheless emotionally very difficult and distressing at times. This period of therapy therefore provided an opportunity for James to risk reducing some of his general emotional avoidance and a safe environment in which to challenge his beliefs about the catastrophic impact of emotions (i.e. 'If I let myself feel anything I won't be able to take it and will go mad').

It was also a useful time to label and normalise the trauma-related intrusions he was experiencing. Collaboratively developing a developmental formulation of his psychosis helped to provide an alternative, more adaptive explanation of the strange experiences he was having.

The final few sessions focused on specific relapse prevention strategies. This involved James identifying thoughts he would typically hold regarding relapse (e.g. 'This proves I'm a failure', 'This is never going to end', 'I deserve this', 'These feeling are the result of someone attacking my brain') and generating alternative, more adaptive statements that resonated with him, based on the preceding schema and formulation work (e.g. 'This is a reminder of what happened', 'It happens to lots of people, it doesn't mean I'm going mad', 'If I had 'flu I'd rest – if I look after myself I'm not failing, I'm working to make sure I feel better faster').

CBT outcome

James' community mental health nurse (CMHN) has reported that, three years after the end of therapy, James has returned to work and has not had any further admissions. He had a couple of 'blips' but with his CMHN's help was able to read through his relapse plan and was able to try out a different way of responding to these upsetting early signs of relapse.

Discussion

The three case illustrations highlight some important clinical and theoretical issues for understanding psychosis in the context of a history of traumatic events. Garety et al. (2001), Birchwood (2003) and Fowler et al. (Chapter 5 in this volume) all propose that traumatic early experiences influence schematic beliefs, which then influence the nature and appraisal of intrusions/anomalous experiences. Similarly, Morrison (2001) suggests that faulty self and social knowledge can influence both intrusions and the interpretations of intrusions. For both James and David, beliefs about persecution seemed to develop in the context of early traumatic experiences (abuse, bullying) and the resulting schematic beliefs (I am worthless, I am weak, others are dangerous). Their early experiences and current social-cognitive context may also have influenced the thematic content of their voices. James heard schema-congruent derogatory voices and David heard angry voices. These early experiences and schematic beliefs can also be seen to be influencing the appraisal they make of these experiences. When James first notices perceptual abnormalities for instance, his appraisals are that someone is attacking him, that this will lead to relapse and that he deserves relapse. David interprets interactions with others as threatening and he becomes paranoid.

Morrison (2001) suggests that traumatic events can lead directly to intrusions in psychosis. Hardy et al. (2005) find some evidence of direct content links between traumatic events and hallucinations and there is evidence of this here. James hears voices whose content is the same as words spoken by his attackers.

Simon's beliefs about aliens developed in the immediate context of bullying and the wider social-cognitive context of his extreme positive beliefs about other people. Janoff-Bulman (1985) described the phenomena of 'shattered assumptions' in PTSD after a traumatic event. Simon reported that the bullying left him thinking that 'the world has gone mad', feeling disorientated and confused. It was as if what was happening to him made no sense based on the reference points he had for life, such as 'others will treat you as you treat them'. Morrison (2001) suggests that such a shift in thinking may lead to culturally unacceptable interpretations of events as previous (culturally acceptable) reference points for making sense of life have been lost.

Cognitive models of PTSD (e.g. Ehlers and Clark 2000) emphasise the role of avoidance of reminders of traumatic events in the maintenance of distress and intrusive symptoms. Interestingly, Harrison and Fowler (2004) examined the relationships between negative symptoms, trauma and recovery in psychosis. They found that negative symptoms were significantly associated with avoidance of traumatic memories. Simon, James and David all experienced reminders and intrusions of traumatic events. Social interactions reminded Simon of his bullying and triggered intrusive memories; specific reminders triggered off intrusions of attacks for James; David was reminded of his rape when he came into contact with men. For James and David this process also triggered off voices and overwhelming negative affect. All three men avoided as many reminders as possible. Overcoming such avoidance by gentle discussion and facilitation of disclosure in sessions was a crucial and systematic strategy adopted in the CBT.

Garety et al. (2001) emphasise the role of emotion and reasoning in the development, and importantly the maintenance, of psychotic symptoms. Simon, James and David all experienced intense negative emotions in response to internal (e.g. voices) or external triggers. This arousal impacted on their reasoning style. Simon had developed a cognitive style of anxiously over-analysing social situations for clues of alien activity and had stored up many examples of such events in memory. James' emotional arousal was experienced as another unusual and threatening experience to have to make sense of.

Steel et al. (2005) propose that individuals with schizotypal beliefs, who have experienced trauma, may have more trauma-related intrusions. These intrusions are hypothesised to derive from poorly contextualised and integrated trauma memories intruding into consciousness. All three men experienced trauma-related intrusions. In CBT with Simon it was therefore crucial to link intrusions with real events and memories. If individuals can begin to incorporate their intrusions within a re-narrated autobiographical account, they may be less prone both to experience intrusions and to externalise them. For James, it was important that he understood the intrusions as something related to previous events, rather than a confusing 'out of the blue' experience to be explained in terms of dysfunctional schema.

CBT itself provides a forum in which to overcome avoidance, and allows for discussion and cognitive restructuring of traumatic events. New information can be incorporated into discussions about traumas, and events can start to be placed properly in the past. It is usual in CBT for PTSD for individuals systematically to relive traumatic events to facilitate proper contextualisation and integration into autobiographical memory. This is not always possible or necessary in psychosis. Reliving of his trauma was strongly resisted by Simon, and detailed discussion of bullying led to high arousal and increases in paranoia. Despite this, it was still crucial to reappraise the meaning of the bullying with Simon. Simon's reappraisal was 'I have been bullied by idiots' (arguably a more culturally acceptable appraisal than his original interpretation that this must be the work of an alien force). Similarly, James did not undertake any reliving of his trauma, but focused instead on reappraising it as something that was not his fault, while using the developmental formulation to understand why he might be drawn to make self-blaming attributions. This also gave James the opportunity to learn to tolerate exposure to (previously avoided) emotional distress.

Finally, Simon's bullying was a protracted trauma. James had experienced multiple attacks and abuses, as had David. It may be important for clinicians to attend to prolonged toxic periods of traumatic stress, such as sexual abuse and bullying, as well as more salient traumatic incidents. In support of this, Hardy et al. (2005) found that sexual abuse and bullying were the most common traumatic events in their psychosis cohort. They may also be the most toxic.

Conclusion

These cases illustrate how trauma work can feature in CBT for psychosis. Therapists and clients do not necessarily begin with targeted attempts at positive symptom reduction or trauma reliving. Time is allowed for the development of an alternative explanation of events and experiences that is neither completely biological, medical nor psychotic. CBT interventions provide the opportunity to develop collaboratively alternative explanations of experiences with individuals who are frequently isolated and distressed. A key part of such formulation-driven CBT is the integration of the experience of psychotic disorder into an acceptable explanation that promotes understanding and self-worth. This is different from promoting 'insight' which, on its own, may be associated with depression (Watson et al. 2006). CBT for psychosis should therefore be inherently non-judgemental, validating of experiences and matched to an individual's goals. An alternative, acceptable explanation of psychotic experiences will sometimes include the integration of traumatic events as well as prior beliefs, psychotic experiences, appraisals and subsequent maintenance factors.

Acknowledgement

This work was supported by a programme grant from the Wellcome Trust (No. 062452).

References

Bebbington, P., Wilkins, S., Sham, P., and Jones, P. (1996) Life events before psychotic episodes: Do clinical and social variables affect the relationship? *Social Psychiatry and Psychiatric Epidemiology, 31*, 122–128.

Bebbington, P. E., Bhugra, D., Brugha, T., Farrell, M., Lewis, G., Meltzer, H., et al. (2004) Psychosis, victimisation and childhood disadvantage: Evidence from the Second British National Survey of Psychiatric Epidemiology. *British Journal of Psychiatry, 185*, 220–226.

Beck, A. T., Rush, A. J., Shaw, B. F., and Emery, G. (1979) *Cognitive therapy of depression*. New York: Guilford.

Birchwood, M. (2003) Pathways to emotional dysfunction in first-episode psychosis. *British Journal of Psychiatry, 182*, 373–375.

Brewin, C. R., Dalgleish, T., and Joseph, S. (1996) A dual representation theory of PTSD. *Psychological Review, 103*, 670–686.

Ehlers, A., and Clark, D. M. (2000) A cognitive model of posttraumatic stress disorder. *Behaviour Research and Therapy, 38*, 319–345.

Fowler, D., Garety, P. A., and Kuipers, E. K. (1995) *Cognitive behaviour therapy for psychosis: Theory and practice*. Chichester: John Wiley.

Fowler, D., Freeman, D., Steel, C., Hardy, A., Smith, B., Hackmann, C., et al. (in press) The catastrophic interaction hypothesis: How does stress, trauma, emotion and information processing abnormalities lead to psychosis?

Garety, P. A., Kuipers, E. K., Fowler, D., Freeman, D., and Bebbington, P. E. (2001) A cognitive model of the positive symptoms of psychosis. *Psychological Medicine, 31*, 189–195.

Hardy, A., Fowler, D., Freeman, D., Smith, B., Steel, C., and Evans, J. (2005) Trauma and hallucinatory experience in psychosis. *Journal of Nervous and Mental Disease, 193*, 501–507.

Harrison, L., and Fowler, D. (2004) Negative symptoms, trauma and autobiographical memory: An investigation of individuals recovering from psychosis. *Journal of Nervous and Mental Disease, 192*, 745–753.

Honig, A., Romme, M. A., Ensink, B. J., Esher, S. D., Pennings, M. H., and deVries, M. W. (1998) Auditory hallucinations: A comparison between patients and non-patients. *Journal of Nervous and Mental Disease, 186*, 646–651.

Janoff-Bulman, R. (1985) The aftermath of victimisation: Rebuilding shattered assumptions. In C. R. Figley (ed.) *Trauma and its wake*. New York: Brunner-Mazel.

McGorry, P. D., Chanen, A., McCarthy, E., Van Riel, R., McKenzie, D., and Singh, B. S. (1991) Posttraumatic stress disorder following recent onset psychosis: An unrecognized postpsychotic syndrome. *Journal of Nervous and Mental Disease, 179*, 253–258.

Morrison, A. P. (2001) The interpretation of intrusions in psychosis: An integrative cognitive approach to psychotic symptoms. *Behavioural and Cognitive Psychotherapy, 29*, 257–276.

Morrison, A. P., Frame, L., and Larkin, W. (2003) Relationships between trauma and psychosis: A review and integration. *British Journal of Clinical Psychology, 42*, 331–353.

Mueser, K. T., Trumbetta, S. L., Rosenberg, S. D., Vivader, R., Goodman, L. B., Osher, F. C., et al. (1998) Trauma and post-traumatic stress disorder in severe mental illness. *Journal of Consulting and Clinical Psychology, 66*, 493–499.

Raune, D., Kuipers, E., and Bebbington, P. (1999) Psychosocial stress and delusional and verbal auditory hallucination themes in first episode psychosis: Implications for early intervention. Paper presented at Psychological Treatments of Schizophrenia, Oxford, September.

Read, J. (1997) Child abuse and psychosis: A literature review and implications for professional practice. *Professional Psychology: Research and Practice, 28*, 448–456.

Read, J., Agar, K., Argyle, N., and Aderhold, V. (2003) Sexual and physical abuse during childhood and adulthood as predictors of hallucinations, delusions and thought disorder. *Psychology and Psychotherapy: Theory, Research and Practice, 76*, 1–22.

Romme, M. A. J. and Esher, D. M. A. (1989) Hearing voices. *Schizophrenia Bulletin, 15*, 209–216.

Steel, C., Fowler, D., and Holmes, E. A. (2005) Trauma related intrusions and psychosis: An information processing account. *Behavioural and Cognitive Psychotherapy, 33*, 1–14.

Watson, P. W. B., Garety, P. A., Weinman, J., Dunn, G., Bebbington, P. E., Fowler, D., et al. (2006) Emotional dysfunction in schizophrenia spectrum psychosis: The role of illness perceptions. *Psychological Medicine, 36*(6), 761–70.

Young, J. E. (1990) *Cognitive therapy for personality disorders: A schema focussed approach.* Sarasota, FL: Professional Resource Exchange.

Chapter 12

Relationships between trauma and psychosis

From theory to therapy

Warren Larkin and Anthony P. Morrison

This chapter will examine a cognitive approach to the understanding of the relationship between trauma and psychotic experiences. It will then consider how this approach can be used to guide assessment and the collaborative development of a shared case conceptualisation. Finally, specific intervention strategies will be described that have been found to be useful in reducing distress and improving quality of life in people with psychosis with trauma-related difficulties.

Theory

Possible relationships between trauma and psychosis

There are several relationships that have been identified as possible links between trauma and psychosis (Morrison et al. 2003). These areas have been considered in detail elsewhere within this book, and will be mentioned only briefly. Some argue that the experience of psychosis can be experienced as traumatic and consequently lead to the development of PTSD (e.g. McGorry et al. 1991; see also Bendall, McGorry and Krstev, Chapter 3 in this book). Similarly, others argue that posttraumatic stress disorder and psychosis are separate but intertwined disorders that exacerbate the course of severe mental health difficulties (e.g. Mueser et al. 2002; see also Jankowski, Mueser and Rosenberg, Chapter 4 in this book). Another is the idea that PTSD and psychosis are similar entities and part of a spectrum of possible responses to traumas (Morrison et al. 2003) and that traumatic life events clearly contribute to the development of psychosis (see Read, Rudegeair and Farrelly, Chapter 2 in this book).

A cognitive model of trauma-related psychosis

Our cognitive approach to the understanding of trauma-related psychosis will be outlined, focusing on both the development of psychotic experiences, the maintenance of such experiences and the associated distress.

Trauma and the development of psychosis

Cognitive models of psychosis may help to explain the relationship between the experience of trauma, the development of psychotic experiences and being labelled with a psychotic diagnosis. In fact, there may be several ways in which traumatic experiences may confer vulnerability to psychosis via cognitive and behavioural processes (Morrison et al. 2003). One theory of psychosis (Morrison 2001) suggests that it is the culturally unacceptable nature of appraisals that determines whether a person is viewed as psychotic or not; in relation to trauma, it may be that the transparency of the link between the traumatic event and the content and form of (subsequent difficulties or 'symptoms') psychotic experiences that contributes to this process. For example, if someone describes vivid perceptual experiences as being related to past physical or sexual assault, then this is likely to be regarded as consistent with a flashback experience in PTSD, whereas if they report that the experiences are real, current and unrelated to past experience, then they are likely to be regarded as someone experiencing psychosis.

It is also possible that the cognitive and behavioural consequences of traumatisation may make people vulnerable to psychosis. Negative beliefs about the self, the world and others (such as 'I am vulnerable' and 'Other people are dangerous') have been shown to be associated with psychosis (Bentall et al. 2001; Garety et al. 2001; Morrison 2001). One study has also shown that such beliefs specifically formed as a result of trauma are related to psychotic experiences (Kilcommons and Morrison 2005). Positive beliefs about psychotic experiences, and procedural beliefs that encourage the adoption of paranoia as a strategy for managing interpersonal threat (such as 'Paranoia is a helpful survival strategy'), may also be related to traumatic experience, and have been shown to be associated with the development of psychosis (Morrison et al. 2005). In addition, responses to trauma such as dissociation may also be involved in the development of psychosis (Morrison et al. 2003).

It is likely that psychotic experiences are essentially normal phenomena that occur on a continuum in the general population (Johns and van Os 2001) and that the occurrence of trauma in the life history of a person experiencing such phenomena may represent the difference between patients and non-patients (Honig et al. 1998). It also appears that catastrophic or negative appraisals of psychotic experiences result in the associated distress (Chadwick and Birchwood 1994; Morrison et al. 2004), and that such appraisals are more likely if people have a history of trauma.

Trauma and the maintenance of psychosis

There are many factors that have been demonstrated to be important in the maintenance of both PTSD symptoms and distressing psychotic experiences.

For example, a very common interpretation in both of these disorders is one of 'going mad'. Negative social stereotypes of 'madness' portray people with serious mental disorders as incomprehensible; out of control; threatening to society; inherently 'odd'; and incapable of functional living (Birchwood et al. 1993). Over two-thirds (70 per cent) of those with psychotic diagnoses reported a 'fear of going crazy' as the most common prodromal symptom (Hirsch and Jolley 1989). This is similar to findings that indicate interpreting initial post-trauma symptoms as a sign of impending madness distinguished clients with a diagnosis of PTSD from those without and recovered clients from those with persistent PTSD (Dunmore et al. 1999). Other maintenance processes that have been found to be common to both diagnostic groups include selective attention, which has been implicated in people experiencing persecutory delusions (Bentall and Kaney 1989) and clients with PTSD (Thrasher et al. 1994). Similarly, safety behaviours designed to prevent feared catastrophes but that may also prevent disconfirmation of problematic interpretations have been identified in voice hearers (Morrison 1998), people with persecutory delusions (Freeman et al. 2001) and clients with PTSD (Ehlers and Clark 2000). Similarly, both clients with a diagnosis of PTSD (Reynolds and Wells 1999) and people with a diagnosis of schizophrenia (Morrison and Wells 2000) have been found to use more dysfunctional thought control strategies (particularly punishment and worry) than people with no psychiatric diagnosis. Biases in autobiographical memory have also been found in those experiencing PTSD (Brewin 1998) and people with a psychotic diagnosis (Baddeley et al. 1996). Expressed emotion in family members has also been linked to symptomatology and/or relapse in both people with a diagnosis of schizophrenia (Barrowclough et al. 1994) and PTSD clients (Tarrier et al. 1999). In addition, dissociation has been implicated in the maintenance of both PTSD (Van der Kolk et al. 1996) and psychosis (Allen and Coyne 1995; Ross and Keyes 2004; Spitzer et al. 1997). Other studies have also shown that vivid and recurrent images are associated with PTSD (Ehlers et al. 2002) and psychotic experiences (Morrison et al. 2002).

Summary of the model

These factors have been combined within an integrative cognitive model that suggests that life experience (including trauma) will lead to the development of beliefs about self, world and others (including beliefs about psychotic experiences, dissociation and other information-processing strategies). These beliefs will affect how ongoing intrusions or events are appraised, and it is argued that if trauma-related phenomena are interpreted in a culturally unacceptable manner, then these will be viewed as psychotic; whereas, if they are interpreted as being linked to the trauma, then the experiences are likely to be viewed as symptomatic of PTSD. These appraisals result in emotional distress and physiological arousal, which can lead to the development of vicious circles which maintain the problematic (psychotic) experiences and their culturally unacceptable misinterpretations. In addition, the cognitive and behavioural responses to these experiences and appraisals (including safety behaviours, avoidance, dissociation, thought suppression and selective attention to interpersonal threat) can also contribute to the maintenance cycles. This model is illustrated graphically in Figure 12.1, and a case example will follow, which demonstrates the utilisation of this model for formulation and intervention purposes.

Therapy

Despite the growing body of literature demonstrating the high rates of trauma in individuals who receive a diagnosis of 'schizophrenia' or psychosis and debating the possible relationships between trauma, PTSD and psychosis, there is little empirical research available to inform clinicians regarding best practice in terms of intervention. However, a number of clinical implications clearly arise from the theoretical model outlined above. These will be considered in relation to assessment, formulation and specific intervention strategies.

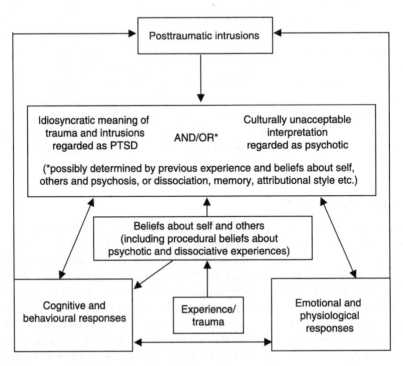

Figure 12.1 An integrative model of trauma and psychosis

Assessment and formulation

The assessment process is a vehicle for engagement with the client and informs the development of a collaborative case formulation. Case formulations aim to explain the development and maintenance of a client's presenting problems in terms of causal relationships between the different aspects of the formulation. In cognitive therapy, case formulations should provide some testable hypothesis about the relationship between environmental, cognitive, affective and behavioural factors in a way that leads us to ideas about how to address identified problems (Beck 1976; Morrison et al, 2004). Butler (1999) describes formulation as 'the tool used by clinicians to relate theory to practice'. Consequently, the assessment process when working with clients where traumatic experience appears to be indicated in the aetiology of their psychosis is guided by the integrative model of trauma and psychosis illustrated in Figure 12.1. The focus of questioning should be influenced by the theoretical models the clinician is using as an explanatory hypothesis to account for the clients' presenting problems. There is no discrete point in therapy where assessment stops and formulation begins; the process is one that is collaborative and continuously evolving. However, to promote clarity in the use of case material, different aspects of the assessment process will be covered in turn.

Gathering information for formulation

When gathering information via the assessment process it is important to be mindful of the model and to elicit information relating to the following areas: developmental factors and life experiences including trauma and abuse, faulty self and social knowledge including beliefs about self and others, meta-cognitive factors including positive and negative beliefs about intrusions or symptoms, intrusions into awareness, interpretation of intrusions, safety behaviours and thought control strategies, emotional and physiological responses.

Ruth: a case example

Presenting problems

Ruth was 36 years old, married and had one child. She was employed as a part-time bookkeeper and worked from home. Ruth had a history of mental health difficulties and had engaged in cognitive therapy on two previous occasions after being referred by her general practitioner (GP) to primary care psychology services. Her initial presentation to services was for severe depression and her second for obsessive-compulsive disorder. A few years after her two referrals to primary care psychology services,

Ruth presented to Accident and Emergency (A&E) in crisis and received a diagnosis of schizophrenia. Ruth was extremely depressed, experiencing paranoia and heard voices criticising her. Ruth was referred to the local community mental health team and was then referred by her community psychiatric nurse (CPN) to a service delivering cognitive therapy to individuals experiencing psychosis. Ruth was prescribed Olanzapine and took this regularly despite feeling that the side effects (weight gain) often outweighed the benefits. Ruth reported a long history of feeling depressed and, more recently, hearing critical or abusive voices. In addition, Ruth also described a range of frightening experiences ranging from feeling panicky and 'spaced out', to distressing intrusive recollections relating to experiences of being bullied while at school. The strong feelings of paranoia she experienced meant Ruth would avoid social situations wherever possible, preferring to 'keep busy' at home. Ruth also described problems getting off to sleep with early waking most days as well as feelings of exhaustion.

Cognitive behavioural assessment, problem list and goals

It is vital that both service user and therapist have a shared understanding of the problems that are going to be addressed in therapy and arrive at therapy goals in a collaborative way. Ruth described her problems and prioritised them as follows:

1   Depression
2   Feeling paranoid and that people would harm her
3   Flashbacks related to bullying
4   Critical voices
5   Feeling useless.

The problem list was discussed and specific, measurable, achievable, realistic and time-limited (SMART) goals were set in relation to each problem. For example, in relation to the depression, Ruth stated that she wanted to feel 'normal again'. It was agreed that an overall reduction in depressive mood, measured by the Beck Depression Inventory (BDI: Beck et al. 1988) would be one aspect of this goal. Ruth stated that initially, 'feeling able to go out' would be an important step as the worst part of the depression was that she felt trapped at home because it was the only place she felt safe. It was agreed that in order to develop SMART goals, a first step would be for her to understand better what triggered depressive thoughts (she would later keep a mood diary). This was to allow further analysis of the triggers which would be valuable in assessing the cognitive-behavioural factors contributing to the maintenance of the problem. It was collaboratively agreed that the overall goal would be to improve

Ruth's low mood to a score of 15 or less on the BDI (the 'mild depression' category). It was also agreed that a more realistic goal initially would be to see any reduction in BDI scores from her initial score of 52 (indicating the presence of 'severe' depressive symptomatology).

Risk issues

Ruth did experience suicidal thoughts and had taken one serious over-dose, which required hospital admission when she was a teenager. She did not have any definite plans at the start of therapy and protective factors included: not wanting to hurt her family, the thought that her mother relied on her since her father had died and the belief that suicide was morally wrong. Risk was monitored during the session each week via the BDI (items 2 and 9), while an agreement was made with her CPN to formally assess risk on a weekly basis, thus freeing up some therapy time. It is useful to have a team approach when working with individuals experiencing trauma-related psychosis (see Jankowski, Meuser and Rosenberg, Chapter 4 in this book).

Individuals who have experienced childhood emotional, physical and/or sexual abuse are at high risk of suicide (see Read, Rudegeair and Farrelly, Chapter 2 in this book). In addition, the process of therapy may lead to temporary increases in affect and intrusive recollections for traumatised individuals. Consequently, close collaboration and liaison with multidisciplinary team members and the service user, regarding how best they can be supported at times of increased risk, is highly desirable.

The development of Ruth's problems: traumatic experiences

Ruth described having a good idea of what led to her current difficulties. She said it was because of the bullying and the fact that no one stopped it from happening. Ruth also disclosed experiences of emotional abuse and neglect at home. Her Mum was described as an 'alcoholic' and her Dad was described as being 'either at work or in the pub'.

Ruth described severe, prolonged bullying which involved her being physically and emotionally abused almost daily by a group of girls at both junior and senior schools. This physical and emotional abuse started when she was 8 years old and went on until she left school at 16, during which time Ruth described receiving little or no support from teachers, the police, her head teacher or the school governors. The friends Ruth had were described as being too few and too afraid to 'stick up' for her. She attended A&E on numerous occasions due to the injuries she sustained. Ruth described frequent and distressing flashback experiences relating to the bullying. During this interview the therapist administered the Davidson Trauma Scale (DTS: Davidson et al. 1997) in order to assess current post-trauma symptomatology, and the Post Traumatic Cognitions Inventory (PTCI: Foa et al. 1999) to provide valuable information regarding thoughts and beliefs that mediate the development and maintenance of PTSD.

Ruth experienced extremely severe and frequent intrusions, avoidance and arousal symptoms in relation to the bullying. The PTCI revealed that Ruth held a number of strongly held negative cognitions in relation to herself (e.g. 'If I think about the event I will not be able to handle it' and 'There is something wrong with me as a person'), self-blaming attributions (e.g. 'The event happened because of the sort of person I am' and 'Somebody else would have stopped the event from happening') and negative cognitions about the world (e.g. 'The world is a dangerous place' and 'You can never know who will harm you').

Initial basic formulation, dissociation and selling the model

Cognitive interventions should be guided by a formulation of the factors that have contributed to the development and maintenance of a problem. At the initial session, Ruth explained that she had given up on previous attempts at therapy because she tended to get 'spaced out' when she thought about her past traumatic life events, or was reminded of them. Ruth described one occasion with her previous therapist when she experienced intrusive recollections of the bullying and literally ran out of the room. When the therapist enquired further, it appeared that in the past when bullying was brought up, Ruth would experience depersonalisation, have vivid recollections of past bullying and physical abuse and find sessions intolerable (see Figure 12.2). The therapist took this opportunity to share with Ruth some normalising information about trauma and dissociation (including some literature to read for homework) and to arrange the next appointment at a venue Ruth felt more comfortable with (she was understandably reluctant to attend appointments at a mental health centre). The next appointment was made at Ruth's GP's surgery, which was a two-minute walk from her home and was somewhere she felt was safe and non-stigmatising.

At the next session, Ruth reprioritised her problem list and it was

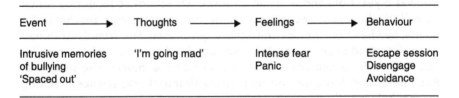

Event	→	Thoughts	→	Feelings	→	Behaviour
Intrusive memories of bullying 'Spaced out'		'I'm going mad'		Intense fear Panic		Escape session Disengage Avoidance

Figure 12.2 Basic formulation of Ruth's previous experience of therapy

agreed the initial focus would be dissociation in order to maximise her chances of engaging in therapy. The change of venue helped Ruth feel more in control and her reading about traumatic reactions, PTSD and dissociation had helped her view her experiences as part of a coping process that was in no way a sign of her 'going mad'. Detailed discussion regarding her posttraumatic reactions followed, allowing the therapist to further share normalising information about trauma reactions and the idea that dissociation can be viewed as a way of coping when we are faced with situations or events that may otherwise be intolerable. Ruth explained that this made sense as she recalled coping with the violent assaults by distancing herself from what was happening to her. After a while, Ruth reported being able to get through the assaults by feeling nothing and numbing herself to what was happening. Ruth recalled that after a while she didn't feel anything (emotionally or physically) while being assaulted and that it was only some time after the assault that she would become upset and distressed. Through a process of collaborative discussion and guided discovery, Ruth's experience of 'spacing out' and her intrusive recollections were explored. Recent specific examples were drawn out on paper using the event–thought–feeling–behaviour format which allowed Ruth to engage with the therapist in a collaborative way and facilitated socialisation into the general cognitive model.

The triggers for Ruth appeared to be feelings of fear and painful memories, which led her to believe she would 'go mad', never be able to cope or feel 'normal'. Some situations in particular reminded her of the bullying; for example, picking her son up from outside his school. Also, Ruth feared bumping into the bullies, some of whom were still living in her local area. Last time she did see one of them, this triggered strong feelings of fear and anger, which led her to feel 'spaced out'.

Over the next weeks, Ruth read Helen Kennerley's article on dissociation (Kennerley 1996) and valuable time was spent discussing and normalising Ruth's dissociative and posttraumatic reactions. Consequently, the therapist was able to utilise Ruth's theoretical and first-hand knowledge of dissociation in a way that allowed her to 'lead' the next few sessions. Ruth was clear that avoidance was contributing to the maintenance of the problem, but it was agreed that 'planned avoidance', as suggested by Kennerley (1996), was a sensible first-line strategy. Furthermore, it was collaboratively agreed that although dissociation had helped Ruth cope when she was the victim of bullying, and part of a continuum of normal experience, it was unhelpful in the way she currently experienced it. Ruth was aware of the maintaining role of safety behaviours and therefore, that this was not intended to be a long-term strategy, but rather a way of helping develop confidence and a sense of control. Time was taken around collaboratively planning the next few sessions, and it was agreed that if Ruth was to cope more effectively with the flashbacks and to feel less distressed by them, she would need skills in managing her 'spacing out' coping response. She would basically need to manage her dissociative reaction when exposed to the stimuli that triggered this response.

A contract was agreed for sessions which stated that:

- The therapist would always ask for consent to approach the subject of bullying.
- Ruth could ask to change the subject or stop the session and have 'time out'.
- Sessions addressing bullying specifically would be planned in advance.
- Ruth would practise her grounding techniques between sessions and bring grounding objects with her.

In between each session, Ruth practised grounding techniques. Refocusing on the environment was found to be useful in helping Ruth to focus less on her internal experiences and thereby avert the 'spacing out' episodes. This seemed to work on two levels: first, the distraction or externalisation of attentional focus, and second, it allowed her to remain in the 'here and now'. A grounding word or phrase in conjunction with this refocusing of attention proved especially successful for Ruth (e.g. 'I am Mrs Ruth Jones and I am a strong and capable wife and mother'). Ruth also began to wear her favourite perfume and bring it to sessions. The perfume reminded her of being married as her husband had first bought it for her on their honeymoon.

The benefit of this work, focusing on managing dissociation in session was that Ruth no longer reported fearing 'spacing out' and instead likened it to daydreaming, which was a much more normalising appraisal. Once she understood the function, triggers and had a range of practised coping strategies for her dissociative reaction, Ruth did not actually experience another dissociative experience in session. The few sessions spent on this phase of the therapy proved extremely engaging in that she reported increased confidence, less frequent thoughts about 'going mad' and gained valuable trust in the therapist and the cognitive therapy approach.

Integrative case formulation

During the course of therapy, the guided discovery approach was employed allowing Ruth to conclude that the 'paranoia', flashbacks and 'spacing out', as well as the 'critical voices', were all in some way related to her experiences of bullying and, in turn, these had a negative effect on her mood. Consequently, it was agreed that being able to see the various factors contributing to both the maintenance and development of her difficulties would be helpful in guiding the decision about which area of her difficulties to tackle next as Ruth felt each of the remaining items on her problem list were equally distressing in different ways. Each box in the formulation diagram was drawn out on a sheet of flipchart paper and labelled with terms Ruth was comfortable with. For example, the first box was labelled 'Intrusions or events', the one underneath labelled 'Making sense/interpretations/thoughts' and so on. The different areas of this formulation diagram were already familiar to Ruth in terms of the event–thought–feelings–behaviour cycle which had already proved useful. The life experiences box and the beliefs about self and others, rules and strategies box were discussed in terms of factors, which would have contributed to the development of her problems. The different problem areas were also labelled (a), (b) and (c) in order to ensure the formulation remained clear and comprehensible to both client and therapist. Over the course of the next few sessions this integrative model of trauma and psychosis was adapted to offer an idiosyncratic formulation of Ruth's difficulties via a process of guided discovery, which incorporated both developmental and maintaining factors (see Figure 12.3). The process of developing this shared formulation proved helpful in a number of ways. First, it suggested that a number of problems could be understood in a unified and coherent manner, which Ruth found reassuring. Second, it consolidated more acceptable and compassionate alternative explanations for some of Ruth's problematic interpretations such as 'I'm going mad', 'I'm not normal'. Third, it allowed Ruth to identify the next area for intervention.

Intervention

As clinicians faced with the dilemma of how best to offer support and intervention to individuals experiencing psychosis as a consequence of trauma, those traumatised by the experience of psychosis and those who do not have a clear diagnosis, but have a history of traumatic experience either as a child or subsequently as an adult, it is important to be pragmatic. However, it is also important to ensure that such approaches are derived from the case conceptualisation and that an informed choice to consent to specific strategies is made by the service user in each instance. As the above work on dissociation illustrates, there is not necessarily a clear distinction between assessment, formulation and treatment; rather, these processes are interrelated, fluid and evolving. However, we shall now describe specific intervention strategies in relation to Ruth's case example.

Emotional consequences and distress

In subsequent sessions, Ruth often identified her low mood, feelings of paranoia and fear as a focus for the main agenda item (it is often the case

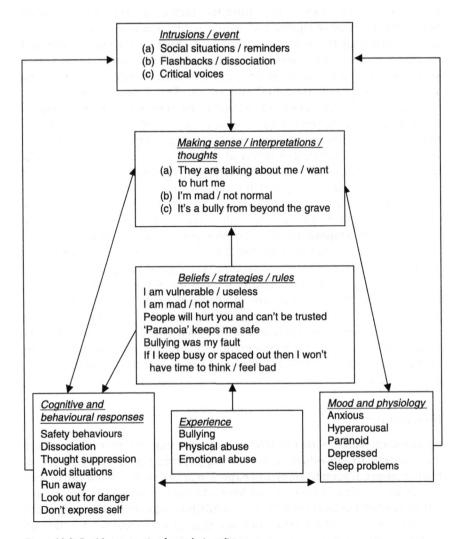

Figure 12.3 Ruth's integrative formulation diagram

that people prioritise the emotional consequences of psychotic experiences, rather than the experiences themselves). Socratic questioning was
used to explore recent events and the subsequent effect on Ruth's emotions. A series of maintenance formulations were constructed using the
event–thought–feeling–behaviour format (Table 12.1).

The therapist then used these examples to socialise Ruth into the general cognitive model in relation to factors that influenced her emotions.
This process is illustrated by the dialogue below:

Table 12.1 Basic maintenance formulation of one of Ruth's episodes of 'paranoia'

Events $\longrightarrow$	Thoughts $\longrightarrow$	Feelings $\longrightarrow$	Behaviours
Standing with other mums at school waiting for son	They always look at me funny	Anxious 'Paranoid'	Prepare self for trouble
	They are going to gang up on me	Frightened	Move away from them
Flashback to bullying at school	It is happening again	Panic	Wait in car with doors locked
	I'm useless, I'll never live a normal life	Depressed Hopeless	Avoid people Do less

Therapist: So whenever you are standing outside your son's school with lots of other mums you get very panicky because you think that the way they look at you and talk among themselves indicates some kind of threat to you. Is that an accurate summary?

Ruth: Yes, and I get all panicky and before I know it it's happening all over again.

Therapist: What's happening again?

Ruth: The bullying. It's like I'm back at school and it's all still happening.

Therapist: What do you think was happening to you when you felt like you were back at school being bullied?

Ruth: I think I'm going mad.

Therapist: Do you have any other explanations for what might be happening?

Ruth: Well, I sometimes think going to pick up my son from school brings it all back to me. I try not to go there if I can help it but sometimes if my husband is working late I have no choice.

Therapist: Do you usually try to avoid things that remind you of the bullying?

Ruth: Yes. I won't even drive past certain areas because it brings it all back to me and then I'll feel really low.

Therapist: How did you feel when you got home from this particular trip to collect your son from school?

Ruth: I felt frightened, then later, I felt depressed and useless. I feel like I'm never going to live a normal life and that I should be over the bullying by now.

Therapist: Let me summarise just to make sure I understand this properly. You feel threatened and afraid when you go to pick your son up from school. If one of the other mums looks at you or they are talking together, you interpret this as a sign that they are planning to gang up on you. You feel increasingly frightened and become panicky, at which point you experience flashbacks of being bullied at school. Then you remove yourself from the situation. Later, when you get home you feel depressed, hopeless about the future and give yourself a hard time. Does this sound accurate?

Ruth: Yes. That's how it happened.

Therapist: If you wanted to feel differently in this situation, what would you need to do?

Ruth: Well, I could wait in the car.

Therapist: Anything else?

Ruth: I could try telling myself that I'll be OK because I'm an adult now and try to distract myself.

Therapist: And have you tried this?

Ruth: Yes. It does help a bit.

Therapist: Why do you think reminding yourself that you are an adult helps?

Ruth: Because it means I'm not likely to be bullied by a bunch of other mums outside a school next to a main road.

Therapist: How do you mean?

Ruth: Well, I've never been bullied as an adult and besides if they tried anything, I'd report them to the police.

Therapist: Is there anything else that might make you feel less distressed in this situation?

Ruth: Well, if I knew they weren't planning together to hurt me, I might feel better about it.

Therapist: Can you think of any explanation for why the other mums might be looking over at you and talking in a group?

Ruth: Well, I suppose they might know each other and just be passing the time of day.

Therapist: Yes, go on.

Ruth: I suppose they might look over out of curiosity. They might be wondering who I am.

Therapist: Why's that?

Ruth: Well, my son has recently started a new school and I've only been there a few times.

Therapist: Is there anything else that might explain why the other mums stood together looked over at you?

Ruth: Well, I suppose they might have wondered whose mum I was. It's sometimes nice to know the parents of the kids your child is friends with at school.

Therapist: Which of these possibilities sounds most likely? That the

	other mums will band together and bully you or one of the others you just came up with?
Ruth:	They are probably a bit curious and are just chatting to pass the time. I expect they might wonder who I am. Come to think of it, someone did say hello to me last time I was there. I think they wanted to start a conversation, but I avoided looking over again.
Therapist:	If you were able to think through these different explanations at the time, and decide that the other mums were just chatting or curious to meet you, would you still feel distressed?
Ruth:	Probably not. And I wouldn't go home feeling useless and depressed either.
Therapist:	So what part of this pattern needs to change for you to feel differently about the situation?
Ruth:	It's the way I look at the situation, it's how I interpret the other mums' behaviour that needs to change.

Over the course of the next three sessions, specific incidents when Ruth felt paranoid were examined using this framework. The therapist discussed with Ruth her positive and negative beliefs about paranoia as well the pros and cons of paranoia as a coping strategy, before collaboratively discussing a normalising rationale for selective attention to interpersonal threat as a reaction to trauma. Consequently, it was agreed that 'paranoia' was possibly inaccurate as a description for what she experienced and was reframed as her attempts to 'stay on guard in order to keep safe'. Ruth became skilled at using thought records, completed several as homework tasks that involved examining evidence for and against her thoughts and the generation of alternative explanations for events in order to help her to evaluate the accuracy of her paranoid and depressive thoughts. She began to see some improvement in her low mood, as well as noticing some reduction in the frequency of her 'paranoid' thoughts, how much she believed them to be true and the distress experienced as a consequence of them. Similarly, Ruth's thoughts that she was 'going mad' became infrequent, less convincing and less distressing.

Examining evidence and generating alternative explanations

The process of examining evidence and generating alternative explanations was also applied to her self-blaming thoughts, in relation to her traumatic experiences. In addition to generating alternative appraisals and evaluating the evidence for each of these alternatives, a pie chart was used to examine responsibility for the bullying occurring and continuing for so long. The result was that Ruth realised she was not to blame for the initiation of the bullying, in that not wanting to be part of the bullies' group was a reasonable choice. With some guided discovery, she concluded that they must have felt threatened that she chose not to be part of their gang and that she did everything she could to put an end to the bullying; from fighting back to trying to avoid them, recruiting allies, telling three separate teachers and the head teacher as well as reporting the bullies to the police. Ruth recalled during the course of this exercise that she did succeed in stopping the bullying for variable periods of time, and she did get some limited support from one teacher, but that it always started again. Under the pie chart Ruth wrote,

> If there is not enough room on this pie chart to fit in all the people who should shoulder the blame before me, then it proves beyond a doubt that it was not my fault. My defiance in not breaking down in front of them [the bullies], even while getting beaten, probably made them feel even more inadequate.

Behavioural experiments

Ruth was keen to test out her hypotheses about why the other mums looked at her and put some of her new coping skills into practice. For example, she went to collect her son from school and predicted that if the other mums were just curious about her, which was one possibility, they would respond warmly if she said hello or smiled at them. A review of the available evidence for each of her alternatives to 'they will gang up on me/want to hurt me' was conducted during the session. This, in addition to exploring any potential obstacles to the experiment, gave Ruth the confidence to carry out the experiment. Ruth did pick her son up from school and smiled at one of the other mums waiting outside the school. The outcome was that the other mum introduced herself and struck up a conversation. On subsequent trips to collect her son, Ruth chatted to the same woman and was soon introduced to the other mums who Ruth had originally felt threatened by. This resulted in a drastic reduction in her belief that she was at any risk from other mums while collecting her son. Similarly, other specific incidents where Ruth had felt 'paranoid' were discussed and addressed in session and via homework tasks, which resulted in a great reduction in feelings of threat from other women in a variety of social situations and a decrease in the frequency of dissociative phenomena.

Safety behaviours were also identified and manipulated via behavioural experiments. For example, because Ruth appraised her intrusive experiences as signs of her 'going mad', she engaged in thought suppression. A simple thought suppression experiment and discussion during session was sufficient to help her to understand that attempting to push intrusive images out of her mind was likely to increase the frequency of intrusions.

A detached-mindfulness approach (Wells and Matthews 1994), similar to that advocated by Ehlers and Clark (2000) was discussed as a home-task and proved extremely effective in reducing both the frequency of intrusions and the appraisals of impending madness. As Wells (1997: 272) points out, 'detached mindfulness is not an attempt "not to think" a thought; it is an attempt to disengage the elaborative ruminative or analytical processing from intruding thoughts. A further aim of detached mindfulness is an increase in meta-cognitive awareness'.

Mastery and pleasure

Activity scheduling was discussed in relation to the formulation as Ruth had little opportunity to engage in activities that gave her a sense of pleasure or achievement. Apart from the obvious mood enhancement aspect of this intervention, the secondary aim was to address the feeling that her life was 'on hold'. Ehlers and Clark (2000) suggest encouraging clients to 'reclaim' their former selves by reinstating previously valued activities with the aim of contextualising memories and to provide the feeling that life is moving forward. However, Ruth stated that she had no real sense of who she was prior to the trauma as she was 8 when it started and 16 when it stopped. Therefore, part of this intervention was to help Ruth re-engage in activities she enjoyed during periods of feeling well and exploring new activities and interests she could associate with her recovery.

Re-examining the meaning of the trauma: bullying and what it meant to Ruth

Initially, Ruth was provided with some educational material about the nature of PTSD (criteria, treatment options and possible outcomes). Following a discussion of treatment approaches to PTSD and the consequences of trauma, it was collaboratively agreed that the therapy would focus on examining the meaning of the trauma, as opposed to imaginal exposure. The process of formulation allowed for a shared understanding to be reached about the development of Ruth's difficulties. The bullying she experienced over the years led her to believe that others were not to be trusted and would harm her. Her first experience of bullying was by other girls who were previously friends and this began when she was only 8 years old. Her parents, teachers and friends were all confided in regarding the bullying, but no one stopped it. The bullying continued. Consequently Ruth came to the conclusion that the bullying happened because of something about her as a person and that somehow it must have been her fault. Ruth's mother told her to 'stick up' for herself and was frequently critical of her. Ruth's school work suffered due to difficulty concentrating and truancy, and over the years she fell behind her peers in terms of academic achievement. Ruth developed the belief that she was useless and vulnerable. The development of the 'spacing out' episodes, although initially part of her coping repertoire, later became distressing and unhelpful. Similarly, the intrusive recollections or flashbacks became distressing and led Ruth to engage in a pattern of avoidance that severely restricted her lifestyle. Ruth interpreted these dissociative phenomena as signs of impending madness and indications that she wasn't 'normal'.

With reference to the shared formulation, the therapist used guided discovery to explore options with Ruth. It was agreed that it was how she made sense of the bullying and the intrusive recollections that led to her distress and that the strategies she adopted were maintaining the problem.

Standard cognitive therapy techniques were employed, such as providing a normalising rationale for her difficulties and using guided discovery to assist in modifying the main problematic appraisals related to the bullying and its consequences. For example, an alternative to 'I'm not normal and never will be' was 'I might have struggled with these experiences, but they are normal reactions to severe trauma and I am learning to cope with them'; 'I should have stuck up for myself' became 'No one could have fought off a group that big'; 'I'm vulnerable' became 'I'm no more vulnerable than anyone else; in fact, I'm a strong, resilient person'.

Dealing with avoidance

Ruth was avoiding areas of town, such as the precinct and the market for fear of bumping into any of the bullies. Ruth had seen one of the perpetrators of the violence (Gina) on the street in the past couple of years. This historical evidence was examined using the familiar event–thought–feeling–behaviour format:

Therapist: So, Gina looked 'on edge' when she saw you. What do you think was the reason for this?
Ruth: I saw it as a sign that she might attack me.
Therapist: How did that make you feel?
Ruth: I felt spaced out and totally panicked
Therapist: What did you do as a consequence of this?
Ruth: I was really scared; I rushed back to the car and locked myself in. When I got home I ruminated about it. I soon convinced myself that if I hadn't escaped so quickly, she would have attacked me.
Therapist: Can you imagine why Gina looked on edge?
Ruth: She might have been deciding whether she could get away with having a go at me in public.
Therapist: Are there any other possible reasons?

Ruth: I'm not sure really.
Therapist: Do you ever feel on edge?
Ruth: Yes.
Therapist: What are some of the reasons you feel on edge?
Ruth: If I'm embarrassed or uncomfortable. Or if I feel anxious.
Therapist: Could any of these reasons apply to Gina?
Ruth: I suppose so.
Therapist: Can you imagine why she might feel embarrassed, uncomfortable or anxious?
Ruth: She might have felt embarrassed or guilty about what she did. In fact she might have even thought I was going to have a go at her for what she did.
Therapist: If at the time you were able to think of these different possibilities, do you think you would have felt so upset?
Ruth: No. I think I would have felt OK.

Some work practising assertiveness skills and in-session role-playing combined with some visualisation was conducted. Ruth would imagine bumping into one of the bullies and role-play her response in this situation. Her avoidance of situations associated with the bullying was reduced and Ruth began shopping in the precinct again with her Mum. By now it appeared that Ruth possessed greater meta-cognitive awareness, a good understanding of the role and consequences of her appraisals, was able to generate alternative appraisals and was very competent at gathering and evaluating evidence. She was experiencing less frequent and distressing intrusive recollections and rarely felt 'spaced out'. Her mood had improved and she no longer experienced suicidal thoughts, although she was still moderately depressed. Overall, she reported less avoidance of either intrusions or situations that reminded her of the bullying.

She also agreed to visit her old school site and was surprised at how much smaller everything looked. Because everything looked very different (several buildings had been knocked down and an annexe had been built), this appeared to facilitate the process of contextualising the bullying as part of her past.

Self-esteem and critical voices

The final problem area prioritised on the agenda was that of critical voices. Ruth described hearing critical voices inside her head. The voices were described as critical, abusive and derogatory in the most part. Ruth reported this experience usually when she was tired, following periods of poor sleep, when her mood was particularly low. The maintenance formulation and her list of possible explanations indicated that this experience was viewed as either Ruth being contacted by the spirit of the 'ring leader' of the girls who bullied her (who had died in an accident five years ago), a sign that she was 'going mad', or 'something to do with being bullied'.

After examining several thought records and voice diary examples, it became clear that a number of internal and external events were reliable triggers for the voices. These were social situations (involving groups of people), feeling like she had made a mistake or 'said the wrong thing' in social situations, and sleep deprivation. Trying to suppress the voices made them worse and reading seemed to help significantly. This information was discussed collaboratively in relation to each of the possible explanations for the voices. A home task was agreed, which involved Ruth researching the experience of 'voice hearing'. At the next session, her research (on the internet) had yielded additional explanations. These were:

1   Confusing thoughts and memories related to bullying
2   My own unrecognised thoughts
3   Me remembering things that people said to me
4   Me giving myself a hard time, but feeling guilty about wishing Sandra dead.

Each alternative was listed and, once more, evidence evaluated in relation to each possible explanation. After much discussion and further investigations for homework tasks, involving diaries and behavioural experiments, Ruth came to view the voices as 'self-critical intrusive thoughts' and acknowledge that her self-esteem was low, which made sense to her considering the experiences she had growing up.

Self-esteem

Because Ruth's core beliefs about herself were negative, this was causing biases in her attention and information-processing strategies, meaning she was unlikely to process any information that wasn't congruent with her negative beliefs about herself. Positive data collection (described by Padesky 1994) was utilised as a method of collecting evidence in support of Ruth's worthwhile attributes and counteracting her negatively biased data collection style. Consequently, in subsequent sessions, Ruth was able to challenge her long-held views that she was 'useless' and 'not likeable' and replace them with more balanced and accurate beliefs which were consistent with the evidence she had been gathering via the positive data log.

Relapse prevention

The usual therapy blueprint was collaboratively discussed and the format was agreed. The blueprint was completed in session and as homework tasks. This consisted of an 'Action plan for the future' as suggested by Fennell (1999). This included a summary of the most useful aspects of the therapy and in addition, copies of the following:

- The formulation diagrams, maintenance, developmental, self-esteem and integrative formulations.
- Pie chart of actual blame.
- List of triggers for problems addressed.
- List of new core beliefs.
- List of new rules and strategies.
- Lists of positive qualities generated by her son, husband, friend and self.

Ruth was able to reflect on the evidence and conclude through a process of guided discovery that she actually coped better with stressful life events and the impact they had upon her mental health than she gave herself credit for. Ruth had experienced several 'set-backs' in relation to her mental health, but had continued to cope with the demands of caring for her family, serious physical health problems, the death of her father and having her driving licence revoked. During this stressful time Ruth had avoided hospital admission, made significant progress in therapy and sought appropriate support from the community mental health team.

Summary

This chapter has outlined a theoretical approach to understanding the relationship between the experience of traumatic life events and the development and maintenance of psychotic experiences. It has also described how such a cognitive model can be utilised to guide the assessment process and develop idiosyncratic case conceptualisations, which, in turn, determine the selection of intervention strategies. This approach has been illustrated using a case example, which, while clearly not exhaustive, demonstrates the therapeutic approach. The case example also serves to illustrate several common difficulties, such as managing dissociative experiences, the links between paranoid ideation as a method for managing interpersonal threat and previous traumatic experiences, and the links between the content of critical and abusive voices and abusive life experiences. Similarly, the case illustrates common treatment strategies such as re-examining the meaning of the trauma, verbal reattribution (including evidence for and against a belief and the generation of alternative explanations) and behavioural reattribution (including behavioural experiments and reduction of avoidance).

References

Allen, J. G., and Coyne, L. (1995) Dissociation and vulnerability to psychotic experiences. *Journal of Nervous and Mental Disease, 183*, 615–622.

Baddeley, A., Thornton, A., Chua, S. E., and McKenna, P. (1996) Schizophrenic delusions and the construction of autobiographical memory. In D. C. Rubin (ed.) *Remembering our past: Studies in autobiographical memory* (pp. 384–428). New York: Cambridge University Press.

Barrowclough, C., Johnston, M., and Tarrier, N. (1994) Attributions, expressed emotion and patient relapse: An attributional model of relatives' response to schizophrenic illness. *Behavior Therapy, 25*, 67–88.

Beck, A. T. (1976) *Cognitive therapy and the emotional disorders.* New York: International Universities Press.

Beck, A. T., Steer, R. A., and Garbin, G. M. (1988) Psychometric properties of the Beck Depression Inventory: Twenty-five years of evaluation. *Clinical Psychology Review, 8*, 77–100.

Bentall, R. P., and Kaney, S. (1989) Content-specific information processing and persecutory delusions: An investigation using the emotional Stroop test. *British Journal of Medical Psychology, 62*, 355–364.

Bentall, R. P., Corcoran, R., Howard, R., Blackwood, R., and Kinderman, P. (2001) Persecutory delusions: A review and theoretical integration. *Clinical Psychology Review, 22*, 1–50.

Birchwood, M., Mason, R., MacMillan, F., and Healy, J. (1993) Depression, demoralization and control over psychotic illness: A comparison of depressed and non-depressed patients with a chronic psychosis. *Psychological Medicine, 23*, 387–395.

Brewin, C. R. (1998) Intrusive autobiographical memories in depression and posttraumatic stress disorder. *Applied Cognitive Psychology, 12*, 359–370.

Butler, G. (1999) Clinical formulation. In A. S. Bellack and M. Hersen (eds) *Comprehensive clinical psychology*, Volume 6, *Adults: Clinical formulation and treatment.* New York: Pergamon.

Chadwick, P., and Birchwood, M. (1994) The omnipotence of voices: A cognitive approach to auditory hallucinations. *British Journal of Psychiatry, 164*, 190–201.

Davidson, J., Book, S. W., Colket, J. T., Tupler, L. A., Roth, S., Hertzberg, M., et al. (1997) Assessment of a new rating scale for post-traumatic stress disorder. *Psychological Medicine, 27*, 153–160.

Dunmore, E., Clark, D. M., and Ehlers, A. (1999) Cognitive factors involved in the onset and maintenance of posttraumatic stress disorder (PTSD) after physical or sexual assault. *Behaviour Research and Therapy, 37*, 809–829.

Ehlers, A., and Clark, D. M. (2000) A cognitive model of posttraumatic stress disorder. *Behaviour Research and Therapy, 38*, 319–345.

Ehlers, A., Hackmann, A., Steil, R., Clohessy, S., Wenninger, K., and Winter, H. (2002) The nature of intrusive memories after trauma: The warning signal hypothesis. *Behaviour Research and Therapy, 40*, 995–1002.

Fennell, M. (1999) *Overcoming low self-esteem.* London: Robinson.

Foa, E. B., Ehlers, A., Clark, D. M., Tolin, D. F., and Orsillo, S. M. (1999) The Posttraumatic Cognitions Inventory (PTCI): Development and validation. *Psychological Assessment, 11*, 303–314.

Freeman, D., Garety, P. A., and Kuipers, E. (2001) Persecutory delusions: Developing the understanding of belief maintenance and emotional distress. *Psychological Medicine, 31*, 1293–1306.

Garety, P. A., Kuipers, E., Fowler, D., Freeman, D., and Bebbington, P. E. (2001) A cognitive model of the positive symptoms of psychosis. *Psychological Medicine, 31*, 189–195.

Hirsch, S. R., and Jolley, A. G. (1989) The dysphoric syndrome in schizophrenia and its implications for relapse. *British Journal of Psychiatry, 155* (Suppl. 5), 46–50.

Honig, A., Romme, M. A. J., Ensink, B. J., Escher, S. D. M., Pennings, M. H. A., and DeVries, M. W. (1998) Auditory hallucinations: A comparison between patients and nonpatients. *Journal of Nervous and Mental Disease, 186*, 646–651.

Johns, L. C., and Van Os, J. (2001) The continuity of psychotic experiences in the general population. *Clinical Psychology Review, 21*, 1125–1141.

Kennerley, H. (1996) Cognitive therapy for dissociative symptoms associated with trauma. *British Journal of Clinical Psychology, 35*, 325–340.

Kilcommons, A. M., and Morrison, A. P. (2005) Relationships between trauma and psychosis: An exploration of cognitive factors. *Acta Psychiatrica Scandinavica, 112*, 351–359.

McGorry, P. D., Chanen, A., McCarthy, E., van Riel, R., McKenzie, D., and Singh, B. S. (1991) Post traumatic stress disorder following recent onset psychosis. *Journal of Nervous and Mental Disease, 179*, 253–258.

Morrison, A. P. (1998) A cognitive analysis of the maintenance of auditory hallucinations: Are voices to schizophrenia what bodily sensations are to panic? *Behavioural and Cognitive Psychotherapy, 26*, 289–302.

Morrison, A. P. (2001) The interpretation of intrusions in psychosis: An integrative cognitive approach to hallucinations and delusions. *Behavioural and Cognitive Psychotherapy, 29*, 257–276.

Morrison, A. P., and Wells, A. (2000) Thought control strategies in schizophrenia: A comparison with non-patients. *Behaviour Research and Therapy, 38*, 1205–1209.

Morrison, A. P., Beck, A. T., Glentworth, D., Dunn, H., Reid, G., Larkin, W., and Williams, S. (2002) Imagery and psychotic symptoms: A preliminary investigation. *Behaviour Research and Therapy, 40*, 1063–1072.

Morrison, A. P., Frame, L., and Larkin, W. (2003) Relationships between trauma and psychosis: A review and integration. *British Journal of Clinical Psychology, 42*, 331–353.

Morrison, A. P., Nothard, S., Bowe, S. E., and Wells, A. (2004) Interpretations of voices in patients with hallucinations and non-patient controls: A comparison and predictors of distress in patients. *Behaviour Research and Therapy, 42*, 1315–1323.

Morrison, A. P., Renten, J. C., Dunn, H., Williams, S., and Bentall, R. P. (2004) *Cognitive Therapy for Psychosis: A formulation-based approach*. Hove: Brunner-Routledge.

Morrison, A. P., Gumley, A. I., Schwannauer, M., Campbell, M., Gleeson, A., Griffin, E., and Gillan, K. (2005) The beliefs about paranoia scale: Preliminary validation of a metacognitive approach to conceptualising paranoia. *Behavioural and Cognitive Psychotherapy, 33*, 153–164.

Mueser, K. T., Rosenberg, S. D., Goodman, L. A., and Trumbetta, S. L. (2002) Trauma, PTSD and the course of severe mental illness: An interactive model. *Schizophrenia Research, 53*, 123–143.

Padesky, C. A. (1994) Schema change processes in cognitive therapy. *Clinical Psychology and Psychotherapy, 1*, 267–278.

Reynolds, M., and Wells, A. (1999) The thought control questionnaire: Psychometric properties in a clinical sample, and relationships with PTSD and depression. *Psychological Medicine, 29*, 1089–1099.

Ross, C. A., and Keyes, B. (2004) Dissociation and schizophrenia. *Journal of Trauma and Dissociation, 5*, 69–83.

Spitzer, C., Haug, H.-J., and Freyberger, H. J. (1997) Dissociative symptoms in schizophrenic patients with positive and negative symptoms. *Psychopathology, 30*, 67–75.

Tarrier, N., Sommerfield, C., and Pilgrim, H. (1999) Relatives' expressed emotion (EE) and PTSD treatment outcome. *Psychological Medicine, 29*, 801–811.

Thrasher, S. M., Dalgleish, T., and Yule, W. (1994) Information processing in post-traumatic stress disorder. *Behaviour Research and Therapy, 32*, 247–254.

van der Kolk, B. A., Pelcovitz, D., Roth, S., Mandel, F. S., McFarlane, A., and Herman, J. L. (1996) Dissociation, somatization, and affect dysregulation: The complexity of adaptation of trauma. *American Journal of Psychiatry, 153* (7 Suppl.), 83–93.

Wells, A. (1997) *Cognitive therapy for anxiety disorders*. Chichester: John Wiley.

Wells, A., and Matthews, G. (1994) *Attention and emotion*. Hove: Lawrence Erlbaum.

Chapter 13

A trauma-based model of relapse in psychosis

Andrew I. Gumley and Angus MacBeth

The chaos and trauma is intense. My perception of everything around me becomes much more heightened. My relations with other people, while they seem to be normal and usual to those who interact with me are problematic. I have no control. My mind becomes bombarded with thoughts, I have beliefs about myself, which are totally unfounded, the paranoia is intense. I worry about the slightest thing from did I say the right thing, did I frighten or harm that person, or do they think I'm mad. I think that my psychosis is inherently evil; a manifestation of the devil. It attacked and nearly destroyed me, and that's why I believed that the devil had taken my soul.

Introduction

This personal testimony encapsulates the major theme that permeates this chapter. That is, this account illustrates the personal significance, meaning and trauma attached to the subjective experience of acute psychosis. Indeed, it is proposed that understanding the personal meaning and trauma attached to the experience of psychosis are critical stages in the development of a compassionate approach to the conceptualisation of psychological interventions aimed at enabling recovery from, and staying well after, psychosis. In this conceptualisation, it is also of great import to recognise psychosis as being a highly significant, frightening and distressing life event, with potentially ongoing ramifications. Relapse has been commonly defined as a recurrence or a deterioration of positive psychotic symptoms, which are associated with increased impairment in day-to-day functioning. There is little doubt that the recurrence of psychosis is a distressing and traumatic experience for individuals, families and loved ones. Thus, it is hardly surprising that relapse is often associated with hospital readmission, slower and less complete recovery, greater loss of social networks, vocational opportunities, and increased personal disability. Furthermore, and intrinsic within the definition of 'relapse', is the experience of an event repeating itself, carrying a corresponding appraisal that the event can no longer be rationalised as a 'one-off'.

Life event dimensions

In psychological terms, Birchwood and colleagues (Birchwood and Iqbal 1998; Birchwood et al. 1993, 2000) have shown that relapse is linked to the development of depressed mood and suicidal thinking. The mechanism for the development of post-psychotic depression (PPD) probably operates via personal appraisals of loss arising from psychosis ('I'll never be able to work again') and entrapment in psychosis ('Relapse just comes out of the blue, there's nothing I can do about it'). This work has also demonstrated that the perception (by the individual) of psychosis as being shameful and humiliating is predictive of the development of PPD (Birchwood et al. 1993, 2000; Rooke and Birchwood 1998). Similar appraisals of psychosis as entrapping, shameful and involving loss have been found in a study of individuals with co-occurring psychosis and social anxiety disorder (Gumley et al. 2004). The dimensions of loss, humiliation, entrapment and danger, when occurring as appraisals of stressful life events, have long been established as important to the development and maintenance of psychopathology (Brown and Harris 1978; Brown et al. 1995). Danger has been an overlooked life event dimension in relation to the appraisals of psychosis. Danger relates to a prospective dimension, which hinges on an individual's perception that, with the occurrence of an event there is an accompanying likelihood of recurrence. Alternatively, the event can also signal the beginning of a series of consequences that are unpleasant or threatening to the individual (Brown and Harris 1996). In psychosis fear of relapse and recurrence are often associated with high levels of anxiety and avoidance. On the other hand, the stigmatising nature of psychosis can mean that the person becomes fearful that friends, family, employers and work colleagues discover that the person has experienced psychosis.

Phenomenology of relapse

A substantial body of evidence from retrospective (e.g. Herz and Melville 1980) and prospective (e.g. Birchwood et al. 1989; Jorgensen 1998) studies of relapse shows that the recurrence or exacerbation of psychotic symptoms is preceded by increases in non-psychotic symptoms, such as anxiety, sleeplessness, preoccupation, irritability and depressed mood. Prospective studies show that, while these 'non-psychotic' symptoms are relatively *sensitive* to relapse, they are not *specific* to relapse: on most occasions when a relapse occurs it is preceded by increases in non-psychotic symptoms, but that is not to say that increases in symptoms such as anxiety and depression always and invariably lead to relapse. In addition, prospective studies show that the specificity of non-psychotic symptoms to relapse is improved when low-level psychotic symptoms such as suspiciousness, paranoia, hearing voices and ideas of reference are incorporated into the formulation of early signs of relapse.

This research base has two important implications. First, it suggests that the non-psychotic symptoms, which have been observed during the early stages of relapse, are likely to represent an individual's idiosyncratic emotional response to the emergence of subtle and covert changes in low-level psychotic experiences. Second, the lack of specificity of non-psychotic symptoms to relapse, suggests that early signs are not indicative of an inevitable trajectory towards relapse. Instead, transition to relapse may depend on other factors including, but not limited to, the magnitude or intensity of individuals' emotional and psycho-physiological responses to low-level psychotic experiences.

In light of these points, this chapter proposes that individuals' emotional, physiological, behavioural and interpersonal responses to changes in existing or recurring low-level psychotic experiences are, first, mediated by their cognitive and emotional appraisal of both these current experiences and the influence of pre-existing core developmental schemata. We also propose that, second, a 'trauma-based' perspective may be helpful in understanding the pathway to transition into relapse for a significant group of individuals with psychosis. In this chapter, trauma refers to experiences that may occur during psychosis, or via early developmental experiences (including abuse and neglect in the context of attachment security) influence their adaptation to psychosis, recovery style and help-seeking in the context of emotional distress.

Subjective experience and psychosis

Many investigators have identified autobiographical memories portraying subtle changes in attention, perception and awareness of movement, thinking and emotion that characterise the early stages of psychosis (Bowers 1968; Cutting 1985; Docherty et al. 1978; Freedman 1974; Freedman and Chapman 1973; Heinrichs and Carpenter 1985; McGhie and Chapman 1961). Boker et al. (1984) investigated naturally occurring coping strategies associated with these basic experiences among forty inpatient individuals during their acute psychosis. Most of the coping strategies reported by participants were active problem-solving-based ones, as opposed to more passive strategies such as avoidance or withdrawal. Such experiences were interpreted by many participants as 'danger signals'. In this sense the subjective experience of cognitive and perceptual dysregulation is by no means a passive experience. Individuals actively attempted to make sense of their experiences, and pursue coping strategies to ameliorate these experiences. The feeling that an internal or external experience signals 'danger' is also implicated in the maintenance of posttraumatic stress disorder (Ehlers and Clark 2000).

Appraisals and relapse

Characteristic experiences associated with early signs of relapse include fear of losing control, puzzlement and perplexity, and fear of going crazy (Hirsch and Jolley 1989). These appraisals represent an individual's cognitive response to signals towards the possible (but not inevitable) recurrence of psychosis (Birchwood 1995; Gumley et al. 1999). These appraisals are understandable given the highly distressing nature of psychosis and hospitalisation reported by individuals. Indeed, as discussed above, these appraisals are likely to be further moulded by pertinent autobiographical memories and experiences.

Compounding these memories and threat appraisals, and consistent with the rich evidence on the dimensions of threatening and unpleasant life events (e.g. Brown et al. 1995; Kendler et al. 2003), the experience of psychosis also encapsulates feelings of loss, entrapment, humiliation and defeat (Iqbal et al. 2000; Rooke and Birchwood 1998). In this context both anxiogenic and depressogenic appraisals such as danger, loss, humiliation and entrapment are relevant to individuals' cognitive responses to the threat of recurrence of psychosis. This is also consistent with relapse phenomenology where symptoms of both anxiety and depression are commonplace. However, it is notable that, as yet, the role of danger appraisals in influencing relapse has not been directly researched. We propose that as relapse is commonly appraised as an event with potential for recurrence, it is wholly consistent with the criteria for a 'danger'-related event. Furthermore, we also contend that this is consistent with existing cognitive models of trauma (e.g. Ehlers and Clark 2000).

Central to this model of relapse is the proposal that individuals have excessively negative, catastrophic and idiosyncratic appraisals of relapse itself and of the sequelae of relapse including associated or residual symptoms, other people's reactions and behaviour, and the social, interpersonal and vocational consequences of symptom recurrence and rehospitalisation. These appraisals generate a sense of external (e.g. 'People want to put me in hospital') and/or internal (e.g. 'I am defective and mentally ill') threat. For some individuals, this may also reflect adverse and threatening interpersonal experiences that have occurred in their earlier development, such as abuse and neglect. Some appraisals may produce a state of persisting and constant fear of relapse. First, the characteristic experiences of psychosis involving dramatic changes in thinking and perceiving may generate catastrophic appraisals of individuals' cognitive perceptual experience. Individuals may perceive changes in the content (e.g. having a suspicious thought) or nature of their own thinking (e.g. thoughts becoming faster) and perceptions (e.g. hearing a voice) as evidence of catastrophic loss of control. In this sense normal cognitive-perceptual processes become 'contaminated' via associative memories of previous episodes of psychosis. These appraisals generate a state of elevated vigilance and threat monitoring.

Psychosis as a traumatic event

There is growing evidence that psychosis is also experienced as a traumatic event. Eight studies have investigated the prevalence of posttraumatic stress disorder symptomatology following psychosis (Frame and Morrison 2001; Jackson et al. 2004; Kennedy et al. 2002; McGorry et al. 1991; Meyer et al. 1999; Priebe et al. 1998; Shaw et al. 1997; Shaw et al. 2002). These studies reported that between 11 and 67 per cent of individuals meet criteria for PTSD following an acute episode of psychosis, although the prevalence of trauma-related symptom clusters such as recurrent intrusive memories is considerably higher in some studies (e.g. Meyer et al. 1999). Most studies indicated that the experience of the psychotic symptoms themselves was primarily responsible for patients' trauma (Frame and Morrison 2001; Kennedy et al. 2002; Meyer et al. 1999; Shaw et al. 2002); however, some studies have suggested that the methods used to treat psychosis may also be partly responsible (Frame and Morrison 2001; McGorry et al. 1991). Although the methodology of these studies has been criticised (Morrison et al. 2003) and despite the fact that acute psychosis is not formally recognised as an event which fulfils DSM-IV (APA 1994) criterion A for PTSD, the findings still appear to indicate that many patients experience significant posttraumatic stress symptomatology which arises following the treatment and experience of acute psychosis. Participants in these studies reported intrusive recollections of stressful hospital-isation events such as police involvement, or symptom-based experiences including uncontrollable auditory hallucinations, persecutory paranoia, thought broadcasting and passivity phenomena. Individuals with a 'sealing over' recovery style were more likely to report fewer intrusions and greater avoidance using the Impact of Events Scale (Jackson et al. 2004). Those participants with greater levels of peri-traumatic depersonalisation, dereali-sation and numbing also had greater levels of intrusions and avoidance (Shaw et al. 2002).

Trauma theory

Ehlers and Clark (2000) have proposed a cognitive model of individuals' reactions to trauma, which specifies multiple sources of appraisal to explain the persistence of traumatic reactions. Ehlers and Clark (2000) propose that PTSD becomes persistent when individuals process a trauma in a way that leads to a sense of serious and current threat. This sense of threat arises from disturbances in personal appraisals and autobiographical memories. First, appraisals responsible for the maintenance of a sense of current threat include excessively negative interpretations of the traumatic event itself and negative interpretations of the sequelae of the traumatic event. These appraisals include interpretations of specific symptoms (e.g. flashbacks), other people's reactions in the aftermath of the event (e.g. anger, horror) and the consequences of the traumatic event for one's life domains (e.g. being able to work, finance) and quality (e.g. pain and disability). Second, disturbances in autobiographical memory characterised by poor elaboration and contextualisation, strong associative memories and strong perceptual priming are also hypothesised to maintain a sense of current threat (see also Brewin 2001). Ehlers and Clark (2000) also hypothesise that behavioural strategies (e.g. avoidance of friends, planning, going outside, carrying a weapon) and cognitive processing styles (e.g. thought suppression, rumination, cognitive avoidance) become maladaptive and problematic because they directly produce PTSD symptoms (e.g. rumination leading to increased intrusions), prevent disconfirmation of negative interpretations of trauma and associated sequelae, and prevent change in the nature of traumatic memories. For the purposes of the model of relapse outlined below, the focus on the threatening nature of traumatic memories, and the concurrent sense of *danger* that the traumatic event may recur is particularly salient.

A trauma-based model of relapse

A trauma-based psychological model of relapse conceptualises one potential pathway to understanding the phenomenology of relapse and the potential psychological mechanisms behind the recurrence of distressing psychotic symptoms. This model updates previous psychological conceptualisations of relapse (Gumley et al. 1999), and suggests a number of important predictions for experimental studies and implications for psychological therapies aimed at promoting staying well after psychosis. Low-level psychotic experiences or cognitive perceptual events that are reminiscent of previous episodes of psychosis create a sense of reliving. This sense of reliving is enhanced by a rich experiential evidence base of intrusive autobiographical memories of previous episodes of psychosis. This leads to the activation of negative, catastrophic threat beliefs leading to emotional distress and affect dysregulation. Individuals' attempts to regulate the above cognitive perceptual experiences and associated emotional distress may lead to the acceleration of relapse via maladaptive coping. This is illustrated in Figure 13.1.

Shaw et al. (1997) found experiences representing loss of control were rated the most distressing by individuals. These 'loss of control' experiences including enforced seclusion, experiencing the self being controlled by external forces, visual hallucinations and thought insertion were associated with the highest levels of distress. Frame and Morrison (2001) found that having controlled for symptoms severity experience of psychosis accounted for a substantial proportion of the variance (24 per cent) in PTSD symptoms, whereas experience of hospitalisation accounted for only 7 per cent of the variance. Therefore, it is possible that certain internal processes and events such as particular symptoms or configurations of symptoms cue intrusive vivid visual memories of previous relapses or events that are associated with

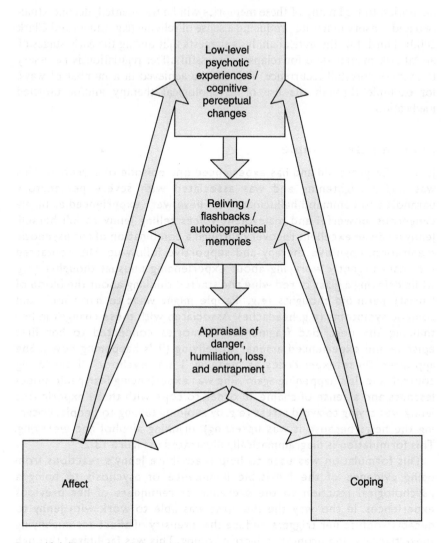

Figure 13.1 Trauma-based model of relapse

relapse. These memories are likely to form the basis for important experiential meanings and appraisals relevant to relapse.

Clinical implications of the model

There are a number of important implications of this model of relapse. First, the model emphasises relapse as an unfolding process the outcome of which is not predetermined. Second, affect and coping during relapse are mediated by personal experiential meanings that are closely related to autobiographical memories. Indeed many of these memories will be fragmented, decontextual-ised and sensory in nature producing a sense of reliving (e.g. Ehlers and Clark 2000). Third, this theoretical analysis suggests that during the early stages of an 'at risk mental state for relapse' successful affect regulation is necessary to avert or forestall recurrence. This can be achieved in a number of ways, for example through the use of psychological therapy and/or targeted medication.

Jenny: a case example

Jenny is 23 years old and has experienced one episode of psychosis. This was highly frightening and was associated with severe persecutory paranoia and command hallucinations. These were experienced as highly dangerous, powerful and malevolent voices telling Jenny to kill herself. Jenny made an excellent recovery through a combination of antipsychotic medication, cognitive therapy and supportive follow-up. She contacted the team urgently worrying about experiencing unusual thoughts (e.g. while drinking a glass of red wine she started thinking about the blood of Christ), paranoid thoughts (e.g. 'People might want to harm me') and somatic symptoms (e.g. headache). Associated with these changes in her thinking she described fragmented memories connected to her first episode and experienced a sense of reliving ('It's happening now'). She appraised these experiences as meaning 'I am psychotic', 'I am losing control' and 'It's happening again'. She was experiencing fear, panic, hope-lessness and a sense of shame. In order to cope with these experiences Jenny was trying to avoid stress (e.g. by avoiding talking to people, watch-ing the news because it was upsetting), drinking alcohol and worrying. This formulation is diagrammatically illustrated in Figure 13.2.

This formulation was used to help reattribute Jenny's reactions from being evidence of the inevitable imminence of psychosis to being a psychological reaction to the presence of reminders of her previous experiences. In this way the therapist was able to work with Jenny to decatastrophise her triggers, reduce the intensity of affect accompanying these triggers, and promote adaptive coping. This was facilitated through increasing support from her keyworker, promoting access to supportive social contacts, self-monitoring triggers and using normalising informa-tion to counter her catastrophic appraisals. Following this crisis period, Jenny was able to explore the specific traumatic autobiographical memor-ies that appeared to fuel her affective and cognitive responses during the crisis period. This allowed Jenny and the therapist to explore and develop alternative perspectives on her psychotic experiences.

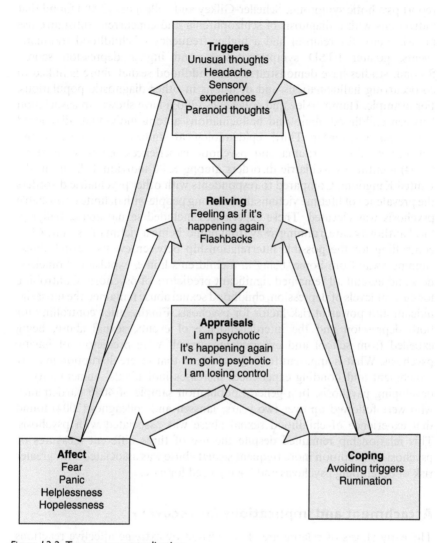

Figure 13.2 Trauma conceptualisation

Role of early development experiences in vulnerability to relapse

Morrison and colleagues (2003) have argued that rates of childhood trauma are elevated among individuals with psychosis. This is based on several lines of evidence. First, studies have demonstrated that there is a high rate of trauma in the lifetimes of those individuals who have established psychosis. For example, in a case-note review of 200 individuals, Read and colleagues (2003) found that those who had experienced sexual abuse were more likely to report psychotic symptoms. Scheller-Gilkey and colleagues (2004) found that individuals with a diagnosis of schizophrenia and concurrent substance use (a risk factor for relapse) had a higher frequency of childhood traumatic events, greater PTSD symptomatology, and higher depression scores. Second, studies have demonstrated that childhood sexual abuse is linked to co-occurring hallucinations and delusions in other diagnostic populations. For example, Hammersley and colleagues (2003) have shown an association between childhood abuse and hallucinations among individuals diagnosed with bipolar disorder. Third, epidemiological studies have shown a link between childhood trauma and psychotic experiences. Bebbington et al. (2004) identified psychiatric disorders among 8580 individuals living in the United Kingdom. Compared to respondents with other psychiatric disorders the prevalence of lifetime victimisation among people with definite or probable psychosis was elevated. These experiences included sexual abuse, bullying, local authority care, running away from home, being a victim of assault. After controlling for the possible interrelationship between events, sexual abuse, running away from home, being in a children's home, expulsion, homelessness and assault all remained significant predictors of psychosis. Controlling for current levels of depression, childhood sexual abuse remained the most significant and powerful risk factor for psychosis. Finally, after controlling for both depression and the interdependence of events, sexual abuse, being expelled from school and experiencing assault were predictors of having psychosis. What is apparent from these data is that severe disruption in early attachment and bonding experiences increases individuals' vulnerability to developing psychosis. In a general population sample of 4045 participants, who were followed up over two years, Janssen and colleagues (2004) found that experience of childhood sexual abuse was associated with psychosis. This relationship remained despite the use of three different measures of psychosis. In addition more frequent sexual abuse was associated with greater risk of developing psychosis and having need for care.

Attachment and implications for recovery

The early stages of relapse are characterised by extreme affective reactions including fear, horror, helplessness, hopelessness, shame and depression. It is in this context we expect individuals to monitor signs of possible relapse and then seek help from a service that may not have provided effective help in the past. Therefore relapse prevention starts with the person's emotional status after psychosis and their interpersonal response to emotional distress. For example, our experience has been that individuals with an avoidant style of recovery do not seek help in the context of increased risk of relapse. This narrows the window of opportunity for early detection and intervention. The impact of this avoidant strategy on families and mental health teams can lead to more coercive strategies of intervention. Coercive strategies such as involuntary hospitalisation are likely to reinforce avoidant self-regulatory strategies, increasing the probability of relapse and reducing the probability of emotional recovery. One theory that has already been developed to explain the link between emotional distress and help seeking is attachment theory (Bowlby 1969, 1973, 1980). Attachment theory is in essence a regulatory theory that is the basis for our developmental understanding of patterns of emotion regulation and proximity seeking.

Following the initial resolution of an acute psychotic episode individuals are often found to withdraw from services and active treatments. Tait and her colleagues (2003) have explored this phenomenon among sixty-two persons recovering from acute psychosis. Tendency towards sealing over or the avoidance of the personally painful and difficult experiences linked to psychosis was predictive of subsequent levels of engagement at six months. Indeed as symptoms and insight improved, individuals tended to become more sealing over. In a subsequent analysis of these data, Tait et al. (2004) explored the hypothesis that individuals who seal over have greater psychological vulnerability and lowered resilience, defined by more negative beliefs about themselves, more problematic early parenting experiences and a less secure self-reported attachment attitude. Compared to integrators, individuals who sealed over had more negative views of themselves, felt more insecure, and rated their mothers and fathers as less caring and more abusive. In addition, individuals who used a sealing over recovery style described their attitudes to attachment as less close, less dependable and rated themselves as having greater fear of rejection by others. Insecure attachment attitudes were related to service engagement; that is those who felt less close, had greater fear of rejection and saw others as less dependable were less engaged with services.

Individuals who 'seal over' their experiences of psychosis isolate these experiences from other domains of their life and thus may not experience explicit memories of previous episodes. In this case the associations may be more implicit. Therefore certain internal events reminiscent of relapse may cue feelings of fear and dread. Similar to findings in the trauma literature (Ehlers and Clark 2000; Schacter et al. 1997), individuals are likely to struggle to source the origins these feelings ('affect without recollection') and therefore they may become vigilant for other forms of threat, for example scanning for interpersonal danger. Meyer et al. (1999) found that psychotic symptoms seemed to be minimised by participants. Individuals were often reluctant to discuss them, a response suggestive of avoidance, embarrassment, denial and efforts to avoid being seen as 'crazy'. Psychotic experiences were consistently rated as distressing, particularly persecutory thoughts, visual hallucinations and passivity phenomena and the patients also reported associated intrusive and recurring thoughts about these experiences. Jackson et al. (2004) also found a relationship between recovery style and intrusion and avoidance symptoms. Those who had a tendency to 'seal over' their psychotic experiences reported lower levels of intrusions and higher levels of avoidance.

Insecure attachment and help seeking

Insecure attachment is not a single construct and those who use sealing over may have very different and contrasting states of mind with respect to adult attachment. Those with an insecure attachment organisation may be preoccupied with attachment relationships or, in contrast, dismissing or minimising of attachment. Often adults with preoccupied attachment states of mind are actively concerned with themes of abandonment and rejection. In contrast, dismissing/avoidant adults minimise and avoid attachment-related experiences and therefore autobiographical memories related to attachment experiences tend to be under-elaborated. The dismissing adult's ability to reflect on his or her own affective experience, and attune to the minds, intentions and mental states of others is diminished. Each of these subgroups acknowledges and responds to distress in quite different ways. Individuals who are securely attached develop meta-cognitive knowledge that emotions can be experienced and safely regulated, and indeed have greater competence in regulating emotion. However, individuals who are insecurely attached tend to have experienced inconsistent or rejecting responses to their negative emotions. These experiences interfere with the development of meta-cognitive knowledge and emotion regulation competencies. Those who develop a preoccupied attachment organisation, value attachment but often feel conflicted, angry or fearful of closeness and rejection, and tend to see others as less dependable. Individuals with preoccupied attachment styles tend to have experienced inconsistent or rejecting experiences that would draw a child's attention towards attachment. Those with a dismissing or avoidant attachment style avoid close relationships, and minimise or deny emotions and distress. Often, these individuals will have learned that seeking out others during times of distress has been ineffective. Dozier and Lee (1995) investigated seventy-six individuals who were diagnosed with schizophrenia or bipolar disorder in order to examine how attachment organisation as measured by the Adult Attachment Interview (AAI: Main et al. 1985) was associated with individuals' self-report of psychiatric symptoms and quality of life. Those individuals with preoccupied styles tended to report more symptoms and greater distress than those with dismissing/avoidant styles. However, in contrast, raters reported those with dismissing styles as more symptomatic (i.e. more delusional and more likely to hear voices) than those with preoccupied styles. The desynchrony between experience and expression of distress has important implications for recovery style and engagement. It may be that there are two (or more) subgroups of individuals who seal over. One group may seal over because they are anxious and fearful and experience attachment as potentially threatening via fears of rejection. This group is likely to report greater distress but be less likely to seek help and engage. Another group may seal over because they are dismissing and avoidant of attachment and regulate distress by minimising or avoiding others. This group is likely to report not being distressed despite appearances to the contrary, and will be more likely to resist engagement. Dozier (1990) found that this group of dismissing individuals were more rejecting of help and less disclosing of problems. Indeed, it is very interesting that clinicians with heavy caseloads report their dismissing clients as less problematic than their clients who are rated as preoccupied (Dozier 1992).

Cognitive interpersonal schemata

Schemas develop in response to early childhood experiences particularly early relationships with close attachment figures. Segal (1988: 147) defines schema as 'organised elements of past reactions and experience that form a relatively cohesive and persistent body of knowledge capable of guiding subsequent perception and appraisals'. They have also been described as evolutionary and become fixed when they are reinforced and/or modelled by parents (Freeman and Leaf 1989). Later, Young (1994) defines schema as 'broad pervasive themes regarding oneself and one's relationship with others developed during childhood and elaborated throughout one's lifetime'. Young (1994) states that early maladaptive schemata arise out of an interaction between inbuilt temperamental tendencies and negative interpersonal developmental experiences including abuse, criticism, abandonment and/or enmeshment. The emphasis in Young's conceptualisation of schema is an entrenched pattern of distorted thinking, negative affect and problematic behaviours. Earlier Bowlby (1973) had proposed that, over the period of normal childhood development, the experience of interactions with attachment figures becomes internalised and thus carried forward into adulthood as mental models, also known as internal working models (IWMs) or core relational schemata (Alexander 1992; Bretheron 1985). These implicit structures produce expectations about the self and others, and regulate responses in subsequent interpersonal interactions. Early attachment relationships therefore come to form the prototype for interpersonal relationships throughout life, through the internal representation of models of the self and others (e.g. Styron and Janoff-Bulman 1997). Problematic early developmental experiences characterised by attachment disruptions and/or traumatic experience lead to the evolution of IWM's that may be impoverished, underdeveloped and rigid leading to difficulties in self-reflection, affect regulation and understanding the mental states of others. In this context, psychological therapy provides the opportunity for a corrective attachment-related experience that has the potential to reorientate attachment-related behaviours, enhance emotional containment and consequentially update IWMs.

In this context, negative cognitive interpersonal schemas are maintained by the interplay between overdeveloped and excessively rigid intra and interpersonal strategies. For example, the belief 'I am bad' might be associated overdeveloped intrapersonal strategies such as self-harm, self-punitiveness and self-neglect. In addition, this belief might be linked to interpersonal strategies such as submission and subjugation to others, non-assertiveness, and fearful avoidance of attachment. In contrast the belief 'others are untrustworthy' might be expected to be associated with overdeveloped suspiciousness, hostility, avoidance of intimacy, avoidance of attachment and attachment-related memories. Similarly, suspiciousness and hostility may directly contribute to the maintenance of the belief that 'others are untrustworthy' by, for example, eliciting negative interpersonal responses from others. In addition, avoidance of others might contribute indirectly to schema maintenance via reducing possible alternative positive interpersonal experiences. Therapeutically, these overdeveloped strategies can be explored by encouraging the client to consider the impact of their experiences, not just on what they believe, but also on the development of ways of behaving towards themselves (intrapersonal strategies) and ways of behaving towards others (interpersonal strategies).

Therefore psychological therapy aimed at reducing vulnerability to relapse could aim to address this interplay between cognitive interpersonal schemata and intrapersonal and interpersonal behavioural strategies. Cognitive interpersonal strategies could be utilised to address underdeveloped intrapersonal and interpersonal coping. Through the development of new or underdeveloped behavioural strategies, new experiences provide the basis to craft and develop alternative interpersonal schemata.

Debbie: implications for relapse prevention

Debbie is a 25-year-old woman who has experienced two episodes of psychosis. These episodes were both associated with compulsory hospital admission, illicit drug use, serious self-harm, overdosing, command hallucinations, persecutory paranoia, and psychotic experiences characterised by feelings of passivity and loss of control due to the perceived actions of alien forces. Following the first episode Debbie avoided conversations regarding her emotional well-being, reported little or no distress, avoided appointments and finally disengaged from the service. At her second admission, it had transpired that she had continued to experience distressing voices, feelings of fear and persecution by others. Psychological therapy focused on exploring Debbie's personal goals and her ways of coping with adversity and distress. This facilitated an exploration of early traumatic experiences. Debbie had limited memories of her early development. However, she was able to describe a number of specific autobiographical memories that had a profound impact on her beliefs about herself ('I am weak and defective. If I show my feelings other people will harm me') and others ('Others are untrustworthy and potentially dangerous'). Linked to these beliefs, Debbie was suspicious and vigilant for signs of threat, had difficulty forming trusting relationships, avoided getting close to others, and used hostility and anger to keep others away. Figure 13.3 provides a cognitive interpersonal formulation of a clinical case.

Therapy initially focused on enhancing underdeveloped intrapersonal strategies such as self-nurturance, coping with distressing emotions, developing a compassionate understanding of the impact of earlier experiences on the genesis of punitive self-critical beliefs about herself and others. This allowed her to reflect on her own self-punitive coping behaviour and her distrust of others. Later, therapy focused on helping Debbie work through difficult interpersonal situations that arose after she returned to college. This was achieved through helping her cope with social anxiety, helping her identify expressions of warmth and interest from others, and through identifying evidence of some others being reasonably reliable and trustworthy. Debbie was able to reflect on her own experiences of engagement and help seeking following her second episode as a template for help seeking and relapse prevention in the future.

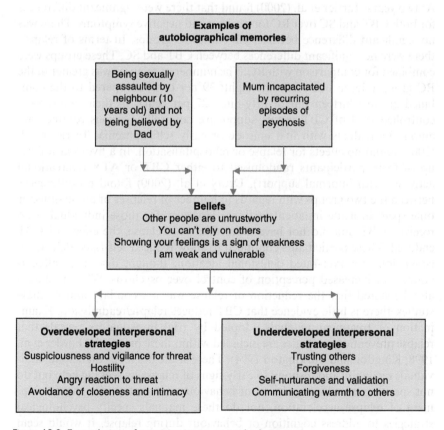

Figure 13.3 Formulation of cognitive interpersonal schemata

Psychological therapies and relapse prevention

Cognitive behaviour therapy is effective in reducing the severity of positive and negative symptoms associated with schizophrenia (Drury et al. 1996a, 1996b; Kuipers et al. 1997; Pinto et al. 1999; Sensky et al. 2000; Tarrier et al. 1993, 1998; Turkington et al. 2002). Five trials provide post-treatment follow-up (Drury et al. 2000; Kuipers et al. 1998; Sensky et al. 2000; Tarrier et al. 1999, 2000, 2004), but Kuipers et al. (1998) and Sensky et al. (2000) do not report relapse rates for their participants. Kuipers et al. (1998) found that at nine months those who had received CBT continued to show improvements in delusional distress and frequency of hallucinations. Sensky et al. (2000) found that the CBT group continued to improve on measures of positive symptoms, depression and negative symptoms. Tarrier et al. (1999) reported twelve-month follow-up results for CBT compared to supportive counselling (SC) or routine care (RC). Participants in CBT continued to show significant treatment effects for both positive and negative symptoms. There were no significant differences between the three groups for relapse at this follow-up. At two years, Tarrier et al. (2000) found that there were significant differences for both CBT and SC over RC for positive and negative symptoms. There was no significant difference between CBT and SC groups. In terms of relapse, there were no significant differences between CBT and SC. These groups were combined for comparison with RC. The number of relapses was greater in the RC group (eleven out of twenty-eight: 39 per cent) compared to the combined group (thirteen out of fifty-nine: 27 per cent). In their randomised controlled trial of CBT versus supportive counselling versus routine care among individuals with first episode or early schizophrenia, Tarrier et al. (2004) found no effects for relapse or rehospitalisation. In a five-year follow-up of forty participants randomised to either CBT or ATY (recreational activities with informal support), Drury et al. (2000) found no differences between the two groups with regards to number of relapses or admissions, or time spent in acute inpatient facilities. However, for those individuals who received CBT and did not have more than one relapse, the effects of CBT endured. These participants continued to show reduced self-rated delusional conviction, observer-rated delusional ideation, thought disorder, hallucinations and increased perception of control over psychosis. While it should also be stated that the reduction of relapse was a secondary aim of these studies, there is little evidence that CBT reduces relapse/readmission. Examination of treatment manuals adopted by trial investigators reveals that relapse prevention strategies are included within these protocols (Fowler et al. 1998; Kingdon and Turkington 1994). These strategies focus on helping individuals recognise and respond to early signs of relapse by seeking help but do not specify particular cognitions or behaviours associated with the development of relapse acceleration, nor do these manuals specify psychological strategies to address cognition or behaviour during relapse. It would seem reasonable to suggest that the results on relapse could, perhaps, be in part due to an inadequacy of existing CBT treatment protocols for relapse in psychosis. The model described in this chapter gives a number of implications for the development of CBT aimed at staying well after psychosis.

This model emphasises the importance of prioritising engagement in relation to recovery and staying well. First, it is important to identify and work with specific concerns and beliefs held by individual patients regarding the consequences of disclosure of symptoms. Patients are likely to have a wealth of experiential evidence attesting to the negative consequences of help seeking and disclosure of symptoms. Second, normalisation strategies have particular importance to enabling the development of engagement and facilitating later trauma work. Normally occurring cognitive perceptual experiences and low-level psychotic experiences become associated with catastrophic consequences and therefore excessively negative threat appraisals are likely to accompany these experiences. Normalisation enables the development of an alternative non-catastrophic perspective on the signs and symptoms of potential recurrence. Third, developing hope can be approached via reframing relapse as an opportunity to develop mastery over an apparently uncontrollable and inevitable process. This process of engagement thus enables the development of an individualised, problem-based formulation aimed at supporting individuals' recovery and staying well. Central to this process is the role of the therapist in providing the scaffolding to help individuals work with the appraisals that are linked to their traumatic experiences and memories. In particular, it is important to appreciate how these experiences are linked to problematic appraisals concerning anger towards self and/ or others, interpersonal trust and fear of being dominated by powerful others, fear of losing cognitive perceptual control, helplessness and self-blame. In addition, it is important to be aware that these appraisals *may* also be influenced by difficult interpersonal experiences with important figures in childhood and adolescence. Cognitive restructuring through the writing and revision of trauma narratives and developing alternative, less problematic, safety seeking strategies also aids development of alternative, less distressing, beliefs and appraisals. Psychological therapy also needs to address how negative cognitive interpersonal schemata are maintained by the interplay between these schemata and problematic over-developed intrapersonal and interpersonal strategies (Gumley and Schwannauer 2006).

There is some evidence that optimising engagement, individualising early signs monitoring and providing prompt early psychological intervention at the appearance of early signs reduces relapse and readmission. Gumley et al. (2003) found that targeting CBT during the early stages of relapse resulted in reduced relapse rates (18.1 per cent versus 34.7 per cent) and readmission rates (15.3 per cent versus 26.4 per cent) over twelve months. Consistent with the prediction that catastrophic appraisals of private cognitive perceptual events drive relapse, Bach and Hayes (2002) found that Acceptance and

Commitment Therapy (ACT) reduced relapse from 40 per cent to 20 per cent over four months. In this study individuals were taught to accept unavoidable private events, to identify and focus actions towards valued goals, and to defuse from odd cognition.

Summary and conclusions

In this chapter we have argued that risk of relapse and recurrence is heightened by excessively negative danger-based appraisals of relapse. Further research is required to investigate the nature of memories and appraisals that are linked to relapse. In addition, we have also proposed that disruption in early developmental and attachment experiences is linked to poorer outcome in psychosis and is a vulnerability to future relapse. This vulnerability is likely to be mediated by problematic interpersonal schema and over-developed interpersonal strategies which prevent the development of trust, affiliation and esteem, and also prevent disconfirmation of negative beliefs about self and others. Psychological therapies need to incorporate strategies to address these aspects of relapse if they are to improve our ability to support individuals' recovery and staying well.

References

Alexander, P. C. (1992) Effect of incest on self and social functioning: A developmental psychopathology perspective. *Journal of Consulting and Clinical Psychology, 60*, 185–195.

American Psychiatric Association (1994) *The diagnostic and statistical manual of mental disorders* (4th edn) (DSM-IV). Washington, DC: APA.

Bach, P., and Hayes, S. C. (2002) The use of acceptance and commitment therapy to prevent the rehospitalization of psychotic patients: A randomized controlled trial. *Journal of Consulting and Clinical Psychology, 70*, 1129–1139.

Bebbington, P. E., Bhugra, D., Brugha, T., Singleton, N., Farrell, M., Jenkins, G., and Meltzer, H. (2004) Psychosis, victimisation and childhood disadvantage: Evidence from the second British National Survey of psychiatric morbidity. *British Journal of Psychiatry, 185*, 220–226.

Birchwood, M. (1995) Early intervention in psychotic relapse: Cognitive approaches to detection and management. *Behaviour Change, 12*, 2–19.

Birchwood, M. and Iqbal, Z. (1998) Depression and suicidal thinking in psychosis: A cognitive approach. In T. Wykes, N. Tarrier and S. Lewis (eds) *Outcome and innovation in the psychological treatment of schizophrenia* (pp. 81–100). Chichester: John Wiley.

Birchwood, M., Smith, J., Macmillan, F., Hogg, B., Prasad, R., Harvey, C., and Bering, S. (1989) Predicting relapse in schizophrenia: The development and implementation of an early signs monitoring system using patients and families as observers. *Psychological Medicine, 19*, 649–656.

Birchwood, M., Mason, R., MacMillan, F., and Healy, J. (1993) Depression, demoralisation and control over illness: A comparison of depressed and non-depressed patients with a chronic psychosis. *Psychological Medicine, 23*, 387–395.

Birchwood, M., Iqbal, Z., Chadwick, P., and Trower, P. (2000) Cognitive approach to depression and suicidal thinking in psychosis: 1. Ontogeny of post-psychotic depression. *British Journal of Psychiatry, 177*, 516–521.

Boker, W., Brenner, H. D., Gerstner, G., Keller, F., Muller, J., and Spichtig, L. (1984) Self-healing strategies among schizophrenics: Attempts at compensation for basic disorders. *Acta Psychiatrica Scandinavica, 69*, 373–378.

Bowers, M. B. (1968) Pathogenesis of acute schizophrenic psychosis: An experiential approach. *Archives of General Psychiatry, 19*, 348–355.

Bowlby, J. (1969) *Attachment and loss, Volume 1: Attachment.* London: Hogarth Press.

Bowlby, J. (1973) *Attachment and loss, Volume 2: Separation, anger and anxiety.* London: Hogarth Press.

Bowlby, J. (1980) *Attachment and loss, Volume 3: Loss, sadness and depression.* London: Hogarth Press.

Bretheron, I. (1985) Attachment theory: Retrospect and prospect. In I. Bretherton and E. Waters (eds) *Growing points of attachment theory and research,* Monographs of the Society for Research in Child Development, 50 (1–2, Serial 129), 3–38.

Brewin, C. R. (2001) A cognitive neuroscience account of posttraumatic stress disorder and its treatment. *Behaviour Research and Therapy, 38*, 373–393.

Brown, G. W., and Harris, T. O. (1978) *Social origins of depression: A study of psychiatric disorder in women.* London: Tavistock.

Brown, G. W., and Harris, T. O. (1996) Guidelines, examples and LEDS–2 notes on rating for a new classification scheme for humiliation, loss and danger. Unpublished manual.

Brown, G. W., Harris, T. O., and Hepworth, C. (1995) Loss, humiliation and entrapment among women developing depression: A patient and non-patient comparison. *Psychological Medicine, 25*, 7–21.

Cutting, J. (1985) *The psychology of schizophrenia.* Edinburgh: Churchill Livingstone.

Docherty, J. P., Van Kammen, D. P., Siris, S. G., and Marder, S. R. (1978) Stages of onset of schizophrenic psychosis. *American Journal of Psychiatry, 135*, 420–426.

Dozier, M. (1990) Attachment organization and the treatment use for adults with serious psychopathological disorders. *Development and Psychopathology, 2*, 47–60.

Dozier, M. (1992) When is intervention coercive for adults with serious psychopathological disorder? Paper presented to the meeting of the Society for Life History Research, Philadelphia.

Dozier, M., and Kobak, R. R. (1992) Psychophysiology in attachment interviews: Converging evidence for deactivating strategies. *Child Development, 63*, 1473–1480.

Dozier, M., and Lee, S. W. (1995) Discrepancies between self and other report of psychiatric symptomatology: Effects of dismissing attachment strategies. *Development and Psychopathology, 7*, 217–226.

Drury, V., Birchwood, M., Cochrane, R., and Macmillan, F. (1996a) Cognitive therapy and recovery from acute psychosis: A controlled trial I. Impact on psychotic symptoms. *British Journal of Psychiatry, 169*, 593–601.

Drury, V., Birchwood, M., Cochrane, R., and Macmillan, F. (1996b) Cognitive therapy and recovery from acute psychosis: A controlled trial II. Impact on recovery time. *British Journal of Psychiatry, 169*, 602–607.

Drury, V., Birchwood, M., and Cochrane, R. (2000) Cognitive therapy and recovery from acute psychosis: A controlled trial III. Five-year follow-up. *British Journal of Psychiatry, 177*, 8–14.

Ehlers, A., and Clark, D. M. (2000) A cognitive model of posttraumatic stress disorder. *Behaviour Research Therapy, 38*, 319–345.

Fowler, D., Garety, P., and Kuipers, E. (1998) Understanding the inexplicable: An individually formulated cognitive approach to delusional beliefs. In C. Perris and P. D. McGorry (eds) *Cognitive psychotherapy of psychotic and personality disorders: Handbook of theory and practice* (pp. 129–146). Chichester: John Wiley.

Frame, L., and Morrison, A. P., (2001) Causes of posttraumatic stress disorder in psychotic patients. *Archives of General Psychiatry, 58*, 305–306.

Freedman, B. J. (1974) The subjective experience of perceptual and cognitive disturbances in schizophrenia. *Archives of General Psychiatry, 30*, 333–340.

Freedman, B. J., and Chapman, L. J. (1973) Early subjective experience in schizophrenic episode. *Journal of Abnormal Psychology, 82*, 46–54.

Freeman, A., and Leaf, R. C. (1989) Cognitive therapy applied to personality disorders. In A. Freeman, K. M. Simon, L. E. Bleutler and H. Arkowitz (eds) *Comprehensive handbook of cognitive therapy* (pp. 403–433). New York: Plenum.

Gumley, A., and Schwannauer, M. (2006) *Staying well after psychosis: A cognitive interpersonal approach to recovery and relapse prevention.* Chichester: John Wiley.

Gumley, A., White, C. A., and Power, K. (1999) An interacting cognitive subsystems model of relapse and the course of psychosis. *Clinical Psychology and Psychotherapy, 6*, 261–279.

Gumley, A., O'Grady, M., McNay, L., Reilly, J., Power, K., and Norrie, J. (2003) Early intervention for relapse in schizophrenia: Results of a 12-month randomized controlled trial of cognitive behavioural therapy. *Psychological Medicine, 33*, 419–431.

Gumley, A., O'Grady, M., Power, K., and Schwannauer, M. (2004) Negative beliefs about self and illness: A comparison of individuals with or without comorbid social anxiety disorder. *Australian and New Zealand Journal of Psychiatry, 38*, 960–964.

Hammersley, P., Dias, A., Todd, G., Bowen-Jones, K., Reilly, B., and Bentall, R. P. (2003) Childhood trauma and hallucinations in bipolar affective disorder: Preliminary investigation. *British Journal of Psychiatry, 182*, 543–547.

Heinrichs, D. W., and Carpenter, W. T., Jr (1985) Prospective study of prodromal symptoms in schizophrenic relapse. *American Journal of Psychiatry, 142*, 371–373.

Herz, M. I., and Melville, C. (1980) Relapse in schizophrenia. *American Journal of Psychiatry, 137*, 801–5.

Hirsch, S. R., and Jolley, A. G. (1989) The dysphoric syndrome in schizophrenia and its implications for relapse. *British Journal of Psychiatry, 155* (suppl. 5), 46–50.

Iqbal, Z., Birchwood, M., Chadwick, P., and Trower, P. (2000) Cognitive approach to depression and suicidal thinking in psychosis 2: Testing the validity of the social ranking model. *British Journal of Psychiatry, 177*, 522–528.

Jackson, C., Knott, C., Skeate, A., and Birchwood, M. (2004) The trauma of first episode psychosis: The role of cognitive mediation. *Australian and New Zealand Journal of Psychiatry, 38*, 327–333.

Janssen, I., Krabbendam, L., Bak, M., Hanssen, M., Vollebergh, W., de Graaf, R., and Van Os, J. (2004) Childhood abuse as a risk factor for psychotic experiences. *Acta Psychiatrica Scandinavica, 109*, 38–45.

Jorgensen, P. (1998) Early signs of psychotic relapse in schizophrenia. *British Journal of Psychiatry, 172*, 327–330.

Kendler, K. S., Hettema, J. M., Butera, F., Gardner, C. O., and Prescott, C. A. (2003) Life event dimensions of loss, humiliation, entrapment, and danger in the prediction of onsets of major depression and generalized anxiety. *Archives of General Psychiatry, 60*, 789–796.

Kennedy, B. L., Dhaliwal, N., Pedley, L., Sahner, C., Greenberg, R., and Manshadi, M. S. (2002) Post-traumatic stress disorder in subjects with schizophrenia and bipolar disorder. *Journal of Kentucky Medical Association, 100*, 395–399.

Kingdon, D., and Turkington, D. (1994) *Cognitive behavioural therapy of schizophrenia*. Hove: Lawrence Erlbaum.

Kuipers, E., Garety, P., Fowler, D., Dunn, G., Bebbington, P., Freeman, D., and Hadley, C. (1997) London-East Anglia randomised controlled trial of cognitive-behavioural therapy for psychosis, I: Effects of the treatment phase. *British Journal of Psychiatry, 171*, 319–327.

Kuipers, E., Fowler, D., Garety, P., Chisholm, D., Freeman, D., Dunn, G., et al. (1998) London-East Anglia randomised controlled trial of cognitive-behavioural therapy for psychosis, III: Follow-up and economic evaluation at 18 months. *British Journal of Psychiatry, 173*, 61–68.

McGhie, A., and Chapman, J. (1961) Disorders of attention and perception in early schizophrenia. *British Journal of Medical Psychology, 34*, 103–116.

McGorry, P. D., Chanen, A., McCarthy, E., Van Riel, R., McKenzie, D., and Singh, B. S. (1991) Posttraumatic stress disorder following recent-onset psychosis: An unrecognised postpsychotic syndrome. *Journal of Nervous and Mental Disease, 179*, 253–258.

Main, M., Kaplan, N., and Cassidy, J. (1985) Security in infancy, childhood and adulthood: A move to the level of representation. *Monographs of the Society for Research in Child Development, 50*, 66–104.

Meyer, H., Taiminen, T., Vuori, T., Aeijaelae, A., and Helenius, H. (1999) Post-traumatic stress disorder symptoms related to psychosis and acute involuntary hospitalisation in schizophrenic and delusional patients. *Journal of Nervous and Mental Disease, 187*, 343–352.

Morrison, A. P., Frame, L., and Larkin, W. (2003) Relationships between trauma and psychosis: A review and integration. *British Journal of Clinical Psychology, 42*, 331–353.

Pinto, A., La Pia, S., Manella, R., Giorgio, D., and DiSimone, L. (1999) Cognitive behavioural therapy and clozapine for clients with treatment refractory schizophrenia. *Psychiatric Services, 50*, 901–904.

Priebe, S., Broker, M., and Gunkel, S. (1998) Involuntary admission and post-traumatic stress disorder symptoms in schizophrenia patients. *Comprehensive Psychiatry, 39*, 220–224.

Read, J., Agar, K., Argyle, N., and Aderhold, V. (2003). Sexual and physical abuse during childhood and adulthood as predictors of hallucinations, delusions and thought disorder. *Psychological Psychotherapy, 76*, 1–22.

Rooke, O., and Birchwood, M. (1998) Loss, humiliation and entrapment as appraisals of schizophrenic illness: A prospective study of depressed and non-depressed patients. *British Journal of Clinical Psychology, 37*, 259–268.

Schacter, D. L., Norman, K. A., and Koutstaal, W. (1997) The recovered memories debate: A cognitive neuroscience perspective. In M. A. Conway (ed.) *Recovered memories and false memories* (pp. 63–99). Oxford: Oxford University Press.

Scheller-Gilkey, G., Moynes, K., Cooper, I., Kant, C., and Miller, A. H. (2004) Early life stress and PTSD symptoms in patients with comorbid schizophrenia and substance abuse. *Schizophrenia Research, 69*, 67–74.

Segal, Z. V. (1988) Appraisal of the self-schema construct in cognitive models of depression. *Psychological Bulletin, 103*, 147–162.

Sensky, T., Turkington, D., Kingdon, D., Scott, J. L., Scott, J., Siddle, R., et al. (2000) A randomised controlled trial of cognitive behavioural therapy in schizophrenia resistant to medication. *Archives of General Psychiatry, 57*, 165–172.

Shaw, K., McFarlane, A., and Bookless, C. (1997) The phenomenology of traumatic reactions to psychotic illness. *Journal of Nervous and Mental Disease, 185*, 434–441.

Shaw, K., McFarlane, A., Bookless, C., and Air, T. (2002) The aetiology of postpsychotic posttraumatic stress disorder following a psychotic episode. *Journal of Traumatic Stress, 15*, 39–47.

Styron, T., and Janoff-Bulman, R. (1997) Childhood attachment and abuse: Long-term effects on adult attachent, depression and conflict resolution. *Child Abuse and Neglect, 21*, 1015–1023.

Tait, L., Birchwood, M., and Trower, P. (2003) Predicting engagement with services for psychosis: Insight, symptoms and recovery style. *British Journal of Psychiatry, 182*, 123–128.

Tait, L., Birchwood, M., and Trower, P. (2004) Adapting to the challenge of psychosis: Personal resilience and the use of sealing-over (avoidant) coping strategies. *British Journal of Psychiatry, 185*, 410–415.

Tarrier, N., Beckett, R., Harwood, S., Baker, A., Yusupoff, L., and Ugarteburu, I. (1993) A trial of two cognitive-behavioural methods of treating drug-residual psychotic symptoms in schizophrenic patients: Outcome. *British Journal of Psychiatry, 162*, 524–532.

Tarrier, N., Yusupoff, L., Kinney, C., McCarthy, E., Gledhill, A., Haddock, G., and Morris, J. (1998) Randomised controlled trial of intensive cognitive behaviour therapy for patients with chronic schizophrenia. *British Medical Journal, 317*, 303–307.

Tarrier, N., Wittkowsky, A., Kinney, C., McCarthy, E., Morris, J., and Humphreys, L. (1999) Durability of the effects of cognitive-behavioural therapy in the treatment of chronic schizophrenia: 12-month follow-up. *British Journal of Psychiatry, 174*, 500–504.

Tarrier, N., Kinney, C., McCarthy, E., Humphreys, L., and Wittkowsky, A. (2000) Two-year follow-up of cognitive behavioural therapy and supportive counselling in the treatment of persistent symptoms in chronic schizophrenia. *Journal of Consulting and Clinical Psychology, 68*, 917–922.

Tarrier, N., Lewis, S., Haddock, G., Bentall, R., Drake, R., and Kinderman, P., et al. (2004) Cognitive-behavioural therapy in first-episode and early schizophrenia. *British Journal of Psychiatry, 184*, 231–239.

Turkington, D., Kingdon, D., Turner, T., and Insight into Schizophrenia Research Group (2002) Effectiveness of a brief cognitive-behavioural therapy intervention in the treatment of schizophrenia. *British Journal of Psychiatry, 18*, 523–527.

Young, J. E. (1994) *Cognitive therapy for personality disorders: A schema focused approach* (rev. edn). Sarasota, FL: Professional Resource Press.

Index

For Product Safety Concerns and Information please contact our
EU representative GPSR@taylorandfrancis.com Taylor & Francis
Verlag GmbH, Kaufingerstraße 24, 80331 München, Germany